Dedicated to

Miki, Natasha, Alexei and Katya

for their encouragement and support

and to

Dr Joseph Petelin, teacher and friend

without whom none of this would have been possible

Contents

List of Authors

Sarah Cheslyn-Curtis, Hammersmith Hospital, London

Timothy Christmas, Charing Cross Hospital, London

Frank Cross, The Royal London Hospital, London

Wadi Gedroyc, St Mary's Hospital, London

Stephen Grochmal, New Jersey Laser Institute, New Jersey

Michael Hershman, Royal Liverpool University Hospital, Liverpool

David Hunt, St Mary's Hospital, London

Roger Kirby, St Bartholomew's Hospital, London

David Rosin, St Mary's Hospital, London

Paul Salmon, Harley Street, London

Hans Troidl, Cologne University, Germany

Justin Vale, Charing Cross Hospital, London

John Waldron, Royal United Hospital, Bath

Hugh Whitfield, St Bartholomew's Hospital, London

Foreword

The rapid rise in the use of minimal access techniques over the last few years has resulted in many new types of operation becoming established. As this book describes so well, this revolution has involved all types of surgery; and the future of minimal access therapy involves full integration with all the specialties.

This is the first book in Radcliffe Medical Press' series, and has contributions from many of the leaders in this exciting new field. It is explicit, relevant and highly authoritative, and provides essential reading for surgeons and physicians alike. It is well balanced, concise and comprehensive, and will provide ideal training material for hospital specialists.

Each chapter opens an Aladdin's cave which is thoroughly enjoyable as well as informative and, I believe, each book in this specialist minimal access series will become *the* reference book for this rapidly expanding subject.

As President of the Society of Minimally Invasive General Surgeons, I am delighted that one of the founders of the Society has launched a series which will extend far beyond the confines of general surgery and lead the way to closer co-operation between health professionals and a more efficient and effective service for our patients.

Lord McColl
March 1993

Preface

'An important phase of medicine is the ability to appraise the
literature correctly.' Hippocrates

Laparoscopic cholecystectomy exploded onto the general surgical scene like
no other procedure before it. Embraced by the public, and promoted by
technological advances, it rejuvenated general surgery. Although there were
a few sceptics, the rush to learn minimal access surgical techniques was phe-
nomenal and took surgical trainers by storm. However, we must remember
that minimal access therapy has been practised by other specialties without
the same excitement or exposure. Gastroenterologists utilizing endoscopy,
urologists, gynaecologists and radiologists have all paved the way for these
new technological advances of video-enhanced surgery and medicine.

No book or series would therefore be complete unless it started by including
all the spheres of influence of minimal access medicine and surgery.

Since witnessing and learning this type of surgery in February 1990, I have
wanted to write not just an article or book, but a series encompassing all
aspects of minimal access therapy. However, the early days were spent in
learning and perfecting the new techniques and, as surgical tradition and
teaching has always done, in passing these as best as I was able on to others.

There are already books and atlases on laparoscopic surgical techniques and
even books on single operations, but I decided early on that what was needed
in this new field was an all-encompassing book, or indeed series of books,
which separately would be useful to specialists, but as a series would serve as
the reference books for all minimal access therapy that centres practising these
techniques, and training young doctors in them, would need.

Obviously, these could not be produced by a single author, or indeed a
single editor, so I have gathered together a brilliant and innovative team of
co-editors who, in turn, have collected internationally recognized leaders
in each specialty. The result, I believe, is the ultimate reference source for
all clinicians and teachers.

The first book, by design, is an introduction to minimal access therapy. To
have covered every specialty would have lost its compactness and possibly

its clarity. However, future books on subjects not included, such as minimal access surgical oncology, clinical anatomy and emergency surgery, as well as minimal access surgery for theatre personnel, are in preparation.

I am truly delighted with the result of this first book in the series and thank my contributors not only for their superb chapters but also for their ability to produce them rapidly. From conception to delivery has been extremely short, for which I am indebted to Andrew Bax and his team at Radcliffe Medical Press.

'It is astonishing with how little reading a doctor can practise medicine, but it is not astonishing how badly he can do it.' William Osler

R David Rosin
March 1993

History

DAVID ROSIN

It was written during the time of Hippocrates, although probably not by Hippocrates himself, that *'the things relating to surgery are the patient; the operator; the assistants; the instruments; the light; where and how; how many things, and how; where the body and instruments; the time, the manner; the place.'* It is interesting to reflect how accurate these predictions were with respect to minimal access surgery, specifically 'the instruments, the light; where and how and the manner.'

The surgeon and the barber

The surgery of the early Middle Ages has been described as meddlesome. In the late Middle Ages when medicine was producing nothing new, surgery was the branch that began to advance. Surgery was separated from medicine during the time of Galen (c. AD 130–200) or even before, and the two branches of medicine took quite different paths in the subsequent 1500 years.

From the beginning of the 13th century, there is little doubt that surgeons existed as separate practitioners. They were to be found in the cities where they joined guilds. Sometimes, they were admitted to universities but, as time passed, they were excluded and thus formed their own colleges such as the College de St Côme in Paris. Along with the surgeons of the long robe, some of whom were clerics, came the barbers – less learned surgeons. Interestingly, physicians usually favoured the barbers because, barbers being the simpler men, they were more likely to be willing to take their orders from these so called learned doctors.

The barbers and surgeons of England had belonged to separate guilds from the 14th century. In 1540, a compromise about rights and duties of each was reached and a single company of barbers, the Worshipful Company of Barber Surgeons was formed. The surgeons agreed to do no barbering and the barbers restricted their surgery to dentistry. This union lasted more than

200 years, but in 1745 it was dissolved and a surgeons' company again existed independently. In 1800, the College of Surgeons of London was formed and it received its Royal Charter from Queen Victoria in 1843 becoming the Royal College of Surgeons of England.

The development of surgery

The real development of surgery depended upon knowledge of anatomy. The surgeon-anatomist Vesalius played an increasingly important role as the knowledge of anatomy advanced. Thomas Vicary in his anatomy text quoted Galen's saying that *'it is as possible for a surgeon not knowing anatomy to work in man's body without error as it is for a blind man to carve an image and make it perfect.'* The teaching of both surgery and anatomy was performed by the professors of surgery in medical schools until the early 20th century. In this century, surgery has been characterized by *'a lifting of the eyes from the local lesion and the operation designed to deal with it to regard the more general aspects of surgical disorders'* according to Churchill. However, Henry J Bigelow told his students back in 1849 that the basis of surgery *'are its settled principles.'*

These principles were exceptionally general, but a discussion of constitution and disease was not entirely neglected by surgeons of this time. In the field of operative surgery, Bigelow confessed *'we occupy more directly what is properly considered to be the province of the surgeon. The surgeon, with the public, is associated with surgical operations; and his notoriety is in measure with the belief which the world may entertain of the number and magnitude of the operations he may perform.'* The public may be impressed, warned Bigelow, and the surgeon should *'guard against much of the exaggerated sense of worth and of drama.'*

In the 1880s, Matas recalled, the head, chest and abdomen were still sanctuaries not to be opened, unless by accident. It has often been stressed that the development of anaesthesia and antisepsis greatly increased the numbers of operations performed, but a look at the statistics reveals that the increase was very slow. Halsted showed in 1904 that in the decade following the widespread acceptance of the theory of antisepsis in the USA (1889–1898), the number of operations performed increased only slightly. In the decade after Lister's momentous papers on the efficacy of antisepsis, there was still a lot of reticence about accepting the method as well as its theoretical foundation, the germ theory of disease. There was also a reluctance to hope for much improvement in the art of surgery.

After the Napoleonic wars at the beginning of the 19th century, French surgeon and author of a surgical text, Alexis Boyer, is supposed to have said *'surgery seems to have obtained the highest degree of perfection of which it is capable.'* Despite anaesthesia and the development of many new techniques, and despite the promise of antisepsis, John Eric Erichsen, one of the most perceptive and influential surgeons of the late 19th century, came to similar conclusions in 1873 – *'That there must be a final limit to development in this department of our profession, there can be no doubt ... Like every other art, be it manipulative, plastic, or imitative, it can only be carried to a certain definite point of excellence. The art may be modified, it may be varied, though it cannot be perfected beyond certain attainable limits ... There cannot always be fresh fields for conquest by the knife; there must be portions of the human frame that will ever remain sacred from intrusion at least in surgeons' hands. That we have nearly, if not quite, reached these final limits, there can be little question.'*

It did not take long to disprove them, and Erichsen along with others proved to be a poor prophet.

In 1900, abdominal surgery was not something undertaken lightly by most doctors or patients. The successful drainage of an appendix abscess of King Edward VII of England, forcing the delay of his coronation in 1902, helped make appendicitis a fashionable disease, and also helped to break down further the resistance to surgery. And now, in this century, surgeons deal with a variety of physiological problems almost every time they operate.

The arrival of endoscopy

Basic disease processes confronting surgeons have changed very little. However, the techniques used and the outcome that a patient and his surgeon can reasonably expect, have changed a great deal. It is technique and outcome that have increasingly turned physicians and surgeons towards minimal access medicine and surgery. This has been made possible by the advent of endoscopy.

By the late 19th century, the roots of modern microscopy, radiology and later endoscopy, had been established. The seeds of electronic technology had been planted combining X-ray imaging devices with television and videotape equipment. Image intensifiers and high speed motion picture cameras have greatly extended the usefulness of endoscopy as a valuable diagnostic tool.

The use of tubes in medicine dates from the earliest days of civilization. Clysters for enemas were known to the ancient Egyptians, Greeks and Romans. Later, tubes were used to introduce nutrients into very ill patients. It was only natural, therefore, that physicians would investigate the use of tubular devices for diagnostic purposes. Hippocrates was reported to have used a clyster with a candle as the light source to examine the rectum. However, the efficient devices used today had to await technological advances in optics, light sources, transmission and miniaturization.

There were three phases in the development of endoscopy: first the rigid phase from 1805–1932; second the semi-flexible phase from 1932–1957 and third the fibre-endoscope phase from 1957 to the present time. The oldest forerunner of the modern endoscope was devised by Phillipe Bozzini, an obstetrician, who practised in Frankfurt am Main and developed an instrument for seeing into the bladder and rectum with candlelight reflected by mirrors (Figure 1.1). It was demonstrated to the Alert Faculty in Vienna, yet they rejected it as a 'magic lantern', and it was apparently never put into practice.

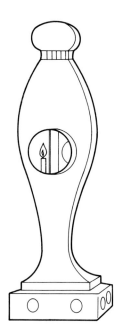

Figure 1.1: Bozzini's cystoscope consisting of a lamp, mirror, and candle. (Reprinted with permission of J.B. Lippincott & Co.)

Antonin J Desormeaux developed an alcohol lamp and lens system, but although the endoscope reached the stomach, the light source was insufficient (Figures 1.2 and 1.3). However, it was used to view the urinary bladder, cervix and uterus. The first internal light source was invented by Bruck, a dentist from Breslau, who in 1867 examined the mouth of a patient using an electrically-plated platinum wire as the light source. As there was the risk of burning the tissue, he later developed a water jacket for cooling the platinum wire. It was not until Edison invented the incandescent light bulb in 1880, and

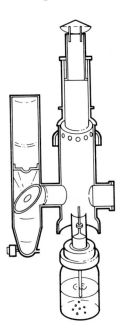

Figure 1.2: Desormeaux's endoscope incorporating kerosene lamp, mirror, and chimney vent. (Reprinted with permission of J.B. Lippincott & Co.)

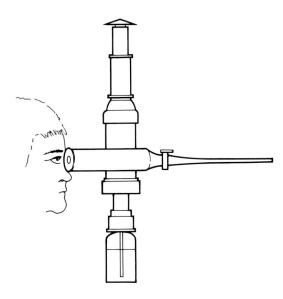

Figure 1.3: The Desormeaux endoscope used as a cystoscope in 1853. (Reprinted with permission of J.B. Lippincott & Co.)

the Germans improved optical systems in the 1890s, that endoscopy became a practical procedure.

The first gastroscope was introduced by Adolf Kussmaul in 1868, apparently after watching a sword swallowing exhibition.

In 1897, Max Nitze, a urologist from Berlin, produced the first usable cystoscope with lenses and electric lighting (Figure 1.4). He was helped by a German optician, Beneche, and a Viennese electro-optician, Joseph Leiter. A few years later in 1901, Kelling reported using a cystoscope to inspect the peritoneal cavity of a dog after insufflation with air. He then coined the term 'celioscopy' to describe this technique. At this time, cystoscopy and other open-cavity endoscopic procedures such as oesophagoscopy, proctoscopy, and laryngoscopy were well established. 'Closed-cavity' procedures had not yet been tried, but the stage was set for the development of laparoscopy. Von Ott performed the first laparoscopy without the benefit of new endoscopes. In 1910, Jacobaeus, a Swedish surgeon, performed the first laparoscopy and thoracoscopy in a human. He is credited with coining the terms 'laparoscopy' and 'thoracoscopy'. The importance of pneumoperitoneum was recognized a

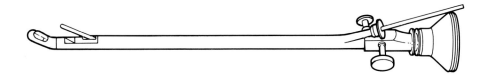

Figure 1.4: The Nitze cystoscope showing bulb illuminator and ureteral probe through probe channel. (Reprinted with permission of J.B. Lippincott & Co.)

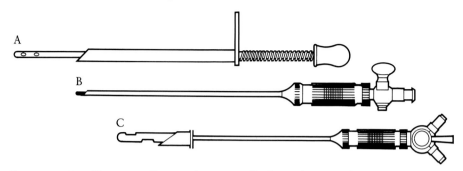

Figure 1.5: Insufflation needles. A: Goetze needle for induction of pneumoperitoneum. B: Veress needle to induce pneumothorax. C: Semm modification for monitoring of intra-abdominal gas pressure. (Reprinted with permission of Springer-Verlag.)

short time later, and prompted Goetze to introduce his insufflation needle in 1918. In 1938 Veress of Budapest wrote about his insufflation needle for producing a pneumothorax. This needle is still used today (Figure 1.5). The first laparoscopic lysis of adhesions was performed by Fervers in 1933, and Boesch of Switzerland is credited with the first tubal sterilization in 1936.

The development of instruments

Meanwhile, Johann Von Mickulicz-Reddecki in 1881, developed an instrument which could be angled by 30° near its lower third. During the next 50 years, improvements in electric light sources, ocular systems and photographic methods resulted in the creation of more advanced instruments. In 1952, Rudolph Schindler introduced a new semi-flexible gastroscope based upon the optical principle proposed by Lang in 1917 (who had discovered that clear images could be transmitted by a series of convex lenses around a gentle curve provided the curvature was not too great).

Heinrich Lamm demonstrated in 1930, that fine threads of glass fibres could be bundled together to act as a conduit for a light source, and that the bundle could be flexed or bent without losing its transmission capabilities. No-one knows why the idea languished for nearly 25 years, but it was in 1954 that the most significant advance was made by Harold H Hopkins and NS Kapany, who pointed out the potential application for endoscopy (Figure 1.6). Three years later, Hirschowitz and his group created the prototype, a genuine breakthrough in the examination of the oesophagus, stomach and duodenum.

The first instruments provided a lateral view and used a distal electric bulb as their light source. Subsequent modifications have provided the practitioner with a straightforward (0°) view, while the lateral viewing device is now reserved for special examinations. Changes in light source from the distal electric bulb to the external light unit and sophisticated light-conducting fibreglass bundles eliminated excessive heat production and occasional burns caused by the distal light bulb in the stomach.

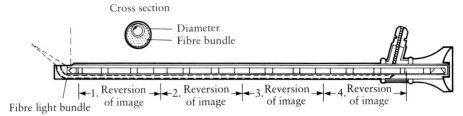

Figure 1.6: Cross section of laparoscope showing Hopkins' rod-lens system (and fiber-optic light illumination). (Reprinted with permission of J.B. Lippincott & Co.)

Prior to this insufflation, the introduction of an endoscope through the abdominal wall had been associated with many major and minor complications. There was a risk to the underlying bowel and vascular structures and this still exists despite insufflation. It is interesting that in 1946, Decker introduced an alternative method by inserting the laparoscope into the abdominal cavity through the cul-de-sac of the vagina because of the dangers to underlying structures during laparoscopy and named the procedure culdoscopy. Raoul Palmer in Paris stressed the importance in 1944 of monitoring intra-abdominal pressure.

However, it was another 20 years before Kurt Semm in Kiel, Germany, developed an automatic insufflation device that monitored abdominal pressure and gas flow. Previously, air had been introduced into the peritoneal cavity by means of a syringe. With the development of safe insufflation needles, as well as instruments for controlling gas flow during pneumoperitoneum, complications were significantly reduced. However, because laparoscopy was considered a 'blind' procedure with the risk of injury to intraperitoneal structures, acceptance was slow throughout the world.

Laparoscopy

Diagnostic laparoscopy was performed by many gynaecologists but only a few general surgeons. It was the gynaecologists and urologists who breached the frontiers of minimal access surgery during the second half of this century. Surgeons in both these specialties soon added operative skills to this minimal access approach for diagnosis. Semm must take much of the credit for the development of laparoscopic instruments such as needle holders, microscissors, clip applicators and atraumatic forceps.

Laparoscopic visualization of the peritoneal cavity was at first restricted to the surgeon, and participation by other members of the team was limited. Therefore, complicated operative procedures proved to be tedious because of the inability of assistants to interact with the surgeons, although articulated attachments containing a series of mirrors could split the image from the instrument; however, these proved to be inefficient and cumbersome.

In 1986, this problem was solved with the development of the computer chip TV camera which could be attached to instruments. Thus began the era of video-guided surgery. Elaborate developments in the area of video imaging resulted in high resolution video monitors affording greater clarity and definition, as well as improved magnification of the operative field, making fine dissection more simple.

Lasers

The first surgical lasers were introduced in the mid 1960s. Early uses of this energy source by ophthalmologists for retinal detachment, and by otolaryngologists for vocal cord surgery, opened the way for its applicability in other fields. In the peritoneal cavity, the fear of uncontrolled bowel injuries from monopolar coagulation also prompted many gynaecologists to adopt the laser as a dissecting and coagulating device. The first clinical report describing laser energy for operative pelvioscopy was by Bruhat, Mage and Manhes in 1979.

Subsequently, laser light has been used for the coagulation and enucleation of endometrial implants, treatment of ectopic pregnancy with preservation of the affected adnexa, adhesiolysis, as well as in cholecystectomy. The theoretical benefits of laser treatment are improved haemostasis, greater precision during tissue dissection and decreased complications from inadvertent burns distant from the operative field. Support for the superiority of this modality over that of electrocoagulation, however, has not been forthcoming.

General surgeons were slow to take up operative laparoscopy. The first procedures were liver biopsies guided under direct vision in the late 1970s. Diagnostic laparoscopy was increasingly used in the 1980s for the acute abdomen.

It was not until March 1986 that the first laparoscopic cholecystectomy was performed by P Muhe in Germany. Since that time, there has been an explosion in laparoscopic procedures in general surgery.

Conclusion

As this century closes, there is no doubt that our patients are benefiting from minimal access medicine and surgery. Stenting by radiologists, upper and lower gastrointestinal tract (GIT) endoscopy with operative procedures, peritoneoscopy and laparoscopic surgery, arthroscopy and thoracoscopy have all led to less invasive procedures being performed, patient comfort, faster recovery rates and return to normal activities, and improved cosmesis.

Minimal access surgery minimizes the trauma of access, not only by virtual abolition of the wound, but also by allowing the execution of complex operative procedures within a closed physiological environment. The use of micro-instruments, the avoidance of retraction to achieve exposure and the minimal handling of tissues has not only led to the benefits mentioned, but in addition, to the virtual abolition of wound infections and other wound-related complications. Rapid post-operative mobilization means that the common complications such as chest infections, deep vein thrombosis, and in orthopaedic surgery, muscle wasting, should be greatly reduced.

One last advantage which should be mentioned is the reduced contact with the patient's blood and other body fluids which should reduce the risk of transmission of viral disease.

References

Boesch PF (1936) Laparoskopie. *Schweiz A. Krankenhaus Anstaltsw.* 6: 62.

Bozzini P (1806) Lichtleiter, eine Erfindung Zur Anschung Innerer Theile und Krankheiten Nebst Abbildung. *J. Pract. Arzeyhunde.* 24: 107.

Desormeaux AJ (1865) Transactions of the Société de Chirurgie, Paris. *Gazette des Hop.*

Fervers C (1933) Die Laparoskopie mit dem Cystoskope. Ein Beitrag zur Vereinfachung der Technik und zur Endoskopischen Strangdurchtrennung in der Bauchole. *Med. Klinik.* 29: 1042–1045.

Goetze O (1918) Die Rontgendiagnostik bei gasgefullter Bauchohle eine neue Methode. *Munch. Med. Wochenschr.* 65: 1480–1481.

Jacobaeus HC (1910) Uber die Moglichkeit, die Zystoskopie bei Unteruchung seroser Hohlungen anzuwenden. *Munch. Med. Wochenschr.* 57: 2090–2092.

Kelling G (1901) Uber Oesophagoskopies, Gastroskopie und Colioskopie. *Munch. Med. Wochenschr.* 49: 21–24.

Ottenjan R and Elster K (1980) Expanding the power of the senses. In: *Atlas of diseases of the upper gastrointestinal tract.* Smith, Kline & French, Philadelphia.

Palmer R (1947) Instrumentation et technique de la colioscopie gynécologique. *Gynecol. Obstet.* 46: 422.

Semm K (1989) History. In: Sanfilippo JS and Levine RL *et al.*, eds. *Operative gynecologic endoscopy.* Springer-Verlag, New York.

Veress J (1938) Ein neue Instrument zur Ausfuhrung von Brust oder Bauchpunktionen und Pneumothoraxbehandlung. *Deutsche Med. Wochenschr.* 64: 1480–1481.

2

The Philosophy of Patient-friendly Surgery

HANS TROIDL

Introduction

Traumatologists, gynaecologists and urologists 'started' endoscopic surgery. As early as the 1930s a few traumatologists (Watanabe, 1936) had started to use endoscopic surgery for diagnosis and treatment (Ikeuchi, 1988; Schonholtz 1988). However, it was for diagnosis that most clinicians used the procedure.

Very few general surgeons used laparoscopy and most did not recognize the benefits that it could bring. Despite my close association with Semm at the University of Kiel, I too failed to recognize the value of this innovation. Even during the First World Congress of Endoscopic Surgery in Berlin (1988), endoscopic diagnosis and treatment in the abdomen or chest was not a topic for discussion (Troidl, 1990).

There have been several pioneers. In Germany, Dr Wittmoser used endoscopic surgery in the 1950s (without the aid of a video camera) (Wittmoser, 1959). His observations, published in 1956, are particularly interesting: *'who once had the opportunity to watch the typical course after thoracoscopic sympathectomy of the upper extremity without any complication will hardly be able to understand that patients with big pleural effusions (90% of cases) would have to tolerate the big thoracic intervention'*. As can be seen, the comfort of patients was already being considered. Mühe, in 1986, presented to the German Surgical Congress the first laparoscopic cholecystectomy that he had performed (Mühe, 1986). He also spoke about the advantages of much reduced operative trauma and the favourable consequences that this produced. The merits of Dr Wittmoser and Dr Mühe's research were not recognized in Germany for many years.

The real breakthrough for endoscopic surgery came from the French surgeons P Mouret and F Dubois, later followed by J Perissat, when they successfully performed laparoscopic cholecystectomy for gallstone disease in the 1980s, with the help of laparoscopy and a video camera. General surgeons became aware of this type of surgery and it was then that the pioneering work of Semm (Semm, 1982) and Götz (Götz, 1988) was given full credit.

There are several reasons why general surgeons, and particularly thoracic surgeons, did not recognize these innovations, and indeed fought against them.

1   The technical equipment was until recently archaic (Wickham, 1982).
2   In the 1970s and 1980s surgeons were busy developing transplant and cardiac surgical techniques. Oncological surgery was also a 'hot' topic.
3   Conventional endpoints such as operative mortality, complications and survival rates dominated outcome assessment (The Veterans' Administration Systemic Sepsis Cooperative Group, 1987).
4   The attitude of general and thoracic surgeons to patient well-being, quality of life, physical integrity, pain and fatigue was not very well developed (Troidl et al., 1987; Troidl et al, 1990; Wickham, 1982).

Based on my long-term experience of endpoints such as quality of life and acute surgical pain (Troidl et al., 1987; Troidl et al., 1987; Troidl, 1989; Troidl and Neugebauer, 1990; Troidl et al., 1990) and of endoscopy, my visits to Götz, who demonstrated laparoscopic appendectomy in 1988 and Perissat in Bordeaux, reassured me that laparoscopic removal of the gall bladder using a video camera was the most beneficial method with which to treat the patient as a real person.

The concept

When we first removed a gall bladder by laparoscopy on October 23 1989, it was done in the belief that this treatment option would produce increased comfort and less trauma for the patient, but still maintain adequate surgical safety (Troidl, 1990). Characteristics of this patient-friendly surgery are minimal inconvenience to the patient during treatment, and safety.

My research into the endpoints of patient well-being and quality of life had shown that, in defining the concept of minimal access surgery, the view of the individual patient was critically important (Eypasch et al., 1990; The Veterans' Administration Systemic Sepsis Cooperative Group, 1987). The surgeon does play a role here, but a subordinate one (Figure 2.1). The role of the surgeon will become a more important one when patients demand this type of surgery and their demands will have to be met. During the development of our quality of life index, we discovered that the ideas of physicians, medical staff, patients and relatives were different, sometimes even contrary (Eypasch et al., 1990). Even today, some surgeons do not understand that pain induced by diagnostic procedures and surgical interventions always comes first on a list of factors that worry the patient. It is not recognized that patients can also be afraid of anaesthesia, and also want to retain their physical integrity.

The concept of patient-friendly surgery is based on more comfort and

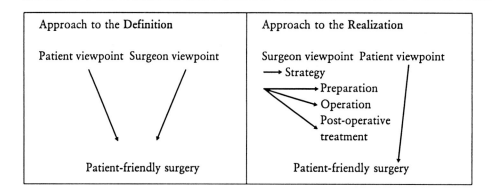

Figure 2.1: Differing roles in patient-friendly surgery.

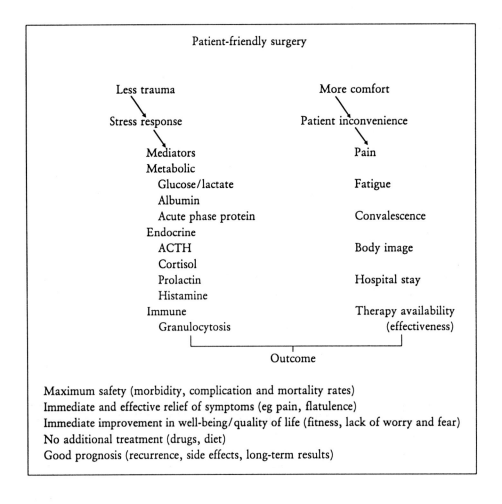

Figure 2.2: Conceptualization of laparoscopic cholecystectomy: using patient-friendly surgery.

less trauma (*see* Figure 2.2). Comfort means a surgical intervention where neither the preparation, the performance nor the post-operative course are inconvenient for the patient. Criteria for this inconvenience have to be defined by the patient. These criteria might include:

- pessaries
- fasting
- invasive diagnostic procedures
- CT scanning
- general anaesthesia
- post-operative pain
- nausea, vomiting
- dressings
- tubes and infusions
- fatigue
- dietary restrictions
- other changes to normal lifestyle.

There is no basic pathophysiological difference between major trauma and a surgical operation (Troidl, 1990). It is therefore important that every surgical treatment is designed to be the least traumatizing, i.e. inducing the least stress response in the body. This can be measured by tests on metabolism, endocrine activity and immunology.

All this is justified by the 'optimal outcome' (*see* Figures 2.2 and 2.3), meaning that the treatment has to be safe, minimally uncomfortable and quick and efficient while ensuring a successful outcome.

Concept = the most patient-friendly surgery = less trauma + more comfort = same or better outcome

Figure 2.3: The hypothesis for endoscopic surgery.

Finally the treatment has to be definitive and should protect the integrity of the physical body without requiring any additional treatment. Endoscopic surgery should have fulfilled this concept.

The need to test the idea

A fascinating idea and theory is born: endoscopic surgery is (the most) patient-friendly surgery. The idea becomes reality, but this is only the first step. The second step is to test this idea according to the stringencies of clinical research. This is a difficult and tedious step which is often neglected. McKinley and Jennett have described this problem very accurately (McKinley, 1981; Jennett, 1986).

McKinley (1981) described the life cycle of a new technology as having five stages of development as unfortunately is the case with so many 'innovations':

1   an enthusiastic and promising single case report. Complications are not observed
2   due to strong competition and the need to be 'in', the idea is adopted by specialized centres and the first news is published in the media
3   professional acceptance of the technique is then driven by public pressure and by companies seeking profit
4   it is proposed that the new technology is accepted as the 'standard procedure'. However, real testing according to current valid criteria of research has not yet taken place
5   the proposal is then discussed, for example in editorials by 'specialists in the field'. An argument between the 'champions' and the trialists is started and single negative aspects of the new technology are used for professional denunciation. Real testing of the innovation has still not taken place.

It is not uncommon for the innovation to attract the public attention before real testing has taken place. The fear of the truth and the labour of a controlled trial have prevented a real evaluation from taking place.

This life cycle of innovation (McKinley, 1981) has to be prevented. According to Sir Karl Popper the most promising way to come closer to the truth is to generate a hypothesis and try to falsify it with available methods. Brian Jennett (1986) suggests that in medicine we do not deal with testing for truth, but changes or exact differences between techniques. The appropriate testing mechanism, the 'gold standard' is the controlled clinical trial (Troidl et al., 1990). Selby and Friedman (1989) have defined three grades of evidence.

Grade I: is testing by controlled clinical trial.

Grade II: is testing by analytical study designed, for example, as an uncontrolled prospective cohort study.

Grade III: is testing by descriptive study.

The disadvantage of uncontrolled observational and descriptive studies is the danger of systematic bias at different levels.

Several authors (Jennett, 1986; Troidl, 1989) have emphasized that testing by controlled clinical trials in surgery can be extremely difficult. From a surgical point of view, the claim that the first patient has to be randomized is sheer nonsense.

From the very beginning it has been my declared intention that the hypothesis that endoscopic surgery is the most patient-friendly surgery has to be tested by controlled clinical trial using the relevant endpoints (Neugebauer et al., 1991). However, I have not been able to achieve this aim (Neugebauer et al., 1991). By testing the hypothesis we realized that a new classification of complications was necessary (see Table 2.1). Our alternative to the controlled clinical trial was the uncontrolled clinical cohort study which we performed with close attention to detail. Another possible alternative could be to use a computerized database in which all patient variables are entered.

A further way to collect relevant information is by failure analysis. This procedure is routine in technical disciplines like aviation where it has

Class I	Incident-free surgery: no technical problems during surgery and no negative outcome for the patient
Class II	Inconsequential incident surgery: one or more technical problems during surgery, but no negative outcome for the patient (intra–abdominal weight loss, bleeding)
Class III	Consequential non-incident surgery: no surgical problems, but one or more negative outcomes for the patient (haematoma, wound infection)
Class IV	Incidents: one or more technical problems during surgery with corresponding negative outcomes for the patient (changing operative method, re-laparotomy)
Class V	Incidents: death related to the operation

Table 2.1: Classification of incidents from the patient viewpoint.

been applied with great success. Sir Karl Popper strongly recommends this procedure for medical technologies (Popper, 1972). Failure analysis is:

1 the general exploration and description of the clinical situation, followed by
2 an analysis of what actually happened, followed by
3 an investigation of the reasons why something has happened, followed by
4 a conclusion of how failure can be avoided and fixed.

This methodological procedure can collect information in single cases and in a whole population of patients under treatment.

Relevant endpoints for endoscopic surgery

It must be clearly stated that the controlled clinical trial with its necessarily high grade of evidence can only function when a detailed study protocol has described and defined the patient population and listed the relevant endpoints under test (Troidl, 1990; Troidl *et al.*, 1990).

In the definition of our concept (the most patient-friendly surgery), the relevant endpoints are:

• the discomfort and inconvenience caused to the patient during treatment
• the intensity and quality of pain suffered
• the fatigue and other side effects suffered
• the recovery rate
• physical body integrity (Troidl, 1989). *See* Figure 2.2.

All these endpoints can be analysed by empirical research methods (Troidl *et al.*, 1990). Instruments like visual analogue scales and quality of life questionnaires can be used. The measurement of quality of life is important in so far as symptoms are not everything, ie the same symptoms can be coped with by individual patients in completely different ways (Eypasch *et al.*, 1990; Troidl *et al.*, 1990). This important information about coping with symptoms and emotions can only be measured and addressed by a global assessment of well-being or quality of life (Troidl *et al.*, 1990).

The use of the same endpoints for the assessment of different treatment strategies such as symptomatic gallstone disease-like fragmentation, gallbladder function, the possibility of passage concretion, a number of residual calculi, complete or incomplete disappearance of calculi, complicates the measurement of outcomes. A sick patient with gallstones seeks medical attention for pain relief, a relief of symptoms such as colic and an end to dietary restrictions. Two different degrees of these symptoms influence the patient's well-being. The patient is absolutely right to ask for safe and quick relief from this very commonplace problem which is impairing his well-being. He is right to want the treatment to be successful without additional long-term treatment and without side effects. Looking at symptomatic gallstone disease these can be seen to be the relevant endpoints for surgical treatment.

The feasibility (Jennett, 1986; Troidl *et al.*, 1991) (*see* Table 2.2) of this hypothesis, the first step of technology assessment according to Jennett, is important, was important and will continue to be important in the future. The feasibility of its elements, complications and operative mortality is, however, only the first step of technology assessment. (The Veterans Administration Systemic Sepsis Cooperative Group, 1987.) Of equal, if not more, importance are the efficacy (benefit for the patient) and the effectiveness (the possibility of applying the new technology with equal efficacy on a general level). Lastly, the benefit to the surgeon has to be considered and the cost-benefit analysis viewed (Jennett, 1986; Troidl *et al.*, 1991). *See* Table 2.2.

Criteria	Element (examples)
1. Feasibility	technical applications complications mortality
2. Efficacy	benefit to the patient in special clinics
3. Effectiveness	safety, applicability, suitability for everyday use
4. Benefit to the surgeon	simplification of operation

5. Cost-benefit	cost-benefit analysis
	influences – medicine
	                  – finances
	                  – society

Table 2.2: Technology assessment (accord. to B. Jennett, mod. by H. Troidl).

With patient-friendly surgery it is essential to comply with this claim using the endpoints of comfort and minimal patient trauma. The technical feasibility, operative mortality and complication rate are not sufficient as endpoints (The Veterans Administration Systemic Sepsis Cooperative Group, 1987).

Definition and terminology

For the definition or description of an entity there are two basic possibilities. It can either be descriptive or theoretical (Bassler, 1991). The phrase 'most patient-friendly surgery' which I have used for minimally invasive surgery is a definition which is called theoretical by Bassler (1991). Sir Karl Popper suggests that you have to be very careful with these kinds of definitions. He refuses to accept definitions which are written from left to right, eg democracy is . . . sepsis is . . . Popper finds these types of definitions too narrow because of the inherent danger that, in an argument, only the narrowness of the definition is defended. For Popper it makes more sense to list the reasonable essential components to the left side of the equation and the hypothetical summary of them on the right side, eg fever, tachycardia, leucocytosis = sepsis. With this kind of summary it is possible to modify the definition later on if necessary. In order to solve this problem it is necessary to discuss the question of terminology.

There have already been many variations in terminology used to describe 'endoscopic surgery' (Wittmoser, 1959). *See* Tables 2.3 and 2.4. Nevertheless, it is necessary to think about the terminology used in these new developments. A name should first of all describe the concept and the philosophy as precisely as possible (*see* Table 2.4). The philosophy of endoscopic surgery is the association of maximum comfort with minimal trauma, and that this is defined by the patient. 'Minimally invasive' and 'minimal access' are partial, although important, aspects.

Minimal invasive surgery	J.E.A.Wickham (urologist)
Minimal access surgery	A.Cuschieri (surgeon)
Minimal invasive chirurgle (MIC)	G.Buess (surgeon)
Endoscopic intra-abdominal microsurgery	K.Semm (gynaecologist)
Minimally invasive general surgery	Royal College of Surgeons

Table 2.3: Terminology currently suggested by general surgeons.

There is no doubt that minimal access is an important characteristic of this type of surgery, eg laparoscopic cholecystectomy. With this kind of surgery for removal of the gallbladder, only access to the operative field is now different. The dissection in Calot's triangle and in the gallbladder bed is somewhat sparing and less traumatic, but it is not really different. The effect of this type of surgery on the patient is produced predominantly by the different approaches to the operative field. The exact opposite is true with cholecystostomy, a therapeutic approach which is very popular in English-speaking countries. This technique for cholecystostomy is more or less minimally invasive and always uses minimal access. However, it is extremely uncomfortable for the patient, eg the tube in the abdominal wall discharging bile or pus. Of course patient-friendly surgery is not on a par with a small surgical intervention. Under favourable circumstances even a big operation, eg removal of a lung lobe, can be patient-friendly.

As well as taking the claims of the patient and the scientific concept into account when justifying terminology, an aspect of promotion must also be considered.

- Imaged thoracoscopic surgery (ITS)

- Video-amplified endoscopic thoracic surgery

- Tele-present surgery

- Video-assisted thorascopic surgery (VATS)

Table 2.4: Terminology currently suggested by thoracic surgeons.

The political aspect of terminology should not be underestimated. A new name has to be accepted by the surgical community, and certain names and definitions induce a certain reaction in the public. For example, in Germany, 'minimal' implies that the surgical treatment is smaller, less invasive, less difficult and financially not as well compensated as conventional surgical techniques (see below). In North America thoracoscopic means a smaller charge to the patient. For example, in Canada, a thoracoscopic lung biopsy costs 70 Canadian dollars, in comparison with an open lung biopsy costing 300 Canadian dollars.

Terminology should avoid unnecessary language problems and not be difficult to pronounce. It should be translatable into different languages and a reasonable and understandable abbreviation should be available (see Table 2.4). The name should allow for development and should not be orientated towards daily political aspects. Last, but not least, the name has to be acceptable to the public and the medical community.

Costs

This is not the place for a complete economic evaluation (Drummond et al., 1990) of the developments in endoscopic surgery. Nevertheless, it is a integral part of the technology assessment and will gain further importance in the future. Currently cost-benefit analysis justification for the acceptance or otherwise of a particular technique is not possible, and an acceptable solution needs to be sought.

Western industrialized countries cannot afford another increase in health care expenditure. On the other hand, an excellent service can only be provided with sufficient income. Therefore, if traditional procedures such as open lung biopsy cost the patient ten times as much in North America as patient-friendly endoscopic lung biopsies then alternative treatment procedures will not always be available to the patient. There is also a danger that endoscopic surgery will not be developed as quickly as it should.

In Germany endoscopic surgery can mean bankruptcy for a hospital which uses the technique. Hospitals are paid on a patient per day basis and each year the different hospitals negotiate with health insurance and health maintenance organizations to find a reasonable compromise on the patient per day rate. Out of this rate the hospital has to pay nurses and for medical equipment. The hospital has a financial interest in patients who undergo low-cost surgical procedures, but have to stay a long time in the hospital. Laparoscopic cholecystectomy, with its short hospital stay of two or three days, could mean financial ruin for a German hospital. The cost implications of endoscopic surgery will be different in each country, and therefore each country needs to devise its own strategy for dealing with them.

References

Bässler U (1991) *Irrtum und Erkenntnis*. Naturwissenschaften–Bibliothek. Springer Verlag, Berlin.

Drummond M *et al.*, (1990) *Methods for the economic evaluation of health care*. Oxford Medical Publications, Oxford.

Eypasch E, Troidl H, Wood-Dauphinée S, Williams JI, Reinecke K, Ure B and Neugebauer E (1990) Quality of life and gastrointestinal surgery: a clinimetric approach to developing an instrument for its measurement. *Theor. Surg.* 5: 3–10.

Götz F (1988) Die endoskopische Appendektomie nach Semm bei der akuten und chronischen Appendicitis. *Endoskopie heute.* 2: 5–7.

Ikeuchi H (1988) The early days of arthroscopic surgery in Japan. *J. Arthroscopic Related Surg.* 4 (3): 222–225.

Jennett B (1986) *High technology medicine: benefits and burdens*. Oxford University Press, Oxford.

McKinley J (1981) From 'promising report' to 'standard procedures': seven stages in the career of a medical innovation. *Millbank Mem. Fund.* 59: 374–411.

Mühe E (1986) Die erste Cholezystektomie durch das Laparoskop. *Langenbecks Arch. Chir. Kongreßband.* 804.

Neugebauer E, Troidl II, Spangenberger W, Dietrich A, Lefering R and the cholecystectomy study group (1991) Laparoscopic versus conventional cholecystectomy and the randomized controlled trial. *Br. J. Surg.* 78: 150–154.

Popper K (1987) *Auf der Suche nach einer besseren Welt*. Piper Verlag München, Zürich.

Popper K (1972) *Objektive Erkenntnis: Ein evolutionärer Entwurf*. Verlag Hoffmann und Kampe, Hamburg.

Schonholtz GJ (1988) Arthroscopic surgery: past, present and future. *J. Arthroscopic Related Surg*. 4 (3): 226–229.

Schuster HP (1981) Sepsis: Klinische Definition und Inzidenz. In: *Sepsis, eine interdisziplinäre Herausforderung*. Hrsg: Reinhard K und Eyrich K. Springer-Verlag Berlin, Heidelberg.

Selby JV and Friedman GD (1989) Sigmoidsocopy in the periodic health examination of asymptomatic adults. *JAMA*. 261: 595.

Semm K (1982) Endoscopic appendectomy. In: *Advances in pelviscopic surgery*. Year Book Medical Publishers, Inc.

The Veterans Administration Systemic Sepsis Cooperative Group (L Hinshaw *et al.*,) (1987) Effect of high-dose glucocorticoid therapy on mortality in patients with clinical signs of systemic sepsis. *N. Eng. J. Med*. 317: 659–665.

Troidl H, Kusche J, Vestweber K-H, Eypasch E, Köppen L and Bouillon B (1987) Quality of life: an important endpoint both in surgical practice and research. *J. Chron. Dis*. 40 (6): 523–528.

Troidl H, Kusche J, Vestweber K-H, Eypasch E and Maul U (1987) Pouch versus esophagojejunostomy after total gastrectomy: a randomized clinical trial. *World J. Surg*. 11: 699–712.

Troidl H (1989) Lebensqualität: Ein relevantes Zielkriterium in der Chirurgie. *Chirurg*. 60: 445–449.

Troidl H (1990) The general surgeon and the trauma surgeon – binding the wounds. *Theor. Surg*. 5: 64–74.

Troidl H und Neugebauer E (1990) Akuter Schmerz in der Chirurgie. *Chirurg*. 61: 485–493.

Troidl H, Spitzer WO, Mulder DS, Wechsler AS, McPeek B, McKneally MF and Balch CM (1990) *Principles and practice of research, Second edition*. Springer Verlag, Heidelberg.

Troidl H (1990) Surgical endoscopy and sonography – surgery at the crossroads. *Surg. Endosc*. 4: 41–46.

Troidl H, Eypasch E, Al-Jaziri A and Spangenberger W, Dietrich A (1991) Laparascopic cholecystectomy in view of medical technology assessment. *Dig. Surg*. 8: 108–113.

Troidl H, Eypasch E, Spangenberger W, Langen R und Holthausen U (1991) Schonendes Operieren – Verfahrenswahl und Strategie: Invasives versus minimal invasives Opericren. *Langenbecks Arch. Chir. Suppl.* 48–56.

Wickham JER (1982) The new surgery. *BMJ.* 295: 1581–1582.

Wittmoser R (1959) Thoraskopische Sympathicotomie bei Durchblutungsstörungen des Armes. *Langenbecks Arch. und Dt. Zeitschr. Chir.* 292: 318–323.

3

Therapeutic Endoscopy in Gastroenterology

PAUL SALMON

Historical background

With the introduction of flexible fibre-optic imaging into medicine in the early 1970s (Ishioka *et al.*, 1970; Jenny *et al.*,1972; Sakita *et al.*, 1971; Salmon *et al.*, 1972), gastroenterologists had the means of making a tissue diagnosis by targeted biopsies from within the tubular digestive tract for the first time. However, it was not long before therapeutic applications became evident. One of the first therapeutic applications was the use of endoscopy in the selection and follow-up of patients treated for peptic ulcer disease (Brown *et al.*, 1972), a technique that rapidly became a routine and mandatory procedure for prospective controlled trials of new ulcer healing agents.

Soon after this, endoscopic sphincterotomy was described (Kawai *et al.*, 1974), and was followed by experimental and clinical studies, initially in Europe, demonstrating the feasibility, value and safety of this procedure in the management of common duct stones and some periampullary tumours (Classen and Safrany, 1975).

Whilst in the early days of diagnostic endoscopy of the gastrointestinal tract there was much debate, especially in the USA, as to whether the increased workload should be undertaken by trained technicians (paramedics), there was never any doubt that therapeutic endoscopy, whether performed by a physician or a surgeon, required an in-depth knowledge of gastrointestinal disease. The importance of clinical judgement during all stages of therapeutic endoscopy (both planning and execution) should not be underestimated.

During the 16 years since the introduction of endoscopic sphincterotomy, the therapeutic applications of endoscopy have rapidly increased so that a whole new subject has evolved. Some therapeutic procedures, such as colonoscopic polypectomy and oesophageal dilatation of oesophageal strictures, have been available for more than 15 years (Williams *et al.*, 1974; Olsen *et al.*, 1977) and are now fully established, whilst other techniques are currently being evaluated. Therapeutic endoscopy in gastroenterology has made considerable advances both in neoplastic and non-neoplastic diseases. Table 3.1 sets out the current options for therapeutic endoscopy in gastrointestinal tumours, whilst Table 3.2 gives an overall perspective of the role of therapeutic endoscopy in gastroenterology.

This chapter will consider the principles and practice of therapeutic endoscopy in this wider context.

Options
- Oesophageal treatment of malignant strictures.
- Endoscopic placement of intestinal tubes.
- Endoscopic thermal haemostasis.
- Endoscopic gastric polypectomy.
- Endoscopic sphincterotomy.
- Endoscopic decompression of the biliary tree.
- Percutaneous cholangioscopy.
- Endoscopic laser treatment (ELT) of gastrointestinal tumours.
- Management of early gastric cancer.

Table 3.1: Therapeutic applications of endoscopy in gastrointestinal tumours (Salmon, 1992).

- Management of oesophageal strictures.
- Placement of intestinal tubes.
- Sclerotherapy.
- Thermal haemostasis.
- Removal of foreign bodies.
- Polypectomy.
- Retrograde sphincterotomy.
- Decompression of the biliary tree.
- Thermal treatment (ETT) of gastrointestinal neoplasms (lasers and BICAP treatment).
- Management of early gastric cancer.

Table 3.2: Therapeutic applications of endoscopy in gastroenterology.

Endoscopic management of oesophageal strictures

Whilst oesophageal dilatation is the primary therapy for benign oesophageal strictures (Benedict, 1966; Olsen *et al.*, 1977; Huchzemeyer *et al.*, 1977), oesophageal dilatation of malignant strictures, together with other procedures, including endoscopic thermal tumour ablation and prosthetic device insertion, are strictly palliative procedures which must be planned in the context of the overall management strategy for the patient (whether surgical or radiotherapy). The prime goal of endoscopic management of oesophageal strictures, whether benign or malignant, is the relief of dysphagia. For that reason, dysphagia, which is a very reliable symptom, should be carefully assessed both before and after treatment.

The usual grading system is as follows: (Earlam and Melo-Cunha, 1981):

Grade 0:   normal swallowing
Grade 1:   occasional difficulty swallowing solids
Grade 2:   unable to swallow solids
Grade 3:   unable to swallow minced food
Grade 4:   unable to swallow puréed or liquid foods
Grade 5:   unable to swallow liquids or saliva.

A simpler system, more directly relevant to endoscopic treatment, and one that I employ, is as follows (Luna, 1983):

Good: Able to swallow a normal diet with occasional dysphagia only, no dilatation needed
Moderate: Occasional or mild dysphagia for solid food, occasional dilatation needed
Severe: Persistent dysphagia even with semi-solid food. Inability to achieve a calibre of 50 French (15–16 mm), frequent dilatation needed.

The nature of the stricture should be comprehensively evaluated prior to treatment. In 80% of cases a detailed history and careful examination will produce the correct diagnosis. This should be followed by contrast radiology by means of a barium swallow which may include a 'solid bolus study' (e.g. a barium-coated marshmallow or barium pill), evaluation of motility in the supine, upright and Trendelenburg's position and in some cases by means of cine-fluoroscopy (three frames per second imaging). Prior diagnostic endoscopy is almost always required with brush cytology and biopsies to establish the nature of the stricture. It is important that prior diagnostic endoscopy should be part of a full upper gastrointestinal (GI) examination, where the stricture will allow this. Use of one of the small diameter endoscopes is recommended to facilitate this requirement. This will allow the endoscopist to exclude a fundal carcinoma, which may cause a lower oesophageal stricture by sub-mucosal invasion of the lower oesophagus, and also to exclude duodenal ulcer disease which may be associated with reflex oesophagitis and peptic stricture formation. For example, if the latter is found, the therapeutic strategy will also include acid-blockade, probably with a proton pump inhibitor (e.g. omeprazole). In some cases, the history and contrast radiology suggest muscular strictures which include achalasia, rings and webs and oesophageal spasm. In these cases, oesophageal manometry may be of additional help. 24-hour ambulatory intra-oesophageal monitoring, with or without manometry (Porro and Pace, 1991), is a further option which may help in establishing whether a stricture is primarily peptic (i.e. due to gastro-oesophageal reflux) in selected patients.

Oesophageal dilatation techniques

Oesophageal dilatation (bougienage) is traditionally performed 'blind', employing a mercury-filled bougie with the patient in the sitting position (Hurst or Maloney bougie). Whilst many cases can be successfully and safely managed in this way, the use of fluoroscopy and endoscopic placement of a guidewire, followed by passage of a hollow-core dilator over the guidewire, is not only safer (McClave *et al.*, 1989), but more applicable to the majority of strictures. Mercury bougies are not suitable for strictures less than 32 French (10 mm diameter), and also carry the risk of possible leakage of mercury from old and worn bougies (environmental and health hazard). They should probably now be replaced by the endoscopic guidewire directed bougies (hollow-core dilators).

Types of dilators used in endoscopic bougienage

Endoscope

Under certain circumstances, such as webs and rings, the endoscope itself may be used to effect some dilatation. The endoscopist should initially ascertain that the stricture is not much smaller than the endoscope. The endoscope should then be gently pushed through the stricture exerting pressure from the thumb and fore-finger only. If the endoscope will not pass the stricture, then another dilator should be employed. The endoscope can also be used to estimate the diameter of the stricture. As a guideline, the Olympus 1T2 OES endoscope has an outside diameter of 11.2 mm (35 French), whilst Pentax endoscopes have the outside diameter (French) included in their name, e.g. Pentax F34JA endoscope (34 French).

Hollow-core dilators

- Savary-Gilliard dilator.
- Celestin stepped dilator.
- Eder-Puestow dilator.
- Triple metal olive dilator.
- Balloon dilator.

All hollow-core dilators are used over a guidewire which should be passed through the biopsy channel of the endoscope into the stomach. Fluoroscopy should be employed wherever possible in order to confirm the position of the guidewire through the stricture. Some endoscopy units and endoscopists do not have fluoroscopy available, in which case special precautions must be taken to avoid perforation of the oesophagus.

Guidewire techniques

Whichever guidewire is used, and there are several types available, it should have a flexible tip. Spring-tip guidewires are provided with the Savary, Eder-Puestow and triple metal olive dilators. The Savary type, with a graduated spring, is more reliable and lasts longer than the Eder-Puestow spring-tip guidewire. Piano wire guidewires with a spring tip are available (Microvasive), and are extremely robust. Angiographic guidewires are also available. The type of guidewire is relatively unimportant, provided it is in good condition, unkinked, has a flexible tip and is used correctly. Correct use of the guidewire involves two people. The assistant must keep the guidewire taut at all times during the introduction of the dilator, and *not* allow it to move with the dilator as the endoscopist passes ('rail-roads') the dilator over the guidewire. If fluoroscopy is not used, and this should only be allowed with short non-neoplastic strictures, the guidewire should be marked after insertion through the stricture, in order to reconfirm the position of the guidewire after insertion of the dilator. Calibrated guidewires are now available and are recommended, especially if fluoroscopy is not employed. The proximal tip of the guidewire, especially with spring steel or piano wire guidewires, is potentially dangerous, as it may flail and cause skin or eye injury to the patient, endoscopist or assistant. For this reason, the exposed wire tip should be protected by a plastic coloured button or other device, so that it can easily be seen by all concerned. For tortuous and very narrow strictures, an angiographic guidewire may be passed into the stricture followed by a straight tapered angiographic catheter. When this has been achieved, the guidewire can be replaced by a torque controlled guidewire to traverse the stricture. The guidewire may then be replaced by a stiff guidewire followed by a suitable hollow-core dilator (McLean *et al.*, 1987).

Guidewire complications include oesophageal perforation and production of a 'false passage'. In the case of malignant strictures the latter complication may not be important. Fluoroscopy is the key to a low complication rate.

Dilator techniques

Rule of threes

This rule dictates that no more than three successively larger dilators should be used above the dilator that first meets resistance. Choice of the initial dilator is by examination of the radiographs and from the endoscopy examination, which can usually estimate the stricture size reasonably accurately.

This rule is especially relevant when employing either metal olive dilators (e.g. Eder-Puestow dilators) or Savary-Gilliard (Savary) dilators.

When using Celestin stepped dilators this rule can be relaxed, as it can with balloon dilators. The principles involved are axial forces with metal olive and Savary dilators (pushing), with radial forces being of more importance in balloon dilatation. The axial forces used in dilatation are potentially dangerous and form the basis of the 'rule of threes'.

Balloon dilators

The great advantage of balloon dilatation is that radial forces are applied to dilate a stricture. The potentially dangerous axial forces, generated by pushing a dilator through a stricture, do not occur. Balloon dilatation of strictures is a developing subject. It is likely that balloon dilatation will soon become the most important form of dilatation of GI strictures (oesophageal, pyloric, biliary and colonic strictures). There are two types of balloon employed:

1. TTS balloon (through the 'scope)

These are size-limited balloons based on the Gruntzig-technique employed in angioplasty. For this reason excess pressure will not cause greater expansion (unlike a latex balloon), and minimal axial force is required for dilatation. The balloons supplied by Microvasive[1] (Rigiflex) are made of an inelastic proprietary polymer, Polytuff 150 or 310. A variety of balloon sizes are available and all can be passed down a biopsy channel of 2.8 mm diameter or greater. For sizes above 1.5 mm (inflated), the rubber biopsy channel valve should be removed. Table 3.3 gives the balloon sizes available with balloon length, recommended inflation pressure and type of syringe recommended both for inflation and deflation.

Balloon size (mm)	Balloon length	Recommended pressure (PSI)	Recommended syringe (Infl)(cc)
4	2 cm	90	20
6	2 cm	75	20
6	8 cm/3 cm	60	20
8	8 cm/3 cm	60	20
10	8 cm/3 cm	50	20
12	8 cm/3 cm	50	20
15	8 cm	45	30
15	3 cm	45	20
18	8 cm	35	30
18	3 cm	35	20
20	8 cm	25	30
25	8 cm	25	30

All balloons should be deflated with a 50 cc syringe

Table 3.3: TTS balloon (Rigiflex) recommended inflation pressures.

Remember that a small syringe gives greater inflation pressure than a large syringe. The recommended inflation pressures should never be exceeded. A Le Veen inflator or Rigiflator (Microvasive) should be employed and the inflation pressure monitored accurately throughout the procedure using a Rigiflex monitor (pressure gauge). Care should be taken in passing the balloon through the biopsy channel. Good lubrication is essential and the balloon should be carefully folded before doing this. The balloon may be filled with dilute contrast medium if required. If so, filling should be done in several stages to remove all the air from the balloon. Similarly, the contrast medium should be carefully removed after use. Fluoroscopy is required to monitor the balloon position. In most cases, a characteristic 'waist effect' is seen prior to dilating the stricture. I personally prefer the 8 cm balloon as the

---

[1]Microvasive, Inc., PO Box 415, Belmont, Massachusetts 02178, USA

short 3 cm balloons are difficult to keep within the stricture unless the stricture is very short.

2. *Pneumatic dilatation (forceful dilatation) in achalasia*

Pneumatic (balloon) dilatation is a time-honoured ('Brusque dilatation' Schindler, 1956), and successful method of treating achalasia and certain cases with oesophageal dysmotility. It involves the use of larger balloons than the TTS balloons previously described. The literature contains a wide variety of balloon dilators (e.g. Sippy dilator, Rider-Moeller dilator) but most of these are now obsolete and have been replaced by low compliance polyethylene balloons. These usually start at 30 mm diameter. The three sizes commonly employed (Microvasive Rigiflex) are 30 mm, 35 mm and 40 mm. A 50 mm balloon is available, but is rarely required. These balloons are hollow-core dilators and must *never* be employed without a guidewire, as the flexible tip can otherwise easily perforate the foregut. Patients with achalasia should be assessed clinically, radiologically and endoscopically by manometry, which will confirm the characteristic mean lower oesophageal pressure of 40 mmHg or greater. The possibility of pseudo-achalasia, due to undiagnosed submucosal gastric carcinoma, should be remembered. Prior endoscopic evaluation should be carried out to confirm whether the oesophagus has retained food residue. If so, this should be removed by oesophageal lavage employing a 12 mm (36 French) tube passed orally. The endoscopist should perform this prior to the balloon dilatation. The balloon dilator should be positioned fluoroscopically across the diaphragm. A check X-ray ensures that the correct position is recorded. The smallest available balloon should be employed in the first place (e.g. 30 mm). Balloon pressures recommended by the manufacturers should not be exceeded (i.e. 15 psi) and the pressure maintained for 1–2 minutes, or less if pain occurs. In most cases, if properly performed, there will be blood on the balloon. The patient should be observed for up to 4 hours and a chest X-ray taken before discharge to detect a pneumomediastinum if perforation has occurred. A normal X-ray does not exclude perforation. Some gastroenterologists carry out a water-soluble contrast-swallow examination before discharging the patient. It is not usually necessary to admit the patient overnight. The perforation rate is probably 5–10% with pneumatic dilatation, although very low perforation rates (e.g. 0.4%) have been recorded (Kozarek, 1981). In a subject where objective measurement is often lacking, I recommend clinical evaluation according to the criteria described by Vantrappen (Vantrappen and Hellemans, 1980), and staging according to Adams (Adams *et al.*, 1961). A recent study has demonstrated that sublingual nifedipine, when administered 30 minutes before food, and in an individualized dose (10–80 mg) is equally effective in reducing symptoms (Coccia *et al.*, 1991).

Oesophageal prosthesis placement

Whereas insertion of an oesophageal prosthesis in malignant dysphagia proved to be a significant advance in the management of mid-oesophageal carcinoma (Atkinson *et al.*, 1978; den Hartog Jager *et al.*, 1979), the development of thermal recanalization by means of laser and bipolar circumactive probe

(BICAP) tumour ablation (*see* page 38) has reduced the need for the technique except in cases of broncho-oesophageal fistula (post-irradiation, tumour invasion or traumatic). Oesophageal stents cannot be employed in the proximal one third of oesophageal neoplasms because of the danger of tracheal compression and asphyxia due to proximal stent migration. Distal ⅓ tumours are also unsuitable, as the stent often becomes blocked, due to angulation. Whilst oesophageal tubes can be manufactured within the GI unit, from either PVC or Tygon (Fischer Scientific) tubing (12–18 mm diameter), commercially available tubes are generally satisfactory. These are made of either latex rubber (Celestin, Proctor-Levinston tube), or silicone rubber (Atkinson tube) and have proximal and distal flanges or cuffs to reduce the risk of proximal or distal migration from the stricture.

Technique

The proximal and distal margins of the oesophageal tumour should be measured from previous radiographs. A suitable length prosthesis should then be chosen, so as to project approximately 3 cm distal to the tumour. The malignant stricture should be dilated up to 54 French (e.g. large size Celestin stepped dilator) and the stent introduced using one of several available methods. The Mark II Nottingham oesophageal tube introducer (KeyMed/Olympus), consisting of a flexible metal staff that is introduced over a flexible spring-steel guidewire, was developed for the Atkinson prosthesis. The flexible over-the-wire staff has a removable expanding olive fitted to grip the oesophageal stent. Care should be taken to avoid lubricant (e.g. KY jelly) getting inside the oesophageal tube which would cause the tube to slip during insertion. The Nottingham introducer is also suitable for Celestin tubes. Graham (1990) employs a paediatric endoscope over which a pusher tube (braided Tygon) and the stent are placed. This allows simultaneous endoscopic control of the tube introduction and is a recommended technique. A suitable hollow-core dilator such as a Savary dilator can also be employed to push the stent into place, providing guidewire control with fluoroscopy is used.

Oesophageal stent placement carries a significant procedural morbidity and 30-day mortality which, although usually quoted as a 10% procedure related mortality (Atkinson et al., 1978), has also been quoted as a 30% 30-day mortality (den Hartog Jager et al., 1979).

Post-stent care

Once the position of the stent has been recorded radiographically, a chest X-ray and water soluble 'barium swallow' should be performed, within a few hours. Provided no perforation has occurred, the patient can be started on clear fluids and graduated to solid food over the next 24–48 hours. All solid food should be well chewed and swallowed with carbonated drinks (e.g. soda-water). Boiled fish and lettuce are common culprits for stent blockage and should not be allowed. Stent blockage can usually be managed by passing a nasogastric tube or clearing the obstruction endoscopically. In patients who survive longer than 6 months, stent change should be considered, as PVC stents lose their plasticizer and therefore flexibility, and latex tubes (e.g. Celestin tubes) may disintegrate (Branicki *et al.*, 1981).

Endoscopic placement of intestinal tubes

Therapeutic intubation of the gastrointestinal tract is an established and clinically proven procedure, which may be indicated in the management of intestinal obstruction, provision of enteral feeding, intestinal decompression, diversion of secretions, and for intestinal stenting.

Long-term naso-enteral intubation, usually for nutritional support, has a number of complications as it predisposes to gastro-oesophageal reflux, aspiration pneumonia, lower oesophageal strictures and rarer complications such as perforation of the stomach or small bowel and jejunal intussusception (Chaffee, 1949). Some of these problems were due to the tubes employed, whether it was the small bore Ryle's tube, the multilumen Miller-Abbott tube or the mercury-loaded Cantor tube. In the critically ill patient, attempts to reduce aspiration pneumonia which remains a major complication of enteral nutrition, have used newly developed endoscopic techniques to form a feeding gastrostomy or jejunostomy, rather than enteral feeding via nasogastric tubes. Percutaneous endoscopic gastrostomy can now replace laparotomy and general anaesthesia in the creation of a feeding gastrostomy (Gauderer and Ponsky, 1980, 1981), and percutaneous endoscopic jejunostomy may be performed, a technique that combines jejunal intubation (for feeding) with gastric decompression (Ponsky and Aszodi, 1984). Neurogenic oropharyngeal dysphagia following a stroke or head injury, critical illness, respiratory failure, septic shock and multiple organ failure comprise the majority of patients requiring nutritional support. Recent reports however, show a relatively high complication rate for percutaneous endoscopic jejunostomy (PEJ) including continued aspiration, gastrointestinal bleeding and catheter problems (leakage, plugging, fracture and tube migration). All recent studies conclude that further improvement in catheter design is needed, that there is insufficient current evidence showing that PEJ is superior to percutaneous endoscopic gastrostomy (PEG) and that the need for nutritional support in these patients persists (Disario *et al.*, 1990; Lazarus *et al.*, 1990; Lowe and Puyana, 1991).

Upper intestinal tube placement

Small bore long intestinal catheters can be readily positioned in the upper small intestine by means of a standard upper GI endoscope. The techniques employed are as follows:

1   A small silk suture loop is tied to the tip of the tube which is then passed into the distal stomach (per-orally). The endoscope is then passed into the stomach, and biopsy forceps are used to grasp the suture loop and push the tube into the duodenum through the pylorus. Care must be taken to avoid pulling the tube out of the duodenum when the endoscope is removed. The

same technique may also be employed to intubate a gastroenterostomy or Billroth II anastomosis.

2   An alternative but similar technique is to pull the silk suture (which must be longer) through the biopsy channel of the endoscope by means of biopsy forceps before the endoscope is passed. The endoscope and the feeding tube are then passed together, the forceps then being used to grasp the suture and push the tube into the small intestine.

3   TTS method. With this technique a large channel endoscope, such as a two channel endoscope with the larger biopsy channel of 3.63 mm, is employed. This will allow a 2.64 mm external diameter feeding tube (e.g. Dobhoff enteric feeding tube) to be passed through the endoscope. A 400 cm 0.035 inch guidewire is also used through the feeding tube, and the wire and tube are then advanced into the small bowel under endoscopic control. The tube tip is checked by fluoroscopy and the endoscope removed when the tube is in position.

Percutaneous endoscopic gastrostomy (PEG)

The principle of PEG is the formation of a feeding gastrostomy without the need for laparotomy or general anaesthesia. The techniques involved are variations of the original 'pull' technique, described by Gauderer and Ponsky (Gauderer and Ponsky, 1980, 1981). In the original 'pull' technique, a 16 French mushroom catheter with the distal flared tip cut off, has a suture placed through the cut tip, which is then threaded through a tapered intravenous catheter. The wide end of the tapered catheter is then pushed over the cut end of the mushroom catheter. This creates a tapered end for the mushroom catheter. The suture is knotted where it comes out of the tapered end. A 3 cm length of soft rubber or plastic tubing is then prepared with two opposite side holes. The tapered catheter is passed through these holes and the 3 cm length of tubing then positioned up against the mushroom tip of the catheter. This cross-piece of tubing will act as a 'bolster' and will be used to pull the gastric wall against the abdominal wall from within the stomach. A second 3 cm rubber or plastic bolster is also prepared. Following a 6-hour fast, gastroscopy is performed under intravenous sedation, and the stomach fully distended with air. The abdominal wall is then punctured at a point two thirds of the distance along a line, drawn from the umbilicus to the mid point of the left costal margin. Transillumination of the abdominal wall from within the air-filled stomach facilitates this procedure. The abdominal wall should be punctured through a small skin incision using an intravenous cannula. The endoscopist then closes a polypectomy snare over the iv cannula following removal of the stylet. At this point, a 150 cm length of silk suture is threaded through the iv cannula into the stomach. After several centimetres of suture have passed into the stomach, the endoscopist closes the snare over the suture and carefully removes the endoscope from the patient, pulling the silk suture with it. Having removed the endoscope, there is now a length of silk suture entering the patient's anterior abdominal wall and passing out of the patient's mouth. The free end of the suture coming out of the patient's mouth is now tied to the suture material coming out of the tapered catheter previously made. Following lubrication of the tapered mushroom catheter, the abdominal wall free end of the suture is gently pulled so that the tapered catheter passes into the patient's mouth and finally out through the abdominal wall puncture site. The gastroscope is then employed to monitor the mushroom catheter and mushroom cross-piece bolster until the bolster is firmly in contact with the gastric mucosa. The second bolster is then positioned over the external end of the mushroom catheter and pushed down on to the anterior abdominal wall. The bolster is then sutured to the skin. The gastrostomy tube can be removed later by gentle traction, leaving the internal bolster within the stomach which is then passed in the stool.

The basic technique described above, originally performed using materials found within a GI unit, has been facilitated by commercial kits now available. A gastrostomy button is available which also contains an anti-reflex device. This button can be introduced, using a stylet to stretch the mushroom through an existing gastrostomy tract.

Modifications of the original 'pull' technique are currently being developed and are required with new catheter design to reduce the significant complication rate. A 'push' technique (Sacks *et al.*, 1983) employs similar preparation of the patient. As previously, an intravenous cannula is employed to puncture the stomach under endoscopic control, and a snare used to grasp a guidewire which is pulled out of the patient's mouth. A gastrostomy tube (e.g. 20 French) is then threaded over the guidewire and pushed down into the stomach and out through the anterior abdominal wall. Gastrostomy tubes are available from Ross, Inc (Columbus, Ohio); AEI Bard, Inc (Mentor, Ohio); Bard International Products UK, and Wilson-Cook Medical, Inc (Winston-Salem, North Carolina). A good description of the use of PEG in oropharyngeal dysphagia following strokes (the most common indication) is given by Allison *et al.*, 1992.

Endoscopic sclerotherapy

Endoscopic sclerotherapy of oesophageal varices has an important role both in the control of acute variceal bleeding and in prevention of recurrent bleeding. It is essential for the endoscopist to employ endoscopic sclerotherapy as part of the overall management of bleeding varices and not as a means to an end. Acute variceal bleeding for example, will require pharmacological control (vasopressin or somatostatin, Resnick, 1990), balloon tamponade, and sometimes emergency surgery in addition to blood transfusion and supportive care. For the prevention of recurrent variceal bleeding, especially in the patient with reasonable liver function (Childs A or B), combined surgery employing one of the newer portal-systemic shunts (Warren *et al.*, 1986) or non-shunt surgery (Sugiura and Futagawa, 1977; Johnston, 1982) with sclerotherapy, may provide the best approach. The precise management remains controversial and will be influenced by local facilities.

Endoscopic sclerotherapy may also be employed in other bleeding lesions including bleeding gastric ulcers.

Oesophageal varices

The value of endoscopic sclerotherapy in the control of variceal bleeding was first established more than 50 years ago (Crafoord and Frenckner, 1939) with few further reports until the large series reported by Johnston and Rogers from Belfast in 1973 (Johnston and Rogers, 1973). These studies, employing general anaesthesia and a rigid oesophagoscope, demonstrated control of bleeding in more than 90% of cases, with a periprocedural complication rate of less than 1%.

The original proponents of rigid-endoscopic sclerotherapy claimed that variceal compression was an essential ingredient of success as it reduced the loss of sclerosant from the injection site. A number of devices and techniques have been introduced to reduce sclerosant loss, but there is now considerable doubt whether variceal stasis is promoted by these compression techniques. Blood flow in oesophageal varices is now thought to be bidirectional between the extrinsic and intrinsic systems of oesophageal veins. Moreover, compression has been shown to have no effect on sclerosant clearance from the injection site, and may in fact increase the clearance rate (Barsoum et al., 1982). The wider use of endoscopic sclerotherapy is due to the use of flexible endoscopes and the development of suitable techniques for their effective use. A randomized study comparing rigid and flexible endoscope use (Bornman et al., 1988) demonstrated a lower incidence of serious complications using a flexible endoscope.

Diagnosis

Oesophageal varices are usually easily recognized endoscopically. A number of classifications have been described as a means of predicting haemorrhage and defining objective change either due to treatment or disease progression.

Whilst accurate grading is desirable, it is essential to define the system employed as there is no agreed international classification but there are numerous published ones. Features that contribute to gradings include: diameter, longitudinal extent, colour and associated findings (e.g. erosions or oesophagitis) (Dagradi, 1972; Beppu et al., 1981). For the endoscopist, predicting factors for bleeding when varices are found are variceal size, presence of red spots ('red colour signs'), and recent variceal bleeding. Variceal size should always be recorded at a specific level, for example, at the oesophagogastric junction (40 cm from the frontal incisors). Varices are usually first seen on the anterior wall of the distal oesophagus and form four columns when fully developed. They may extend proximally for 15 cm when gross.

Sclerotherapy techniques

Numerous techniques are available, the merits of which appear to be largely dictated by local availability of equipment and experience. One of the first published series employing a flexible endoscope, employed a semiflexible overtube with an opening (window or slot) at the distal end. This was used to allow the varix for injection to protrude into the tube and to allow compression (Williams and Dawson, 1979). The overtube method may have some advantages over free-hand injection, both with regard to severity of rebleeding and number of sclerotherapy sessions needed (Westaby *et al.*, 1983). In spite of this, most endoscopists do not employ compression techniques and rely on free-hand injection. Sclerotherapy may be either paravariceal or intravariceal. A number of authors claim that paravariceal injection is preferable (Paquet and Oberhammer, 1978; Fleig *et al.*, 1983; Cello *et al.*, 1984) but most employ intravariceal injection. In many cases, intravariceal injection also includes inadvertant paravasal sclerosant injection (Barsoum *et al.*, 1978; Rose *et al.*, 1983). Intravariceal injection is recommended.

There are a large number of options open to the endoscopist for injection sclerotherapy. Detailed discussion of the relative merits of each is outside the scope of this chapter, but no one combination has been shown to be superior. The options available include: intravariceal or paravariceal injection, choice of sclerosant, volume of sclerosant employed at each injection site, number and site of injections and length of segment employed for injection.

Recommended procedure

Intravariceal injections are employed without compression, commencing distally at the site of maximum varix size (usually at 39–40 cm). 1–3 ml of sclerosant is injected into each varix at this level until blanching is observed. This is repeated at 37–38 cm and then 35–36 cm, repeating every 2 cm in a proximal direction until the varices are of small diameter. Injection volume should be recorded at each level and the total volume injected also recorded. Choice of sclerosant can be made from Table 3.4. Protective goggles should be worn both by the endoscopy nurse and the endoscopist to avoid eye injury from accidental sclerosant spillage during injection. Sclerotherapy needles (flexible) are available from a number of suppliers. They consist of an outer guiding catheter (usually 7 French) and an inner injection catheter (usually 4 French) attached to a 23–25 gauge needle. The entire assembly is 180–200 cm in length.

If sclerotherapy is attempted during variceal bleeding, balloon tamponade and pharmacological control should be employed initially. If these are not available or have not succeeded, more sclerosant than recommended above may be injected into the largest varices, bearing in mind that endoscopy may be very difficult during active bleeding, with only limited vision. In most cases, sclerotherapy will be performed as an interval procedure and a means of reducing rebleeding. Weekly injections may be performed, until the varices are obliterated. This relatively short interval is more acceptable to patients but does increase the chance of finding oesophageal ulceration from the previous treatment. A recent meta-analysis of 26 clinical trials of beta-blockers (e.g.

Sodium tetradecyl sulphate	3%
Ethanolamine oleate	5%
Polidocanol (paravariceal use)	
Phenol and almond oil (paravariceal use)	

Table 3.4: Sclerosants recommended for variceal sclerotherapy.

propranolol) has shown significantly reduced bleeding and overall mortality related to variceal haemorrhage (Hayes *et al.*, 1990). This suggests that the combination of sclerotherapy plus beta-blockers may provide an important combination in reducing recurrent variceal haemorrhage, as suggested by a preliminary report comparing propranolol alone with propranolol plus sclerotherapy (O'Connor *et al.*, 1988).

Complications

Complications due to either local or systemic effects of sclerotherapy occur in 2–20% of cases.

1 **Oesophageal ulceration.** Ulceration at the site(s) of injection probably occurs in the majority of patients. It does not appear to increase significantly the risk of rebleeding, although a large ulcer (which is unusual) may bleed. When this occurs, the bleeding may be difficult to treat. It is not known whether ulcer-healing agents are effective.
2 **Oesophageal strictures.** These occur in about 3% of patients following sclerotherapy. They are more likely to occur following paravariceal sclerotherapy. They are not related to the use of a particular sclerosant since all can cause strictures to develop. Endoscopic dilatation is usually successful.
3 **Oesophageal perforation.** Perforation is described in 1–6% of patients. It usually occurs 5–7 days after sclerotherapy and can be insidious with minor symptoms.
4 **Chest pain.** Substernal discomfort, odynophagia or more severe chest pain due to oesophageal spasm, may occur.
5 **Fever.** A low-grade fever occurs in about 10% of patients and usually resolves spontaneously within 48 hours.
6 **Sepsis.** Whilst bacteraemia has been described in a small number of patients undergoing sclerotherapy, prophylactic antibiotics are not recommended.
7 **Cardiovascular complications.** Bleeding from distal duodenal or colonic varices is described after oesophageal sclerotherapy. Portal venous thrombosis, mesenteric venous thrombosis, and digital ischaemia are also described, presumably due to the systemic effects of sclerosant. Cardiac arrythmias, acute pericarditis and angina (coronary spasm) are also documented.
8 **Pulmonary complications.** Pleural effusions which resolve spontaneously are occasionally found.

Non-variceal sclerotherapy

Injection therapy for non-variceal lesions has been available for about 15 years. Whilst there are many published studies available, most are either uncontrolled or comparative studies, without a control group. In spite of this, it appears that injection of either a vasoconstrictor or vasoconstrictor sclerosant solution, or vasoconstrictor/thrombin solution can control bleeding gastric lesions and reduce recurrent bleeding. (Soehendra *et al.*, 1985; Asaki *et al.*, 1983; Panes *et al.*, 1987; Chung *et al.*, 1991; Balanzo *et al.*, 1990.)

Table 3.4 lists a variety of solutions and regimens employed. The injection technique often employed is to inject in four quadrants around the bleeding vessel or site of haemorrhage. Up to 3 ml can be injected at each site with this technique. A further injection may then be made under the bleeding vessel. The injection needle employed is the supra as used for variceal sclerotherapy.

Complications

Infarction of the stomach or duodenum has been described (Levy *et al.*, 1991; Lopifido *et al.*, 1990). In each case, a sclerosant was employed with adrenaline (sodium tetradecyl sulphate or polidocanol). The use of adrenaline alone, perhaps with hypertonic saline, may prove to be the optimum injection solution.

Injection therapy for non-variceal bleeding is a cheap and relatively safe procedure which should be available to all endoscopists.

Endoscopic thermal haemostasis

Acute haemorrhage from the upper GI tract results in about 25 000 hospital admissions each year in the UK and about 125 000 in the United States. In the UK, 20% of these admissions require emergency surgery and 10% die from loss of blood (Holman *et al.*, 1990), whilst in the US a 7–8% mortality has persisted for the past 40 years, despite great improvements in diagnosis and supportive care.

Pharmacological control of acute upper GI bleeding has proved very disappointing, except in certain sub-groups such as oesophageal varices, portal hypertensive gastropathy and stress ulcer disease. It is, however, inaccurate to consider upper GI bleeding as a single entity, since variceal haemorrhage requires completely different management and has a higher mortality. On the other hand, endoscopic therapy, especially in the case of non-variceal haemorrhage, has resulted in a lower mortality of 3–5%.

Peptic ulceration is the most important cause of non-variceal haemorrhage from the upper GI tract, and has been the subject of research for 20 years with respect to endoscopic methods of haemostasis. A number of methods of endoscopic haemostasis have been developed during this time (*see* Table 3.5), but only thermal haemostasis and injection therapy have so far proved to be promising. A meta-analysis of 25 randomized controlled trials of thermal

Tissue glues (cyanoacrylates)
Clotting factors
Mechanical clips
Sutures
Injection therapy
Thermal haemostasis

Table 3.5: Methods of endoscopic haemostasis.

endoscopic haemostasis, compared with standard therapy in bleeding peptic ulcers, has demonstrated a highly significant benefit with endoscopic thermal haemostasis, resulting in a reduction in rebleeding and need for emergency surgery of more than 60%, and a 30% reduction in mortality (Sacks et al., 1990). In addition, the Consensus Development Panel of the National Institutes of Health (National Institutes of Health Consensus Conference on Therapeutic Endoscopy in Bleeding Ulcers, 1990), broadly confirmed the efficacy of endoscopic thermal haemostasis, especially in high risk patients (large initial bleed, active bleeding, non-bleeding visible vessel at endoscopy). The advances that have taken place are firstly, the application of three thermal techniques: lasers, electrocoagulation and the heater probe; secondly, work that has defined endoscopic criteria that can predict the likelihood of rebleeding; and lastly, a greater understanding of the effects of heat on tissues that has assisted the application of optimum techniques.

Fundamental to endoscopic thermal haemostasis, is the recent appreciation that certain endoscopic criteria can be employed as predictors of further bleeding (stigmata of recent haemorrhage). The so-called 'visible vessel' which consists of a blue/red protruding lesion, in association with an ulcer base, is now recognized as having at least a 50% chance of rebleeding (Swain et al., 1986), although when originally described, it was found that the rebleeding rate was 100% (Griffiths et al., 1979). Spurting arterial bleeding also carries a very high risk of rebleeding but other stigmata of recent haemorrhage, such as an overlying clot, or non-protruding black or red spot, carry a rebleeding risk of 10% or less. Clearly, appreciation of these criteria is essential when planning endoscopic thermal haemostasis.

Laser (light amplification by stimulated emission of radiation)

Two types of laser have been employed for endoscopic haemostasis: the argon laser (wavelength 0.5 μm) and the Nd:YAG (neodymium-yttrium aluminium garnet) laser (wavelength 1.06 μm). Whilst the argon laser is absorbed preferentially in the region of the haemoglobin wavelength, most of the available energy is absorbed at the mucosal surface, giving a penetration of about 1 mm. However, the longer near infra-red wavelength of the Nd:YAG laser penetrates 4 mm with only 10% of the original energy. Seven published trials of Nd:YAG laser haemostasis have confirmed the efficacy and general preference of this type of laser for endoscopic haemostasis (Swain et al., 1986; Krejs et al., 1987; MacLeod et al., 1983; Ihre et al., 1981; Homer et al., 1985; Rutgeerts et al., 1982; Rohde et al., 1980). Suitable commercially available flexible waveguides are provided that can be passed down the biopsy channel of the endoscope. A Nd:YAG filter (visually transparent) is fitted to the eyepiece of the endoscope as a safety measure. The technique employed in the most successful controlled trial of Nd:YAG laser haemostasis provides 8–10 0.5 seconds 80 W pulses around the lesion (Swain et al., 1986). The waveguide tip is positioned about 1 cm from the target. Coaxial CO_2 is employed to clear blood away from the target and to provide some tissue cooling. The importance of the Swain study was the stratification of the patients, randomized to laser therapy in high and low risk cases, as predicted by the endoscopic presence of a non-bleeding visible vessel (50% rebleeding risk) or other stigmata of recent haemorrhage (10% rebleeding risk). Contact tip lasers employing sapphire tip waveguides are becoming available. These may prove important, since they offer the possibility of coaptation (*see* below), an important principle of thermal haemostasis.

Electrocoagulation

The first use of electrocoagulation endoscopically, employed a monopolar-active electrode through a gastrostomy stoma (Youmans *et al.*, 1970). Whilst there are some enthusiastic supporters of monopolar electrocoagulation, whether using the 'dry' technique or liquid monopolar electrodes (electro-hydrothermal method) to reduce tissue charring and adhesion (Papp, 1990), nearly all endoscopists now employ multipolar electrodes. The BICAP (ACMI) electrode has three pairs of electrodes arranged axially at the probe tip. The voltage generated by the BICAP probe is only 10% of that generated by the monopolar electrode, so that sparking (fulguration) and tissue erosion does not usually occur. The six published controlled trials employing bipolar (BICAP) electrodes, showed reduced rebleeding (Goudie *et al.*, 1984; Kernohan *et al.*, 1984; O'Brien *et al.*, 1986; Brearley *et al.*, 1987; Laine, 1987; Laine, 1988), and this has been confirmed by the Consensus Development Panel report previously mentioned. In addition to showing that bipolar electrocoagulation is superior to no endoscopic treatment, the same authors showed that bipolar electrocoagulation reduced the rebleeding rate, requirement for surgery, transfusion requirements and mortality to the same extent as injection therapy with absolute alcohol in 60 high risk patients with bleeding peptic ulcers (Laine, 1990). Irrigation and coaptation are two further important factors in thermal haemostasis, both of which are supplied by electrocoagulation methods. Irrigation refers to the passage of water which is pumped from a small reservoir (e.g. dental irrigation pump) through channels related to the thermal probe tip. This assists the clearing of blood from the probe tip and the target tissues, and may help to prevent excessive heating of tissues. All electrocoagulation probes, except the 'dry' monopolar probe, are employed with irrigation facilities. Coaptation (tamponade) is an inherent property of contact methods of thermal haemostasis (as opposed to non-contact laser haemostasis). The local pressure effect of contact probes appears to limit the local loss of heat due to blood flow ('heat sink effect'), resulting in higher, more localized tissue heating and sealing of blood vessels of 1.5–4 mm in diameter (Sigel and Hatke, 1967; Johnston *et al.*, 1987). Non-contact thermal methods cannot employ coaptation, which explains why vessels larger than 1 mm are not usually effectively sealed by these methods, and why increased arterial bleeding may be induced (Krejs *et al.*, 1987).

Heater probe

This device consists of a Teflon (non-stick) coated metal probe containing a heating element (silicon diode) which also measures the probe temperature which can therefore be set by the operator (endoscopist). As a result, the amount of energy delivered to the tissues (a function of the probe temperature and time) can be pre-set. With a maximum probe temperature of 250°C, 20–30 J is delivered for 3–8 seconds. Both irrigation and coaptation are provided by this thermal technique. There have been a number of recent studies that have confirmed the efficacy of this treatment (Fullarton *et al.*, 1988; Lin *et al.*, 1990), and that haemostasis with the heater probe is comparable to electrocoagulation and laser haemostasis (Chung *et al.*, 1991; Hui *et al.*, 1991). The heater probe is obtained from Olympus (Olympus HPU).

Endoscopic removal of foreign bodies

Ingestion of foreign bodies occurs most often in children aged 1–5 years. In adults, several groups are more prone to foreign body ingestion: alcoholics, prisoners, drug smugglers, the mentally ill and the mentally handicapped form the majority, whilst those with intrinsic disease of the oesophagus or anatomical abnormalities of the GI tract (e.g. webs, diaphragms and diverticula) form the majority of patients with food bolus obstruction in most series (Vizcarrondo *et al.*, 1983). Foreign body ingestion usually occurs in those without intrinsic GI disease.

Applied anatomy

Small and sharp bones may become lodged in the hypopharynx (pyriform fossae or vallecula) and should be examined by indirect laryngoscopy.

Oesophageal foreign bodies usually become lodged at one of four levels: 15, 23, 27 or 40 cm from the frontal incisors, which correspond to the cricopharyngeus muscle, the aortic arch impression, the left main bronchus impression and the lower oesophageal sphincter respectively. Below the oesophagus, the pylorus, fixed duodenal angles (e.g. Treitz ligament), ileocaecal valve, rectosigmoid and anal sphincters are potential levels of obstruction.

Clinical evaluation

Careful clinical assessment is essential in order to plan appropriate intervention. In the case of young children, most accidental ingestion of true foreign bodies involves non-toxic objects, and intervention is not necessary. In the case of sharp or harmful foreign bodies, endoscopic removal may be required, especially if the object is longer than 6 cm (children) or 13 cm (adults) (Murat *et al.*, 1969). In adults, it is easy to identify high risk groups who deliberately ingest foreign bodies. Oesophageal foreign bodies may cause dysphagia or odynophagia, whilst retained gastric foreign bodies are often asymptomatic. The nature of the foreign body should be assessed. Following a careful history and examination, which should include a search for supraclavicular emphysema (indicating pneumomediastinum), plain films should be taken of the neck, chest and abdomen, to include lateral cervical views. In certain cases, soft tissue radiography (xeroradiography) may be necessary. Glass and wood are radiolucent and may be undetected by conventional radiography.

Endoscopic removal

In some cases, endoscopic removal should be attempted as a matter of course. These include:

* alkaline button batteries (toxic contents)
* safety pins and razor blades
* plastic bag clips
* toxic metal objects (e.g. lead).

It should be stated however, that most button batteries pass through the GI tract without problem, and that amongst 600 British gastroenterologists there was no consensus on management (Studley *et al.*, 1990).

Endoscopic removal should not be immediately considered for blunt or non-toxic objects (e.g. most coins), nor for condoms containing narcotics, since endoscopic removal may break the condom resulting in toxic overdose. Most authors writing on endoscopic management of foreign bodies correctly stress the importance of proper clinical assessment before considering interventional management. The surgical maxim: 'Patience, porridge, and peristalsis' should remind us that the majority of foreign bodies can be safely left to pass spontaneously. Although five days is an average bowel transit time for a swallowed foreign body, some may take as long as three weeks, such as the dislodged Celestin tube which the author watched radiographically in a patient until it passed safely in the stools several weeks after dislodgement in the oesophagus.

Endoscopy equipment and technique

A single or double channel forward viewing endoscope should be employed. There are no published studies showing the advantage of a two channel instrument, although there are obvious theoretical advantages. In children, a paediatric endoscope with an outside diameter of less than 1 cm will avoid tracheal compression.

Ancillary equipment available should include:

* 14 mm (42 French), 60 cm length Tygon (or similar) overtube, and
* foreign body forceps (rat-toothed forceps, alligator forceps, tripod (triprong) forceps, polypectomy snare(s), Dormia-type basket).

The use of an overtube is mandatory for sharp objects (e.g. opened safety pins and razor blades). The overtube should be well lubricated on the inside with a silicone aerosol lubricant and passed over the endoscope before insertion up to the control handle. After insertion of the endoscope and visualization of the foreign body, the overtube, which should be lubricated on the outside with a water soluble lubricant (e.g. KY jelly), is passed over the endoscope as far as the foreign body. This will allow the sharp object to be removed through the overtube without damaging the oesophagus or hypopharynx, and will also allow the endoscope to be removed and reinserted repeatedly if necessary. This latter procedure may be necessary in some forms of foreign body ingestion, such as bezoars and food bolus obstruction, where piecemeal removal is necessary.

Sharp or pointed objects should be removed with the sharp edge or point trailing. Glucagon may be administered (0.25–1 mg iv) to relax the oesophagus during removal. Objects with holes, such as keys, may be removed by passing a suture thread through the hole by means of biopsy forceps, and then grasping the free end of the suture with the forceps prior to removal. Alternatively, the biopsy forceps themselves (unopened) can be passed through the key-hole and then opened to trap the key prior to removal. Where possible, coins should be removed in the coronal plane which anatomically gives more space. The clear message is to plan the removal procedure and practise with a similar object (e.g. key) in the endoscopy unit before attempting it on the patient.

Bezoars

Bezoars are aggregates of animal or vegetable fibrous material. Several types are described: phytobezoars (vegetable material), trichobezoars (hair balls) and diospyrobezoars (persimmon bezoar). Nearly all experienced endoscopists encounter cases from time to time. Most of the cases of phytobezoars are associated with a delay in gastric emptying (post-gastroenterostomy or in diabetic autonomic neuropathy). Trichobezoars, which are more common in young women, may cause gastric outflow obstruction or even jejunal obstruction, without any underlying gut motility problem. Phytobezoars may be treated with oral cellulase (75 mg in solution with food) or even by transcatheter injection into the bezoar (Pollard and Block, 1968; Gold et al., 1976). A pro-kinetic agent such as cisapride or metaclopramide may aid distal passage of bezoar fragments. Papain has been used in the past, but should now be reserved for the rare persimmon bezoar (Dann et al., 1959). Further details may be found in monographs (e.g. Brady, 1990) or from original papers.

Complications

Whilst there are theoretical complications with foreign body removal (perforation, haemorrhage and pulmonary aspiration), very few have been reported. It can be assumed that the complication rate is greater than the 1.3 per 1000 for diagnostic upper GI endoscopy (Silvis et al., 1976), but the true figure is not known.

Endoscopic polypectomy

The use of endoscopy to remove projecting mucosal lesions (polyps) by polypectomy, was first described for gastric polyps more than 20 years ago (Tsuneoka and Uchida, 1969; Classen and Demling, 1971), followed by the technique of endoscopic colonic polypectomy (Dehyle et al., 1971).

Endoscopic polypectomy has subsequently become widely accepted and is the standard treatment for gastrointestinal polyps accessible to flexible endoscopes. Fundamental to endoscopic polypectomy, is the realization that it is an invasive technique requiring proper indications, preparation and performance, and should only be performed by an experienced and properly trained endoscopist. Detailed technique is outside the scope of this review which should therefore be read in conjunction with one of the monographed accounts (e.g. Williams, 1990).

Gastric polyps

Hyperplastic polyps, which have a very low malignant potential, comprise 80–90% of epithelial gastric polyps, and therefore endoscopic follow-up after initial removal and histological classification is not so important. Adenomas, although less common in the stomach, *do* need endoscopic follow-up since they have a malignant potential as in the colon.

Submucosal polyps may be mesenchymal neoplasms (leiomyoma, fibroma, lipoma etc) and are not easily removed by conventional endoscopic polypectomy. However, endoscopic ultrasonography may be a superior means of defining, staging and following up these tumours (Tio *et al.*, 1990). In a follow-up study of 80 patients with pernicious anaemia, it was shown that of 12 patients with dysplastic epithelium followed up endoscopically over 14 months, one developed a severely dysplastic adenoma and a further patient developed a carcinoid. These results suggest that dysplasia is an indication for endoscopic follow-up (Armbrecht *et al.*, 1990).

Endoscopic retrograde sphincterotomy (EST)

Endoscopic sphincterotomy (EST) was one of the first modern therapeutic applications of endoscopy to be introduced (Kawai *et al.*, 1974), and has become one of the most valuable and widely accepted therapeutic techniques in endoscopy. Following its introduction in Japan, it was rapidly introduced into Europe, and was evaluated initially by a multicentre study in Germany, representing a collaboration between physicians and surgeons (Reiter *et al.*, 1978). Initial results from the UK, Germany and other centres in Europe confirmed the success, safety, efficacy and acceptability of the technique (Safrany, 1978), as did the first Japanese collective experience (Nakajima *et al.*, 1979), and US experience (Siegel, 1981). EST is the treatment of choice for recurrent common duct stones after cholecystectomy, but the indications should be seen as much wider than this (*see* Table 3.6). EST involves endoscopic electrosurgical incision of the intramural bile duct as it passes through the posteromedial wall of the descending (second part) duodenum. This intramural portion of the common bile duct varies in length from 5–30 mm (Boyden, 1957). Pressure studies have suggested that the sphincter of Oddi is approximately 4 mm in length (LoGiudice *et al.*, 1979).

Choledocholithiasis
    postcholecystectomy
    gall bladder *in situ*
    failed percutaneous extraction
    acute gallstone pancreatitis
Biliary decompression
    endoprosthesis placement
    balloon dilatation
Unresectable periampullary tumour
Papillary stenosis
Sump syndrome

Table 3.6: Main indications for endoscopic sphincterotomy (EST).

EST equipment

Three basic pieces of equipment are required:

* standard side-viewing duodenoscope
* cannulating catheters and sphincterotomes
* an electrosurgery unit.

The duodenoscope should be in good condition with the up/down angling control taut without much play, the fibre bundle (if fibre-optic duodenoscope is used) not yellow and damaged by previous irradiation (X-ray damage) and the elevating bridge in good condition. On no account should endoscopic retrograde cholangiopancreatography (ERCP)/EST duodenoscopes be used by trainees for routine upper GI duodenoscopy. More than one duodenoscope is required for any GI unit performing serious ERCP/EST work. Fully submersible duodenoscopes (e.g. Olympus OES endoscopes) are mandatory, to allow proper sterilization to modern accepted standards (*see* BSG *Good clinical practice* guidelines).

Sphincterotomes (papillotomes) are available in a number of forms. Several types should be available in the endoscopy unit and used as circumstances dictate. The 'pull-type' sphincterotomes are used most frequently. These sphincterotomes are produced in a variety of versions. It is now realized that the short wire sphincterotomes with about 5–15 mm of exposed wire are difficult to orientate correctly in the papilla of Vater, so long wire sphincterotomes are very useful in difficult cases. The long exposed wire allows much easier orientation of the sphincterotome in the papilla, although only 5–8 mm of wire is in contact with the target tissue (roof of ampulla). Over-the-wire sphincterotomes are very useful in difficult cases. These are 7.0 French sphincterotomes with a single or double insulated channel which will take a guidewire. In difficult cases, especially where a standard 5.0 French diagnostic cannula can be passed into the bile duct, a 0.035 inch guidewire is passed down the cannula into the bile duct, the cannula is removed and the over-the-wire sphincterotome is passed over the wire into the bile duct. Specialized sphincterotomes, such as the push-type shark-fin sphincterotome, may be used in certain circumstances. They may help, for example, to produce a pre-cut into the papilla of Vater in difficult cases. Whilst the pre-cut method is controversial, I have found it helpful in some difficult cases whereby a 3–4 mm pre-cut is made and a second stage cannulation is attempted 24–48 hours later. This should allow entry into the bile duct on the second occasion, so that the procedure can be completed. Needle-knife sphincterotomes have a limited but definite value in difficult cases. The exposed wire employed (variable length) should normally be about 4–5 mm. The electrosurgical current employed should be about five times less than for standard EST. With 5 W instead of 30 W power, the needle-knife can be used to open the bile duct when it is clearly visible endoscopically because of an impacted stone. Needle-knife sphincterotomy can also be employed from the papillary orifice to perform a pre-cut in difficult cases, in order to allow a standard 'pull-type' sphincterotome to complete the sphincterotomy. The cut should be made in an upward direction from the papillary orifice for only 5 mm maximum. A large series has shown that this technique can increase sphincterotomy success from 101/190 (53%) in difficult cases to 171/190 (90%) by needle-knife sphincterotomy (Huibregtse et al., 1990), without an increase in complication rate over the standard rate for EST (2.5% and 2.15%). My own experience of 103 cases subjected to needle-knife EST, showed a morbidity of 5.2% and mortality of 2%, suggesting that even in experienced hands needle-knife sphincterotomy has appreciable risks which must be carefully considered (Dowsett et al., 1990). A new sphincterotome catheter has been described which allows both diagnostic ERCP and EST. This is a polytef catheter with an internal current-conducting wire (Feretis et al., 1990).

The endoscopist should understand the basic physics of electrosurgery before performing EST. A good review (e.g. Barlow, 1982) should be available in the endoscopy unit to remind all staff of the principles involved. Electrosurgery generators produce outputs of alternating current between 400 000 and 1 000 000 Hz. Different generators produce different waveforms so that comparison is difficult. In essence, the outputs are described as cutting current (continuous sinusoidal waves or bursts of active current), coagulation current (short, repetitive bursts with inactive periods between bursts) and blended current (a combination of cutting and coagulating current). In order to avoid patient burns, the patient plate (ground plate) should be large and with a large area of contact. This point is sometimes overlooked in elderly, confused and sedated patients. In patients with pacemakers, it is mandatory to check that the pacemaker is properly shielded from radio frequency current (most are). Rarely capacitative coupling can result in a burn to the endoscopist, and if the blocking condenser of the electrosurgery unit (blocks flow of low frequency nerve and muscle stimulating current) is faulty, ventricular fibrillation may occur, especially if the patient has a transvenous cardiac pacemaker in situ. The conclusions are clear:

• have a small dedicated electrosurgery unit in the endoscopy unit
• employ blended current for most EST cases

• understand the principles involved.

The power setting suitable for EST should be noted for the particular generator employed.

EST techniques

Endoscopic sphincterotomy should only be attempted after considerable skill has been acquired with diagnostic ERCP (endoscopic retrograde cholangio-pancreatography). The skills for ERCP depend on meticulous technique, which should be obtained by studying a comprehensive monograph of ERCP methodology (Vennes, 1987; Cotton, 1990), followed by extensive hands-on experience. One of the most important ingredients of success is the trained GI nurse assistant. Two are required for successful ERCP and EST. Prior to performing EST, a full coagulation screen must be performed, and the procedure should be covered by intravenous antibiotics given either one hour before or immediately before the procedure. The first consideration prior to EST is to obtain a cholangiogram. During the initial ERCP, when the cholangiogram is obtained, it is important to remember the angle at which the cannula entered the common bile duct (CBD) and to simulate this with the sphincterotome. Some sphincterotomes make it necessary to work at a distance from the papilla, although 'the nearer the better'. The sphincterotome can be manoeuvred by altering the cannula elevator bridge, moving the sphincterotome in and out, angling the endoscope tip in the 'up' direction and pulling back on the endoscope. The sphincterotomy wire should be orientated between the 11 o'clock and 1 o'clock positions with the CBD at 12 o'clock. Whilst it is preferable to use the long 30–35 mm exposed wire sphincterotomes, it is equally important to have only 5–8 mm of wire in contact with the roof of the ampulla at the time of EST. This means that the sphincterotome wire must be slowly withdrawn from the papilla prior to EST. Having positioned the sphincterotome in the CBD, contrast medium is injected to check its position fluoroscopically. The sphincterotome is then slowly flexed into a bow taking care not to tighten the bow too hard. When the position of the wire has been verified, with regard to orientation and depth of insertion and bowing, short intermittent bursts of current (blended current) are passed. Stepwise sphincterotomy is the correct procedure. A 'zipper' effect due to too high a current should be avoided. The size of sphincterotomy should rarely exceed 1 cm and will be dictated by the size of the common duct stone(s) and the length of the intramural bile duct. Stones larger than 1.5 cm will require lithotripsy prior to removal by EST techniques.

Stone removal techniques

Following EST for choledocholithiasis, stone extraction can be contemplated, but should be preceded by an estimation of sphincterotomy size. This can be carried out either by the use of a flexed sphincterotome pulled out through the sphincterotomy opening, or by a balloon-tipped catheter. Balloon-tipped catheters should be the first choice for endoscopic common duct stone removal since they are safe to use and easy to position above common duct stones. An effective method is to pass the balloon-tipped catheter up the common bile duct to the bifurcation and then to check its position by injection of contrast medium (half strength recommended). Having checked its position and the diameter of the common bile duct, the balloon is then distended to its recommended diameter, or to a smaller diameter if it reaches the diameter of the common duct. The balloon is then trawled down the bile duct by traction, finally extracting it through the sphincterotomy by angling the endoscope tip.

The alternative method is to use a wire basket ('Dormia' type basket) to remove the stones. The stone basket should be opened above the stone and then drawn down in order to trap the stone. This may prove very difficult, especially with rectangular, square or piston-shaped stones. If the stone impacts, or is impossible to remove through the sphincterotomy in view of its size (i.e. more than 1.5 cm), then the basket should be disengaged and removed. A mechanical lithotripsy basket may be used if available (Riemann *et al.*, 1982). Enthusiasts have reported high success rates (94%) with mechanical lithotriptors (Siegel *et al.*, 1990).

For large common duct stones, (more than 2.5 cm), various options are available (Table 3.7). The use of methyltertbutylether (MTBE) for dissolving cholesterol stones is well established and it has been used via transhepatic catheters and nasobiliary catheters, passed surgically through the cystic duct. The development of an ether-resistant balloon entrapment system to retain MTBE in the biliary tract (and avoid anaesthesia) has not yet become fully available.

Endoscopic electrohydraulic lithotripsy, employing a balloon to trap the stone during treatment, has been used in 21 patients with large CBD stones. An 86% success rate for stone fragmentation was achieved (Siegal *et al.*, 1990). Pulsed laser technology (Lux *et al.*, 1986; Cotton *et al.*, 1990) can also be successful with minimal complications. Extracorporeal shockwave lithotripsy (ECWL) has been shown to be successful in 86% of cases where other endoscopic methods had failed to clear the CBD stones. EST and nasobiliary common bile duct drainage was established in these patients prior

Surgery

MTBE (chemical dissolution)

Lithotripsy
    Mechanical
    Electrohydraulic
    Laser
    ECWL

Long-term biliary stents

Table 3.7: Available methods for treating retained large CBD stones.

to ECWL, and bile duct clearance was achieved after fragmentation in 90% of cases (Vandermeeren *et al.*, 1990).

Long-term biliary drainage by means of endoscopic biliary endoprostheses (stents) has been shown to be successful, especially for the elderly patient with difficult retained common duct stones. Two double pig-tailed stents (6–8 French) can be used to trap the stones distally, but a larger straight (Amsterdam) stent is now preferable to provide drainage through the papilla. Follow-up studies have shown that over a three-year period, in 34 patients with a mean age of 81, cholangitis did not reoccur in 80% of the cases, and that stent blockage occurred in only one patient (Soomers *et al.*, 1990).

Nasobiliary catheter drainage

A nasobiliary drainage catheter can be left in the common bile duct to maintain biliary drainage when a stone is left *in situ*, and especially when a patient has severe cholangitis. It is not necessary to perform EST, so that nasobiliary catheter drainage can be performed quickly even if there is a coagulopathy in order to buy time for the patient. 5 or 7 French 250 cm catheters are suitable, and available with 0.035 inch, 480 cm guidewires.

The catheters all have at least six side holes near the tip for drainage. If a standard diagnostic 5 French cannula is placed in the CBD, the 480 cm, 0.035 inch guidewire can be passed down the cannula (provided the tip has been dilated with an 18 gauge needle), which is then removed and replaced over the guidewire with a nasobiliary catheter. Various designs are available, including distal and mid-duct pigtails and other preformed loops, all of which assist in keeping the catheter in place.

Endoscopic decompression of the biliary tree

Biliary decompression was first described following the introduction of percutaneous transhepatic cholangiography (PTC) (Nakayama *et al.*, 1978; Ring *et al.*, 1978), and was rapidly developed to include not only external biliary drainage, but the possibility of inserting a percutaneous transhepatic biliary endoprosthesis for internal biliary drainage (Perieras *et al.*, 1978; Burchanth, 1978).

Whilst both these advances are considerable, PTC is contraindicated if there is an uncorrectable coagulopathy and is made difficult or impossible in some patients with ascites. In addition, the presence of hepatic vascular lesions (e.g. haemangioma) or hydatid cysts, and sensitivity to radiological contrast medium, increase the risks of the procedure. Placement of an external catheter is associated with patient discomfort and pain, and requires support from the family and medical health care team. A percutaneous biliary endoprosthesis whilst providing excellent internal biliary drainage and obviating the need for external drainage, does eventually obstruct, resulting in cholestasis and cholangitis.

There are also a number of possible complications of the external drain/catheter including infection, pain, pneumothorax, biliary leaks and haemorrhage.

It is usually difficult to obtain access to the biliary endoprosthesis once it has become blocked, although a current technique has been described (Jackson *et al.*, 1990; Lee *et al.*, 1990).

Nasobiliary catheter drainage (Cotton *et al.*, 1979) was the first endoscopic method described for providing continuous access to the biliary tract. With this technique (*see* page 47), a catheter at least twice the length of a duodenoscope (i.e. 300–400 cm) is passed over an atraumatic 0.035 inch, 400 cm guidewire into the common bile duct. The advantage of nasobiliary drainage is that it can be safely and quickly introduced in a sick patient with severe ascending cholangitis. No EST is required. The nasobiliary drain provides initial biliary decompression, yet allows continuous access to the biliary tract for serial per-oral cholangiography and instillation of drugs (antibiotics, stone dissolution agents etc).

The best method is to carry out diagnostic retrograde cholangiography, employing the standard 5 French catheter, but with the tip dilated so that it will take the 0.035 inch guidewire, (an 18 gauge needle will dilate the catheter tip). Having introduced the guidewire with the diagnostic catheter, the catheter is carefully withdrawn whilst the guidewire is fed by the endoscopy assistant. This reciprocal movement must be well rehearsed and monitored fluoroscopically to prevent the catheter being dislodged from the bile duct.

Following removal of the catheter, the nasobiliary catheter is introduced over the guidewire into the bile duct. At this stage, the guidewire is withdrawn into the endoscope but no further. The final position of the nasobiliary catheter is then adjusted, by advancing it to form the gastric and duodenal loop required. The wire is then finally withdrawn. The endoscope is then carefully withdrawn with the catheter elevating bridge open, and the endoscopy assistant gently advancing the nasobiliary catheter to maintain the catheter loop required in the gut. 5, 6, 7, 9 and 10 French nasobiliary drains are available (e.g. Wilson-Cook). Various configurations are also available including distal pigtail (Liguory catheter) and mid-duct pigtail.

Endoprosthesis placement (biliary stenting)

Endoscopic stent insertion has proved to be an important development in the palliation of malignant jaundice, and as a palliative measure for high risk patients with biliary stones or non-extractable stones. A randomized trial comparing percutaneous biliary drainage with endoscopic biliary stenting, showed that the side-effects of biliary stenting were substantially less than via the percutaneous route, both in terms of 30-day mortality and associated morbidity (Speer *et al.*, 1987).

Distal and mid-common bile duct stenting has a high success rate (90%), but hilar obstruction can be much more difficult, especially in type III strictures with multiple segment involvement. It has become apparent that the technique offers excellent palliation for the high risk elderly patient who has limited survival (Dowsett *et al.*, 1988). For the younger patient however, surgical bypass is usually the treatment of choice (Hatfield, 1990).

One of the major and continuing problems with biliary stents is stent blockage. This invariably occurs as a late complication, the timing being directly related to stent size. The smaller stents (e.g. 8 French) block within three months, but the larger (10–12 French) last on average for six months before blocking.

Blockage occurs due to a combination of live bacteria, protein and bacterial mucoproteins and enzymes ('biofilms'). The presence of side holes may in fact increase the blockage rate (Coene *et al.*, 1990). In the majority of cases, stent replacement is a relatively simple procedure. The stent is removed endoscopically, employing a stone retrieval basket, or by means of a balloon catheter, especially if the stent has migrated into the bile duct (Wengrower and Goldin, 1990). A good review of biliary sludge is given by Murray and Hawkey (1992).

Metallic biliary endoprostheses: these metallic self-expanding stents are increasingly being used, especially via the percutaneous-transhepatic route. The Wallstent metallic stent appears to be relatively easy to insert, especially as it can be introduced over a 7 French introducing catheter (Adam *et al.*, 1991; Lammer *et al.*, 1990). The disadvantages are related to the fact that these stents are permanent, and that the wire mesh may promote tumour growth. Their precise place in promoting biliary drainage is not yet established.

Biliary stents

Biliary polyethylene stents were originally small (7–8 French) and were positioned over a 0.035 inch guidewire without a guiding-catheter in between. The original models had one or two pigtails (e.g. Zimmon double pigtail stent). These stents are now rarely used and have been replaced by straight stents (Amsterdam stents) or straight stents with a gentle 'bile duct curve' (Cotton-Leung biliary stents). The straight stents now employed are from 10–11.5 French. They have a tapered tip and two side flaps, one being positioned above the stricture, and the other remaining in the duodenum to avoid proximal migration of the stent.

Equipment

A suitable duodenoscope is essential. Whilst a 3.8 mm channel duodenoscope is suitable for the smaller stents (e.g. 8–10 French), the greater use of larger (10–12 French) stents means that a therapeutic endoscope such as the Olympus TJF 4.2 mm channel endoscope must be employed. Electronic endoscopes will undoubtedly replace fibre-optic endoscopes in due course, but the principal mechanical operations employed for stenting are almost identical regardless of the imaging technology.

Biliary stents are available from 6 French up to 11.5 French (12 French) – the largest size that can be passed with a commercially available duodenoscope – most stents used now are 10–11.5 French in size. Biliary stents can be manufactured in the endoscopy unit. The materials needed are:

- 0.035 inch Teflon coated guidewire, 350–400 cm, with a 3 cm floppy tip (William-Cook TSF.35.300)

- 6.5 French guiding catheter tubing, (e.g. Meadox/Surgimed 1.2 x 2.0 mm tubing No 53, or William Cook PERT 6.5 tubing) 250 cm
- 10 French pushing-tube catheter, (e.g. Meadox/Surgimed 2.4 x 3.2 mm tubing No 1) 200 cm
- 8–10 French tubing (stents) with lengths cut from 7–20 cm
- 6.5 French tubing for nasobiliary tubes (William Cook PERT-6.5 radio-paque polyethylene tubing).

Whilst the materials required have been listed, many companies now supply excellent biliary stent sets. These include Wilson-Cook, Olympus, Meadox Surgimed, Microvasive and MTW.

Technique

The stents usually employed now (the 10–11.5 French stents) are introduced employing a three-layer technique. This technique involves the inner layer, a 0.035 inch atraumatic (Teflon coated) guidewire, the intermediate layer, a 6.5 French guiding-catheter, and the outer layer, the stent with a pushing-tube, usually 10 French. The 10–11.5 French stent is placed over the guiding-catheter and is pushed down the guiding-catheter within the endoscope channel.

The first task is to perform diagnostic ERCP, in order to identify the precise position and length of the biliary obstruction (stricture). The most important point is to use a catheter that will take the 0.035 inch guidewire, in order to avoid cannulating the stricture twice. The catheter employed should be primed with contrast medium to avoid injecting air. Having obtained good radiographs and measured the stricture, a suitable stent should be chosen. Stent size (length) is measured between the side flaps. If the stricture is 3 cm in length and 5 cm above the papilla of Vater, i.e. 8 cm above the papilla, then a correction is made for the 1.3 magnification present with most X-ray sets used for ERCP, i.e. 6 cm real length. 2 cm are added, 1 cm for the duodenal end and 1 cm for the proximal end of the stricture. This means that an 8 cm stent (measured between flaps) should be chosen for this example.

After choosing the stent, it may be necessary to aspirate bile and contrast medium in order partially to decompress the biliary tree. If this is carried out, a prior radiograph of the stricture should be obtained in order to facilitate stent placement. The 0.035 inch guidewire must be passed down the catheter, and then the catheter exchanged with the guidewire *in situ*, for the 6.5 French guiding-catheter. Once the guiding-catheter and guidewire are in place through the biliary stricture, then the stent can be placed over the guiding-catheter and pushed down the endoscope channel and into the bile duct, employing the 10 French pushing-tube. It may be necessary to use lubrication at this stage, and liberal lubrication of the guiding-tube with silicone oil will reduce friction between it and the pushing-tube.

There can be difficulties (e.g. due to tortuous strictures, types II and III hilar strictures) where refinement of technique is required. In cases where two stents are required for a complex hilar stricture for example, a steerable guidewire can be employed for gaining access to the difficult left hepatic duct (Hoffman *et al.*, 1990). In any event, the endoscopist should study a monograph account of technique (Cotton 1990; Siegel 1990).

Stricture dilatation

Some endoscopists employ a 7 French tapered dilating catheter (Van Andel catheter, Wilson-Cook) which can take the 0.035 inch guidewire. This will allow sequential dilatation of a tight stricture and will make passage of the 10-11.5 French stent easier.

A TTS Olbert balloon catheter system (Meadox/Surgimed) can also be employed for stricture dilatation (benign and malignant strictures). It is preferred by some endoscopists, since a 'waist' can be seen fluoroscopically with the balloon *in situ* if contrast (dilute) is used to inflate the balloon, in addition to radiological confirmation of dilatation (Rao *et al.*, 1990). Both dilating systems are positioned over guidewires. Very tight strictures will require a tapered dilating catheter.

Strictures that I have found to respond adequately are post-traumatic surgical strictures, dominant strictures in sclerosing cholangitis, strictures following biliary-eneteric anastomosis, and common duct strictures proximal to a sphincterotomy. Hilar biliary strictures following liver transplantation (hepatic artery occlusion, ductopenic arteriopathic rejection, cytomegalovirus infection, idiopathic stricture formation) have been successfully dilated by percutaneous transhepatic dilatation, employing the techniques described, and have been followed successfully by long-term stenting (Ward *et al.*, 1990).

In the Far East, ascariasis and clonorchiasis may be related to benign stricture formation (Leung *et al.*, 1990), and form the basis of a further indication for interventional stricture dilatation. It is recommended that a good review of percutaneous techniques (Gya *et al.*, 1990) and endoscopic techniques (Huibregtse, 1990) be read.

Sphincterotomy

Some endoscopists routinely make a small (3–4 mm) sphincterotomy cut prior to placement of a biliary stent. This is a safe procedure and will allow two stents to be positioned should that be necessary. Other endoscopists rarely employ sphincterotomy. I believe that a small sphincterotomy is a sensible measure when passing stents of 10–11.5 French, and is made easier now that a two channel insulated guidewire sphincterotome is available.

Radiotherapy in bile duct tumours

Iridium 192 can be employed in bile duct tumours and can be delivered endoscopically, either in a pre-loaded 11 French double-lumen endoprosthesis or by means of an afterloading technique via a 10 French nasobiliary catheter. The latter technique reduces radiation exposure to the endoscopist (Siegel, 1990). More results are required in order to place this treatment in perspective.

'Combined procedure'

The development of a combined procedure whereby an interventional radiologist places a percutaneous transhepatic guidewire through a difficult hilar stricture (usually type II or III) or papilla, has proved invaluable in selected cases. The procedure is usually carried out as a planned second-stage procedure after a previous failed endoscopic transpapillary approach. The radiologist passes a 400 cm, 0.035 inch wire via a 6–7 French percutaneous transhepatic catheter, through the stricture (obstruction) and into the duodenum. With the guidewire protruding from the guiding-catheter, the endoscopist secures the guidewire tip with a polypectomy snare or stone retrieval basket, and pulls the wire out through the endoscopy channel (approximately 200 cm should be visible). The guidewire is then employed exactly as for stent placement, being the inner core of the three-layered system described previously.

Points to note are the importance of 'pushing' the radiologist's guide-tube up through the stricture, and the danger of advancing the stent too far which may cause stent impaction and failure to drain. One technique employed to minimize this risk, is for the endoscopist to pull back the 400 cm guidewire under fluoroscopic control until the wire tip is in the common hepatic duct or major suprahilar duct. The wire tip can then be advanced a few centimetres prior to advancing the stent over the guide-tube into a major hepatic duct. The radiologist will replace the withdrawn guidewire with a second guidewire immediately, in order to maintain the possibility of repositioning should this be required.

After stent placement by this technique, the per-oral guidewire, guide-tube and pushing-tube are removed, but the percutaneous catheter is left *in situ* for 24–48 hours for check cholangiography (Hall *et al.*, 1990). Where it is felt that a good team approach could be employed, then the editorial *Biliary perestroika* should be consulted (Liguory and Vitale, 1990).

Post-stent care

All patients prior to stenting are given parenteral antibiotics (usually a cephalosporin and/or gentamycin) which are continued for several days. Adequate hydration is important. It is sensible to perform a 'decompression ultrasound' at 36 hours to confirm stent drainage, but this is not strictly necessary unless stent malfunction is suspected. Early clinical review is essential however. Evidence of good stent function will include return of normal stool and urine colour, clinical and biochemical reduction of bilirubin, and early reduction of pruritus.

Endoscopic thermal treatment (ETT) of gastrointestinal neoplasms (laser and BICAP treatment)

Endoscopic thermal ablation of tumour tissue (debulking) is now an established technique for palliation of advanced malignant disease of the GI tract. In colorectal cancer the Nd:YAG laser has proved to be of value in the palliation of obstructive or bleeding lesions, by recanalizing an obstructed bowel and stopping haemorrhage with resulting reduced in-patient stay (Mathus-Vliegen and Tytgat, 1985). The only limiting factor has been accessibility of the lesion to the endoscope. In the fore gut, malignant dysphagia responds to both Nd:YAG recanalization techniques and to BICAP thermal recanalization, both techniques reducing dysphagia and allowing an oesophageal prosthesis (tube) to be positioned subsequently if indicated.

Emphasis formerly placed on survival in patients with malignant dysphagia is currently being focused on palliation, with relief of dysphagia as a major goal. Whilst surgery must remain the current gold standard for relief of malignant dysphagia, the operative mortality of 10–30% and the high complication rate (30–35%) have stimulated development of endoscopic palliation with its low mortality and complication rate. Endoscopic techniques have already largely replaced palliative bypass, especially in the case of advanced tumours in the elderly or those with concurrent disease.

Thermal treatment of malignant dysphagia can be applied to proximal third oesophageal carcinomas as the sole palliation or, in the case of middle and lower third oesophageal tumours, can be followed by placement of an oesophageal tube.

BICAP

This method employs a series of bougies (3, 9, 12 and 15 mm). Each bougie (BICAP probe) is heated by radial bipolar electrodes. Having passed a guidewire through the malignant stricture under fluoroscopic control, the BICAP probe (start with the smallest) is placed in the stricture and two-second pulses of current are passed into the tumour (unit setting 7–10), whilst the probe is rotated through the tumour. This technique can give satisfactory tumour ablation (Jaffe et al., 1987). It should be reserved for full circumference tumours with at least 5 mm intraluminal narrowing. There is a danger of perforation in asymmetrical tumours, so a careful endoscopic survey of the tumour should be made initially. The BICAP tumour probe is much cheaper than ELT, but the results of BICAP tumour ablation and ELT are probably comparable (Jensen et al., 1988).

Nd:YAG photocoagulation

Since laser photocoagulation was introduced for the relief of malignant dysphagia (Fleischer et al., 1982), a number of studies have verified that ELT is a safe, technically feasible and effective therapy (Swain et al., 1984; Mathus-Vliegen and Tytgat 1986; Rutgeerts et al., 1988). A Nd:YAG laser with a power output of 60–100 W is usually employed. The laser output is transmitted down a flexible waveguide, sheathed within a protective catheter which also allows a flow of coaxial non-inflammable gas (e.g. CO_2) to protect the fibre by blowing away combustible material from the fibre tip. Various techniques have been used, although to date there is no good data to show which method is preferable. The methods are not mutually exclusive.

Antegrade approach

With this method the laser beam is aimed at the centre of the proximal margin of the tumour (from above) and 'drilled' through the obstruction.

Retrograde approach

In this method the endoscope is passed through the tumour, perhaps after bougienage, and ELT is then applied to the distal margin. Treatment then proceeds in a proximal direction.

Non-contact treatment

The non-contact method was the first method employed with the Nd:YAG laser, whereby the laser fibre tip was held about 1 cm away from the target tissue, with the aiming beam (Nd:YAG light is invisible) provided by a helium neon low power laser (cherry red spot).

Contact treatment

Contact laser treatment was introduced (Sankar *et al.*, 1985), whereby a sapphire-tip fibre in contact with the target tissue, transmits the laser output directly into the tissue. The sapphire tip can be constructed in different ways so that the laser output is distributed according to the sapphire tip geometry. The power required for contact methods is less than with non-contact methods but the treatment time is longer.

Interstitial therapy

In this form of treatment a non-specialized waveguide (e.g. the standard quartz laser fibre) is inserted into the tissue.

The chief complication with ELT is perforation, which in many published series is 5–10%. This compares favourably with oesophageal prosthesis insertion and stricture dilatation. Whilst perforation accounts for 50% of the complications, other complications include fistulae (oesophagobronchial), haemorrhage and sepsis.

Endoscopic management of early gastric cancer

Early gastric cancer or EGC as defined by the Japanese, refers to a T1 gastric cancer (N0 or N1, M0) using the International Classification (Spiessl *et al.*, 1985). This type of gastric cancer carries a 5-year survival rate of greater than 90% (Kajitami and Takaji, 1979). Whilst EGC was regarded as a Japanese disease for many years, both European and North American studies have clearly established over the past 15 years that T1 gastric

	Country of Study	% of all stomachs that were gastric cancer	Year
Holdstock and Bruce	UK	1.6	1981
Deakin and Colin-Jones	UK	2.6	1986
Newbold et al.,	UK	6.3	1989
Serck-Hanssen	Norway	9.2	1979
Machado et al.,	UK	9.6	1976
Evans et al.,	UK	10.0	1978
Green et al.,	USA	11.8	1981
Carter et al.,	USA	18.3	1984
Rubio et al.,	Sweden	24.4	1982
Hisamichi et al.,	Japan	66.0	1984

Table 3.8: Early gastric cancer (T1 gastric cancer) in resected gastric tumours.

cancer is widespread, although the detection rate of 1.6–18.3% in resected gastric cancers is much lower than in Japan (Table 3.8). Japanese experience with early gastric cancer (T1 gastric cancer) currently shows that they account for 66% of all resected gastric cancers (Hisamichi and Sugawara, 1984), and account for 30% of all gastric cancers in Japan (Ohta et al., 1981).

The low detection rate of EGC outside Japan, in conjunction with the slow decline of advanced gastric cancer in some countries (Correa, 1986), has probably contributed adversely to the advancement of management techniques. Whilst visual recognition of high risk lesions remains the hallmark of effective endoscopic management, the employment of certain policies can increase the chance of detecting EGC (Salmon, 1981). In addition, there are some recent endoscopic techniques that may eventually prove to be of additional value. In spite of this, some of the following discussion is still philosophical.

Gastric ulcers and the Japanese classification of EGC

50% of all EGC are either type IIc or III or mixed forms. These types are, by definition, depressed or ulcerated forms, and therefore present clinically, endoscopically and radiologically as gastric ulcers. An aggressive, diagnostic approach to gastric ulcers is therefore highly recommended as a means of detecting EGC, even though the yield is low. In general, if the ulcer remains unhealed three months after initial diagnosis, in spite of proper medical treatment (full acid blockade) and monthly negative biopsies (minimum of five biopsies from the ulcer rim, base and surrounding mucosa), then surgery with full excision biopsy of the lesion should be performed (Salmon, 1981).

Recently a new type of early gastric cancer, the penetrating type (PEN) has been described, in which there is deeper invasion of malignant cells in the submucosa and a tendency to pronounced scirrhous proliferation (Hirayama *et al.*, 1991). The significance of the PEN-type EGC is that there is a much greater number of oestrogen receptor-positive tumour cells in PEN-type EGC. Epidermal growth factor (EGF) and transforming growth factor-B (TGF-B) are also involved in this type of gastric cancer. The significance of sex hormones in gastric carcinoma growth may therefore be important, suggesting that immunohistochemical studies (using monoclonal oestrogen-receptor antibodies) on gastric biopsies should be considered (Hirayama *et al.*, 1992). The PEN-type EGC may be the precursor of linitis plastica.

Endoscopic criteria of EGC

Suspicion of EGC should be aroused with discoloured areas (Misumi *et al.*, 1989), well-demarcated depressed areas (Oohara *et al.*, 1984) or depressed areas with convergence of folds or clubbed folds (Iishi *et al.*, 1985). Types I and IIa EGC (projecting and elevated forms) are probably more easily detected endoscopically (Oohara *et al.*, 1984), but even this is contested (Iishi *et al.*, 1985). With the development of electronic endoscopes and the use of colour enhancement techniques, the recognition of subtle colour changes (Misumi *et al.*, 1989) may well assume greater importance.

Endoscopic strip biopsy (SB) and endoscopic gastric mucosal resection (EGMR)

SB and EGMR, which are identical techniques, refer to a procedure that has been practised in Japan for several years. The technique involves endoscopic recognition of a suspicious lesion (raised, flat or depressed) less than 1.5 cm in diameter. Physiological saline is injected into the mucosa in order to elevate and produce a polypoid lesion which can then be removed by endoscopic polypectomy in the usual way.

Histological studies have shown that both mucosa and submucosa are usually present. This means that there is sufficient material for the pathologist to decide whether the lesion is malignant and, if so, whether it has been completely resected. If there is submucosal invasion, then surgery is performed with a local gastric resection. If the mucosa alone is involved, then resection is judged to be complete (Oguro, 1991; Tada *et al.*, 1988; Takechi *et al.*, 1992; Fujimori *et al.*, 1992). It is generally agreed in Japan, that EGC types IIc and III are unsuitable for EGMR, but types IIa and IIb are suitable. Long-term follow up has demonstrated no residual lesion in 45 cases after five years (Tada *et al.*, 1990). Initial success rates in Japanese series for EGMR are quoted as 66% (Tada *et al.*, 1988; Maruyama, 1991). An interesting two-endoscope technique for EGMR is described by Takechi *et al.*, 1992.

Dye-spray (dye-scattering) techniques

Both congo red/methylene blue and indigo carmine can be used to enhance the endoscopic appearance of suspicious gastric lesions. Their use helps in deciding which procedure to carry out next (e.g. multiple biopsies, EGMR, close follow-up policy). Substantial Japanese experience (Tatsuta *et al.*, 1983; Oohara *et al.*, 1984) suggests that dye-spray technique should be more widely used.

Endoscopic tumour ablation

ELT employing either the Nd:YAG laser or photodynamic therapy (PDT) with an N2-dye laser, has been employed successfully to 'cure' mucosal early gastric cancer (Imaoka *et al.*, 1987; Teixeira *et al.*, 1991). In the more recent study, 17 patients over the age of 80 (for ethical reasons) with gastric cancer were treated either by EGMR, Nd:YAG laser therapy or immunotherapy (OK-432). In 13 patients curative treatment was attempted. In 11/13 patients in this group, follow up at two years showed no evidence of histological recurrence. These results suggest that endoscopic therapy has a role in the management of selected cases of gastric cancer.

In spite of the fact that gastric cancer has a poor prognosis, an aggressive diagnostic approach is justified. It should always be remembered that size of tumour is not necessarily equated with a poor prognosis. The use of non-invasive markers such as Ca-50 or Ca-74-2, serum pepsinogen levels and possibly the presence of H. pylori in the stomach, should be remembered. Meanwhile, recent studies of DNA-ploidy, recognition of the mutant p53 gene and measurement of transforming growth factor provide some hope for the future.

References

Adam A *et al.*, (1991) Self-expandable stainless steel endoprotheses for treatment of malignant bile duct obstruction. *AJR Am. J. Roentgenol.* 156: 321–325.

Adams C *et al.*, (1961) Achalasia of the cardia. *Guy's Hospital Reports.* 110: 191–236.

Allison M *et al.*, (1992) Percutaneous endoscopic gastrostomy tube feeding may improve outcome of late rehabilitation following stroke. *J. Roy. Soc. Med.* 85: 147–149.

Armbrecht U *et al.*, (1990) Development of gastric dysplasia in pernicious anaemia: a clinical and endoscopic follow-up study of 80 patients. *Gut:* 31: 1105–1109.

Asaki S *et al.*, (1983) Endoscopic control of gastrointestinal haemorrhage by local injection of absolute alcohol: a basic assessment of the procedure. *Tokoku J. Exp. Med.* 140: 339–352.

Atkinson M *et al.*, (1978) Tube introducer and modified Celestin tube for use in palliative intubation of oesophagogastric neoplasms at fiberoptic endoscopy. *Gut.* 19: 669–671.

Balanzo J et al., (1990) Injection therapy of bleeding peptic ulcer: a prospective, randomized trial using epinephrine and thrombin. *Endosc.* 22: 157–159.

Barlow D (1982) Endoscopic applications of electrosurgery: a view of basic principles. *Gastrointes. Endosc.* 28: 73–82.

Barsoum M et al., (1978) Technical aspects of injection sclerotherapy of acute oesophageal variceal haemorrhage as seen by radiography. *Br. J. Surg.* 65: 588–589.

Barsoum M et al., (1982) Tamponade and injection sclerotherapy in the management of bleeding oesophageal varices. *Br. J. Surg.* 69: 76–78.

Benedict E (1966) Peptic stenosis of the esophagus: a study of 233 patients treated with bougienage, surgery, or both. *Amer. J. Dig. Dis.* 11: 761–770.

Beppu K et al., (1981) Prediction of variceal haemorrhage by esophageal endoscopy. *Gastrointest. Endosc.* 27: 213–218.

Bornman P et al., (1988) Rigid versus fiberoptic endoscopic injection sclerotherapy. *Ann. Surg.* 208: 175–178.

Boyden E (1957) The anatomy of the choledochoduodenal junction in man. *Surg. Gynecol. Obstet* 104: 641–645.

Brady P (1990) Endoscopic removal of foreign bodies. In: *Therapeutic gastrointestinal endoscopy.* Ed. Silvis S, 2nd Ed. 98–125. Igaku-Shoin, Tokyo.

Branicki F et al., (1981) Structural deterioration in Celestin tubes. *Br. J. Surg.* 63: 851–852.

Brearley S et al., (1987) Per-endoscopic bipolar diathermy coagulation of visible vessels using a 3.2 mm probe – a randomized clinical trial. *Endoscopy.* 19: 160–163.

British Society of Gastroenterology (BSG) (1991) Good clinical practice guidelines. *Gut.* 32: 823–827.

Brown P et al., (1972) Double blind trial of carbenoxolone sodium capsules in duodenal ulcer therapy based on endoscopic diagnosis and follow-up. *BMJ.* 3: 661–664.

Burchanth F (1978) A new endoprosthesis for non-operative intubation of the biliary tract in malignant obstructive jaundice. *Surg. Gynecol. Obstet.* 146: 76–78.

Cello J et al., (1984) Endoscopic sclerotherapy versus portacaval shunt in patients with severe cirrhosis and variceal haemorrhage. *New Engl. J. Med.* 311: 1589–1594.

Chung S et al., (1991) Injection or heater probe for bleeding ulcer. *Gastroenterology.* 100: 33–37.

Classen M and Safrany L (1975) Endoscopic papillotomy and removal of gallstones. *BMJ.* 4: 371–375.

Classen M and Demling L (1971) Operative gastrokopie: Fiberendoskopische polypenatrogung in magen. *Dtsch. Med. Wochenschr.* 96: 1466.

Coccia G *et al.*, (1991) Prospective clinical and manometric study comparing pneumatic dilatation and sublingual nifedipine in the treatment of oesophageal achalasia. *Gut.* **32**: 604–606.

Coene P *et al.*, (1990) Clogging of biliary endoprostheses: a new perspective. *Gut.* **31**: 913–917.

Consensus Development Panel National Institutes of Health (1990) Consensus statement on therapeutic endoscopy and bleeding ulcers. *Gastrointest. Endosc.* **36**: S62–S63.

Correa P (1986) Epidemiology of gastric cancer. In: Filipe M and Jass J (Eds) *Gastric carcinoma.* Churchill Livingstone, Edinburgh.

Cotton P *et al.*, (1979) Trans-nasal bile duct catheterisation after endoscopic sphincterotomy. *Gut.* **20**: 285–287.

Cotton P *et al.*, (1990) Endoscopic laser lithotripsy of large bile duct stones. *Gastroenterology.* **97**: 1128–1133.

Cotton P (1990) Therapeutic endoscopic retrograde cholangio-pancreatography (ERCP). In: Cotton P and Williams C. *Practical gastrointestinal endoscopy*, 3rd ed, 118–156.

Crafoord C and Frenckner P (1939) New surgical treatment of varicose veins of the oesophagus. *Acta Otolaryngol.* **27**: 422–429.

Dagradi A (1972) The natural history of esophageal varices in patients with alcoholic liver cirrhosis: an endoscopic and clinical study. *Am. J. Gastroenterol.* **57**: 520–540.

Dann D *et al.*, (1959) The successful medical management of a phytobezoar. *Arch. Intern. Med.* **103**: 598–601.

Dehyle P *et al.*, (1971) Endoscopic polypectomy in the proximal colon. *Endoscopy.* **2**: 103.

den Hartog Jager F *et al.*, (1979) Palliative treatment of abstructing esophagogastric malignancy by endoscopic positioning of a plastic prosthesis. *Gastroenterology.* **77**: 1008–1014.

Disario J *et al.*, (1990) Poor results with percutaneous endoscopic jejunostomy. *Gastrointest. Endosc.* **36**: 257–260.

Dowsett J *et al.*, (1988) Interventional endoscopy in the pancreatico-biliary tree. *Am. J. Gastroenterol.* **83**: 1329–1336.

Dowsett J *et al.*, (1990) Needle knife papillotomy: how safe and how effective? *Gut.* **31**: 905–908.

Earlam R and Melo-Cunha J (1981) Benign oesophageal strictures: historical and technical aspects of dilation. *Br. J. Surg.* **68**: 829–836.

Feretis C *et al.*, (1990) Evaluation of a new catheter (ER-PT) suitable for both diagnostic ERCP and endoscopic papillotomy. *Gastrointest. Endosc.* **36**: 598–599.

Fleig W *et al.*, (1983) Emergency endoscopic sclerotherapy for bleeding esophageal varices: a prospective study in patients not responding to balloon tamponade. *Gastrointest. Endosc.* **29**: 8–14.

Fleischer D *et al.*, (1982) Endoscopic Nd:YAG laser therapy for carcinoma of the esophagus: a new palliative approach. *Amer. J. Surg.*. **143**: 280–283.

Fujimori T *et al.*, (1992) Endoscopic resection of small early gastric cancer by modified strip biopsy. *Endoscopy.* **24**: 230–238.

Fullarton G *et al.*, (1988) Controlled study of heater probe (HP) in bleeding peptic ulcers. *Gastrointes. Endosc.* **94**: A138.

Gauderer M *et al.*, (1980) Gastrostomy without laparotomy: a percutaneous endoscopic technique. *Gastrointest. Endosc.* **27**: 9–11

Gauderer M and Ponsky J (1981) A simplified technique for constructing a feeding gastrostomy. *Surg. Gynecol. Obstet.* **152**: 82–85.

Gold M *et al.*, (1976) Cellulase bezoar injection: a new endoscopic technique. *Gastrointest. Endosc.* **22**: 200–202.

Goudie B *et al.*, (1984) Controlled trial of endoscopic bipolar electrocoagulation in the treatment of bleeding peptic ulcers. *Gut.* **25**: 1185A.

Graham D (1990) Treatment of benign and malignant dysphagia by intubation at endoscopy. *J. Roy. Soc. Med.* **72**: 894–897.

Griffiths WJ *et al.*, (1979) The visible vessel as an indicator of uncontrolled recurrent gastrointestinal hemorrhage. *N. Eng. J. Med.* **300**: 1411–1413.

Gya D *et al.*, (1990) Balloon dilatation of biliary strictures: experience and review of the literature. *Aust. N. Z. J. Surg.* **60**: 316–364.

Hall R *et al.*, (1990) Percutaneous-endoscopic placement of endoprostheses for relief of jaundice caused by inoperable bile duct strictures. *Surgery.* **107**: 224–227.

Hatfield A (1990) Palliation of malignant obstructive jaundice: surgery or stent? *Gut.* **31**: 1339–1340.

Hayes P *et al.*, (1990) Meta-analysis of value of propranolol in prevention of variceal haemorrhage. *The Lancet* **336**: 153–156.

Hirayama D *et al.*, (1991) The specificity of the penetrating and the superficial spreading types of early gastric cancer. *Dig. Endosc.* **3**: 16 – 24.

Hirayama D *et al.*, (1992) Immunohistochemical study of estrogen receptor in the penetrating type of early gastric cancer. *Dig. Endosc.* **4**: 31–36.

Hisamichi S and Sugawara N (1984) Mass screening for gastric cancer by X-ray examination. *Jap. J. Clin. Oncol.* **14**: 211–215.

Hoffman B *et al.*, (1990) Multiple stent placement with a new steerable guidewire. *Gastrointest. Endosc.* **36**: 595–596.

Holman R *et al.*, (1990) Value of a centralized approach in the management of haematemesis and melaena: experience in a district general hospital. *Gut.* **31**: 504–508.

Homer AC *et al.*, (1985) Is Nd:YAG laser treatment for upper gastrointestinal bleeds of benefit in a district general hospital? *Postgrad. Med. J.* **61**: 19–22.

Huchzemeyer H *et al.*, (1977) Dilation of benign esophageal strictures by peroral fiberendoscopic bougienage. *Endoscopy.* **9**: 207–210.

Hui W *et al.*, (1991) A randomized comparative study of laser photocoagulation, heater probe and bipolar electrocoagulation in the treatment of actively bleeding ulcers. *Gastrointest. Endosc.* **37**: 295–298.

Huibregtse K (1990) Endoscopic palliation in malignant bile duct strictures: the Amsterdam experience. *Dig. Endosc.* **2**: 203–206.

Ihre T *et al.*, (1981) Endoscopic YAG laser treatment in massive upper gastrointestinal bleeding. *Scandinav. J. Gastroentol.* **16**: 633–640.

Iishi H *et al.*, (1985) Endoscopic diagnosis of minute gastric cancer of less than 5 mm in diameter. *Cancer.* **56**: 655–659.

Imaoka W *et al.*, (1987) Is curative endoscopic treatment of early gastric cancer possible? *Endoscopy.* **19**: 7–11.

Ishioka K *et al.*, (1970) Direct vision biopsy and cytologic diagnosis. *Stomach and Intestine.* **5**: 829–834.

Jackson J *et al.*, (1990) Biliary endoprosthesis dysfunction in patients with malignant hilar tumors: successful treatment by percutaneous replacement of the stent. *AJR Am. J. Roentgenol.* **155**: 391–395.

Jaffe M *et al.*, (1987) Esophageal malignancy: imaging results and complications of combined endoscopic-radiologic palliation. *Radiology.* **164**: 623–630.

Jenny S *et al.*, (1972) Endoskopisch-radiologische Diagnostik des Bulbus duodeni (Ulkus, Narbe). *Deutsche med. Wochenschr.* **97**: 118–120.

Jensen D *et al.*, (1988) Comparison of low-power YAG laser and BICAP tumor probe for palliation of esophageal cancer strictures. *Gastroenterology.* **94**: 1263–1270.

Johnston G (1982) Six years experience of oesophageal transection for oesophageal varices, using a circular stapling gun. *Gut.* **23**: 770–773.

Johnston J *et al.*, (1987) Experimental comparison of endoscopic YAG laser, electrosurgery, and heater probe for canine gut arterial coagulation. Importance of compression and avoidance of erosion. *Gastroenterology.* 92: 1101–1108.

Johnston G and Rodgers H (1973) A review of 15 years experience in the use of sclerotherapy in the control of acute haemorrhage for oesophageal varices. *Br. J. Surg.* 60: 797–800.

Kajitami J and Takaji K (1979) Cancer of the stomach at Cancer Institute Hospital, Tokyo. *Gann Monograph on Cancer Research.* 22: 77–82.

Kawai K *et al.*, (1974) Endoscopic sphincterotomy of the ampulla of Vater. *Gastrointest. Endosc.* 20: 148.

Kernohan R *et al.*, (1984) A controlled trial of bipolar electrocoagulation in patients with upper gastrointestinal bleeding. *Brit. J. Surg.* 71: 889–891.

Kozarek R *et al.*, (1981) Intraluminal pressures generated during esophageal bougienage. *Gastroenterology.* 81: 833–837.

Krejs G *et al.*, (1987) Laser photocoagulation for the treatment of acute peptic ulcer bleeding. *New Eng. J. Med.* 316: 1618–1621.

Laine L (1987) Multipolar electrocoagulation in the treatment of active upper gastrointestinal haemorrhage. *New Engl. J. Med.* 316: 1613–1617.

Laine L (1988) Multipolar electrocoagulation (MPEC) for the treatment of ulcers with non-bleeding visible vessels (VV): a prospective controlled trial. *Gastroenterology.* 94: A246.

Laine L (1990) Bipolar/multipolar electrocoagulation. *Gastrointest. Endosc* 36: 5S338–5S341.

Lammer J *et al.*, (1990) Obstructive jaundice: use of expandable metal endoprosthesis for biliary drainage: work in progress. *Radiology.* 177: 789 – 792.

Lazarus B *et al.*, (1990) Aspiration associated with long-term gastric versus jejunal feeding: a critical analysis of the literature. *Arch. Phys. Med. Rehabil.* 71: 46–53.

Lee M *et al.*, (1990) Occlusion of biliary endoprostheses: presentation and management. *Radiology.* 176: 531–534.

Leung J *et al.*, (1990) Endoscopic cholangiopancreatography in hepatic clonorchiasis: a follow-up study. *Gastrointest. Endosc.* 36: 360–363.

Levy J *et al.*, (1991) Fatal injection sclerotherapy of a bleeding peptic ulcer (letter). *The Lancet.* 337: 504.

Liguory C and Vitale G (1990) Biliary perestroika (editorial). *Am. J. Surg.* 160: 237–238.

Lin H *et al.*, (1990) Heat probe thermocoagulation and pure alcohol injection in massive peptic ulcer haemorrhage: a prospective randomized controlled trial. *Gut.* **31**: 753–757.

LoGiudice J *et al.*, (1979) Variations in propagation of phasic pressure waves in the human sphincter of Oddi. *Gastroenterology.* **76**: 1187–1192

Lopifido S *et al.*, (1990) Extensive necrosis of gastric mucosa following injection therapy of bleeding peptic ulcer. *Endoscopy.* **22**: 285–286.

Lowe D and Puyana J (1991) Nutritional support in the intensive care unit. *Current Opinion in Gastroenterology.* **7**: 290–298.

Luna L (1983) Endoscopic therapy of benign esophageal stricture. *Endoscopy.* **15**: 203–206.

Lux G *et al.*, (1986) Tumor stenosis of the UGI tract: therapeutic alternatives to laser therapy. *Endoscopy.* **18**: 37–43.

MacLeod IA *et al.*, (1983) Neodymium yttrium aluminium garnet laser photocoagulation for major haemorrhage from peptic ulcers and single vessels: a single blind controlled study. *Brit. Med. J.* **286**: 345–348.

Maruyama (1991) Personal communication.

Mathus-Vliegen E and Tytgat G (1986) Laser photocoagulation in the palliation of colorectal malignancies. *Cancer.* **57**: 2212–2216.

Mathus-Vliegen E and Tytgat G (1985) Nd-YAG laser photocoagulation in gastro-enterology: its role in palliation of colorectal cancer. *Lasers in Medical Science.* **1**: 75–80.

McClave S *et al.*, (1989) Prospective randomized study of Maloney esophageal dilation blinded versus fluoroscopic guidance (abstract). *Gastrointest. Endosc.* **36**: 195.

McLean G *et al.*, (1987) Radiologically guided balloon dilatation of gastrointestinal strictures. Part I. Technique and factors influencing procedural success. *Radiology.* **165**: 35–40.

Misumi A *et al.*, (1989) Endoscopic diagnosis of minute small and flat early gastric cancers. *Endoscopy.* **21**: 159–164.

Murat J *et al.*, (1969) A propos de 108 observations de corps etrangers deglutis du tube digestif a l'exclusion de l'oesophage. *Lyon Chir.* **65**: 379 – 388.

Murray F and Hawkey C (1992) Biliary sludge. *Br. J. Intensive Care.* **2**: 41 – 49.

Nakajima M *et al.*, (1979) Five years experience of endoscopic sphincterotomy in Japan: a collective study from 25 centres. *Endoscopy.* **11**: 138.

Nakayama T *et al.*, (1978) Percutaneous transhepatic drainage of the biliary tract: technique and results in 104 cases. *Endoscopy.* **74**: 554–559.

O'Brien JD *et al.*, (1986) Controlled trial of small bipolar probe in bleeding peptic ulcers. *The Lancet.* **1**: 464–467.

O'Conner K *et al.*, (1988) A comparison between propranolol, propranolol plus endoscopic sclerotherapy, and propranolol plus transhepatic sclerotherapy in preventing major rebleeding and death from esophageal varices. *Gastrointest. Endosc.* **34**: 180–188.

Oguro Y (1991) Endoscopic treatment of early gastric cancer. *Dig. Endosc.* **3**: 3–5.

Ohta H *et al.*, (1981) Studies on the 1000 cases of early gastric cancer–with special reference to microscopic classification. *Jap. J. Gastroenterol. Surg.* **14**: 1399–1406.

Olsen H *et al.*, (1977) The fiberoptic approach to dilation of stenotic lesions of the oesophagus. *Gastrointest. Endosc.* **23**: 201–202.

Oohara T *et al.*, (1984) Clinical diagnosis of minute gastric cancer less than 5 mm in diameter. *Cancer.* **53**: 162–165.

Panes J *et al.*, (1987) Controlled trial of endoscopic sclerosis in bleeding peptic ulcers. *The Lancet.* **2**: 1292–1294.

Papp J (1990) Monopolar and electrohydrothermal treatment of upper gastrointestinal bleeding. *Gastrointest. Endosc.* **36**: 34–37.

Paquet K and Oberhammer E (1978) Sclerotherapy of bleeding oesophageal varices by means of endoscopy. *Endoscopy.* **10**: 7–12.

Perieras R *et al.*, (1978) Relief of malignant obstructive jaundice by percutaneous insertion of a permanent prosthesis in the biliary tree. *Ann. Intern. Med.* **89**: 589–593.

Pollard H and Block G (1968) Rapid dissolution of phytobezoar by cellulase enzyme. *Am. J. Surg.* **116**: 933–936.

Ponsky J and Aszodi A (1984) Percutaneous endoscopic jejunostomy. *Gastroenterology.* **79**: 113–116.

Porro G and Pace F (1991) The role of continuous oesophageal pH monitoring in the diagnosis of gastro-oesophageal reflux. *Euro. J. Gastroent. Hepat.* **3**: 501–509.

Puestow K (1955) Conservative treatment of stenosing diseases of the oesophagus. *Postgrad. Med.* **18**: 6.

Rao K *et al.*, (1990) Use of a modified angioplasty balloon catheter in the dilatation of tight biliary strictures. *Gut.* **31**: 565–567.

Reiter J *et al.*, (1978) Results of endoscopic papillotomy: a collective experience from nine endoscopic centers in West Germany. *World J. Surg.* **2**: 505.

Resnick R (1990) Somatostatin for variceal bleeders. *Gastroenterology.* **99**: 1524–1526.

Riemann J et al., (1982) Clinical application of a new mechanical lithotriptor for smashing common duct stones. *Endoscopy*. 14: 226.

Ring E et al., (1978) Therapeutic application of catheter cholangiography. *Radiology*. 128: 333–338.

Rohde H et al., (1980) Results of a defined therapeutic concept of endoscopic Nd:YAG laser therapy in patients with upper gastrointestinal bleeding. *Brit. J. Surg.* 67: 360.

Rose J et al., (1983) Factors affecting successful endoscopic sclerotherapy for oesophageal varices. *Gut.* 24: 946–949.

Rutgeerts P et al., (1982) Controlled trial of Nd:YAG laser treatment of upper digestive haemorrhage. *Gastroenterology*. 83: 410–416.

Rutgeerts P et al., (1988) Palliative Nd:YAG laser therapy for cancer of the oesophagus and gastroesophageal junction: impact on quality of remaining life. *Gastrointest. Endosc.* 34: 87–90.

Sacks B et al., (1983) A nonoperative technique or establishment of a gastrostomy in the dog. *Invest. Radiol.* 18: 485–487.

Sacks H et al., (1990) Endoscopic haemostasis: an effective therapy for bleeding peptic ulcers. *JAMA*. 264: 494–499.

Safrany L (1978) Endoscopic treatment of biliary-tract diseases: an international study. *The Lancet*. 2: 893.

Sakita J et al., (1971) Observations on the healing of ulcerations in early gastric cancer. *Gastroenterology*. 60: 835–844.

Salmon P et al., (1972) Endoscopic examination of the duodenal bulb. *Gut.* 13: 170–175.

Salmon P (1981) Gastric ulcer in early gastric cancer. *Proceedings of the Second British Society of Gastroenterologists Sk and F International Workshop*, pp 63–64.

Salmon P (1992) Endoscopic treatment for GI tumors. Is surgery necessary? *Endoscopy*. 24: 229–231.

Sankar M et al., (1985) Vagolysis and mucosal antrectomy by contact intragastric Nd:YAG laser photocoagulation. *Gastrointest. Endosc.* 31: 130–138.

Schindler R (1956) Observations on cardiospasm and its treatment by brusque dilatation. *Ann. Intern. Med.* 45: 207–215.

Siegal J (1981) Endoscopic papillotomy in the treatment of biliary tract disease: 258 procedures and results. *Dig. Dis. Sci.* 26: 1057

Siegel J et al., (1990) Endoscopic electrohydraulic lithotripsy. *Gastrointest. Endosc.* 36: 351–356.

Siegal J (1990) Techniques for endoscopic decompression of the biliary tree. In: Sivis S (Ed) *Therapeutic gastrointestinal endoscopy*, 2nd edn. 282–312.

Sigel B and Hatke F (1967) Physical factors in electrocoaptation of blood vessels. *Arch. Surg.* 95: 54–58.

Silvis S *et al.*, (1976) Endoscopic complications: results of the 1974 American Society for Gastrointestinal Endoscop. Survey. *JAMA.* 235: 928 – 930.

Soehendra N *et al.*, (1985) Injection of non-variceal bleeding lesions of the upper gastrointestinal tract. *Endoscopy.* 17: 129–132.

Soomers A *et al.*, (1990) Endoscopic placement of biliary endoprostheses in patients with endoscopically unextractable common bile duct stones: a long term follow-up study of 26 patients. *Endoscopy.* 22: 24–26.

Speer A *et al.*, (1987) Randomized trial of endoscopic versus percutaneous stent insertion in malignant obstructive jaundice. *The Lancet.* 2: 57–61.

Spiessl B *et al.*, (1985) *TNM atlas*, 2nd edn. Springer, Berlin.

Studley J *et al.*, (1990) Swallowed button batteries: is there a consensus on management? *Gut.* 31: 867–870.

Sugiura M and Futugawa S (1977) Further evaluation of the Sugiura procedure in the treatment of esophageal varices. *Arch. Surg.* 112: 1317–1321.

Swain CP *et al.*, (1984) Laser recanalization of obstructing foregut cancer. *Br. J. Surg.* 71: 112–115.

Swain CP *et al.*, (1986) Controlled trial of Nd:YAG laser photocoagulation in bleeding peptic ulcers. *The Lancet.* 1: 113–117.

Swain CP and Mills TN (1986) An endoscopic sewing machine. *Gastrointest. Endosc.* 32: 36–37.

Tada M *et al.*, (1988) Evaluation of endoscopic strip biopsy therapeutically used for early gastric cancer. *Stomach and Intestine.* 23: 373–375.

Tada M *et al.*, (1990) Long term follow-up study of strip biopsy therapy for early gastric cancer. *Endoscopia Digestiva.* 2: 1515–1518 (In Japanese).

Takechi K *et al.*, (1992) A modified technique for endoscopic mucosal resection of small early gastric carcinomas. *Endoscopy.* 24: 232–238.

Tatsuta M *et al.*, (1983) Diagnosis of minute cancer by the endoscopic congo red-methylene blue test. *Endoscopy.* 15: 252–256.

Teixera C (1991) Endoscopic therapy for gastric cancer in patients more than 80 years old. *Am. J. Gastroenterol.* 86: 725–728.

Tio T *et al.*, (1990) Endoscopic ultrasonography for the evaluation of smooth muscle tumors in the upper gastrointestinal tract: an experience with 42 cases. *Gastrointest. Endosc.* 36: 342–350.

Tsuneoka K and Uchida T (1969) Endoscopic polypectomy of the stomach. *Gastroenterol. Endosc.* 11: 174.

Vandermeeren A *et al.*, (1990) The management of giant bile duct stones after endoscopic sphincterotomy (abstract). *Gastroenterology.* A264.

Vantrappen G and Hellemans J (1980) Treatment of achalasia and related motor disorders. *Gastroenterology.* 79: 144–154.

Vennes J (1987) Techniques of ERCP. In: Sivak M (ed) *Gastroenterologic endoscopy.* WB Saunders, Philadelpha, 562–580.

Vizcarrondo F *et al.*, (1983) Foreign bodies of the upper gastrointestinal tract. *Gastrointest. Endosc.* 29: 208–210.

Ward E *et al.*, (1990) Hilar biliary strictures after liver transplantation: cholangiography and percutaneous treatment. *Radiology.* 177: 259–263.

Warren W *et al.*, (1986) Distal splenorenal shunt versus endoscopic sclerotherapy for long term management of variceal bleeding. Preliminary report of a prospective, randomized trial. *Ann. Surg.* 203: 454–462.

Wengrower D and Goldin E (1990) Balloon retrieval of biliary stents. *Gastrointest. Endosc.* 36: 639–640.

Westaby D *et al.*, (1983) A prospective randomized study of two sclerotherapy techniques for esophageal varices. *Hepatology.* 3: 681–684.

Williams C *et al.*, (1974) Colonoscopy in the management of colon polyps. *Br. J. Surg.* 61: 673–682.

Williams C (1990) Colonoscopic polypectomy and therapeutic procedures. In: Cotton P and Williams C *Practical gastrointestinal endoscopy*, 3rd ed. 224 - 242.

Williams K and Dawson J (1979) Fibreoptic injection of oesophageal varices. *BMJ.* 2: 766.

Youmans C *et al.*, (1970) Cystoscopic control of gastric haemorrhage. *Arch. Surg.* 100: 721–723.

4

Interventional Radiology

WADI GEDROYC

Introduction

The last 10 years have seen a huge increase in the scope and application of interventional radiology. Radiologists are now entering many areas that were previously the uncontested domain of surgeons, e.g. percutaneous gallstone dissolution. Many of the procedures described in this chapter have become, over this period of time, standard, commonly-performed radiological procedures.

Interventional radiology has practical applications in a wide variety of medical conditions. The most widely practised procedures fall into the following categories:

- uroradiology
- biliary radiology
- angiointervention
- abscess drainage.

The intention of this chapter is to provide a generalized overview of these areas, plus some of the basic principles of the techniques involved, rather than an exhaustive account of all aspects of interventional work.

There is no single correct way to perform any of the procedures described in this chapter. Where appropriate, some of the alternative techniques available are mentioned, but other variations may be equally successful in experienced hands. Many of the techniques used are common to each branch of interventional radiology. The details of the techniques used will therefore be more comprehensive at the beginning of the chapter than at the end, to minimize repetition.

Uroradiological intervention

Nephrostomy drainage and antegrade pyelography

Indications

Antegrade pyelography

1 Visualization of the urinary tract above the bladder when retrograde pyelography is not possible, and where an intravenous urography (IVU) has not given adequate information.
2 As part of a Whittaker test (*see* page 72).
3 For localized urine sampling for culture and microscopy or cytology specimens.

Nephrostomy drainage

1 Drainage of the obstructed urinary tract.
2 As access for ureteric stent placement.
3 Part of percutaneous renal stone removal, or biopsy or foreign body removal from the upper renal tract.
4 Urinary diversion associated with ureteric and pelvic leaks and fistula formation.
5 For the infusion of pharmacologically active substances, e.g. chemotherapy, stone dissolution therapy.

Contraindications

The only real contraindication to nephrostomy drainage is a bleeding diathesis. Infection is not a contraindication and nephrostomy in patients with obstruction should be covered with antibiotics immediately prior to the procedure.

Technique

The ability to carry out safe and rapid nephrostomy drainage is the basis of all renal interventional procedures. Imaging of the renal collecting system should be carried out prior to drainage. This can be achieved in the following ways:
1 **IV contrast administration.** This is only possible if renal function is adequate, but if the pelvicaliceal systems can be adequately opacified, then renal puncture is relatively easily carried out using only fluoroscopy.
2 **Ultrasound.** This will demonstrate the renal collecting system in the majority of cases and is especially useful when IV contrast will not opacify the affected kidney. However, ultrasound guidance for puncture, requires a significant degree of expertise and experience, using needles and probes simultaneously. Ideally, ultrasound should be used in association with a fine (22 gauge Chiba) puncture to enter the renal collecting system,

which can then be opacified with dilute contrast so that the system is easily visualized with fluoroscopy. An appropriate calyceal puncture with a larger needle that will allow guidewire passage, can then be carried out. Ultrasound is not usually reliable enough to allow puncture into a particular selected calyx.

3 **Blind puncture.** This can be carried out in a non-functioning, non-opacified kidney and can be a highly effective, quick technique of puncturing the kidney, particularly when ultrasound is not available or the operator is not skilled in its use. It is especially useful when there is significant upper tract dilation secondary to obstruction.

The renal position is determined by a combination of plain abdominal films, previous IVUs and appearances on screening. A 22 gauge Chiba needle is used to puncture the area where the collecting system is expected to lie. Once the system is entered, it is opacified with dilute contrast so that the whole system is easily visualized on fluoroscopy and a subsequent further puncture into the calyx of choice can be carried out with a larger needle.

Patient positioning and puncture site

The intention of a nephrostomy puncture is to enter the collecting system through a posterior calyx via the avascular or Brödel's line (Figure 4.1), which is between the interlobular arteries. This allows puncture with a relatively low risk of haemorrhage. The renal pelvis itself should not be punctured directly, other than with a 22 gauge needle, since the potential for vascular trauma (Coleman C et al., 1984), urinoma formation and catheter dislodgement is much greater at this site.

The easiest patient position in which to achieve the above is the prone 30–40° oblique with the affected side uppermost (Figure 4.2). A vertical puncture will then follow along the correct (avascular) line naturally, and a calyx or calyceal neck/infundibular junction should be punctured.

The puncture should ideally be placed at, or just lateral to, the paravertebral musculature since punctures significantly lateral to this may traverse colon, spleen or liver. Punctures should ideally be below the twelfth rib to minimize the chance of pneumothorax.

Catheter placement

1 **Double puncture technique.** Following the initial fine needle puncture, the opacified collecting system is repunctured using an 18 gauge needle in the desired calyx as described above. This needle allows the passage of an 0.35 inch or 0.38 inch guidewire, usually of a J-tip configuration, into the renal pelvis. A nephrostomy catheter is then advanced into the renal pelvis over the guidewire, following initial appropriate track dilation. (Over dilation by 1 French in size is helpful in the renal and biliary system.)
2 **Alternative puncture technique.** Several other techniques are available to achieve the same goal as the above method. They include:
   • single-step puncture techniques using 0.18 inch guidewires which will pass down a 21 gauge needle with subsequent use of concentric dilators

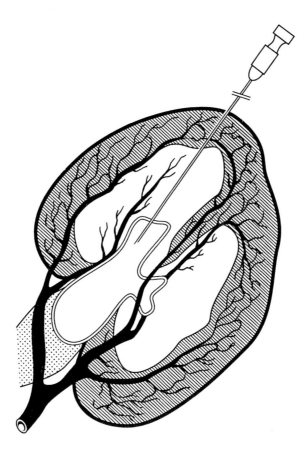

Figure 4.1: Needle inserted into posterior calyx through the avascular Brödel's line.

> which allow a 0.38 inch guidewire to be placed directly into the renal
> collecting system
> • direct punctures with trochar needles carrying nephrostomy catheters
>   on their shafts.

The advantages of the double puncture technique are that it utilizes 'Seldinger-
type' techniques which are familiar to most radiologists, and the equipment
needed is readily available in most X-ray departments.

Once the catheter is in the renal collecting system, it should be positioned

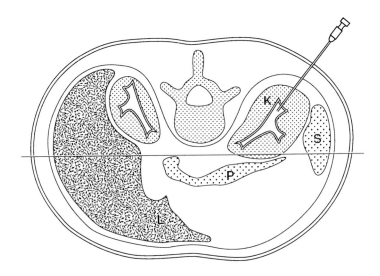

Figure 4.2: A vertical puncture when the patient is placed in a 45° prone oblique position allows the needle to pass through the avascular plane into a posterior calyx.

so that the draining pigtail is in the renal pelvis. Placement of a pigtail drain in the upper ureter is undesirable because of the potential for direct ureteric damage from the catheter. Self-locking drainage catheters of the Cope type have a greatly decreased incidence of dislodgement.

Antegrade pyelograms are performed in the same overall way, but the puncture is carried out using a 22 gauge needle exclusively, and no subsequent catheter placement is usually required. A Whittaker test is a modified type of antegrade puncture where the pressure is measured within the bladder and kidney, and the two pressures are subtracted from each other to provide a gradient across the renal collecting system. This test is regarded as the gold standard for the diagnosis of urinary tract obstruction above the bladder.

Ureteric stenting

Indications

1   Ureteric obstruction, particularly where strictures are close to the vesico-ureteric junction (VUJ), and retrograde manipulation of catheters is very difficult. Benign or malignant lesions may be stented with success.
2   Ureteric tears/fistulae, especially when used in conjunction with nephrostomy drainage of the upper track.
3   As an adjunct to ureteric stricture balloon dilation.

Technique

Puncture of the renal collecting system is carried out as described previously. Ideally, a mid or upper pole calyx is punctured so that it is easier to transmit downward force to the catheter in the ureter, and to prevent coiling of the guidewire and catheter in the renal pelvis. This may necessitate a further puncture in the eleventh to twelfth rib interspace (Mitty *et al.*, 1986). The patient should receive appropriate premedication including sedation, analgesia and antibiotic coverage prior to the start of the procedure.

A guidewire and catheter are manipulated through the pelvo-ureteric junction (PUJ), and down the ureter to the area of obstruction. The intention is to traverse the stricture with a guidewire, followed by a catheter, and subsequently to place a double J internal stent across the lesion (Figure 4.3). Crossing the stenosis/obstruction may be problematic, and the use of different shaped catheters and a selection of guidewires, including 'glide' wires, may be required. The use of such equipment allows the operator to cross the lesion in the majority of cases.

Once a catheter has crossed the stenosis, it is subsequently manoeuvred into the bladder and a heavy-duty, stiff guidewire is positioned with its distal

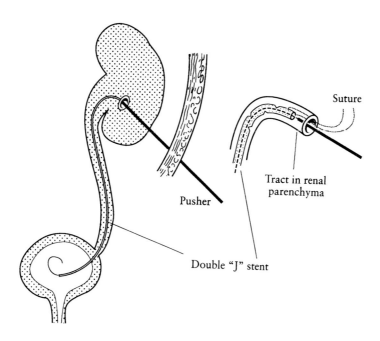

Figure 4.3: Stent placement. The guidewire tip has been placed with one end in the bladder having traversed the ureter. The stent is being advanced along the guidewire by the pusher. A suture in the upper end of the stent allows the stent to be pulled backwards if it is pushed in too far.

end coiled in the bladder and its proximal end externally. The double J stent mounted on a straightening inner catheter, followed by an integral pusher, is advanced along the heavy-duty guidewire so that its distal end comes to lie freely in the bladder, and its proximal end lies in the renal pelvis. An extra safety guidewire is placed in the renal pelvis at an early stage in the procedure, to allow easy placement of a nephrostomy catheter at the end of the procedure.

If at any time during the procedure, the wire and stent start to coil in the renal pelvis, a large sheath should be inserted and further manipulations carried out through this. The sheath supports the stent, preventing coiling and directs it at the PUJ (Salazar *et al.*, 1983). Once the stent is in the correct position, which is ascertained by careful screening, the heavy-duty guidewire is removed, whilst maintaining the stent in place with the pusher – thus freeing the stent. The pusher is then removed and a nephrostomy catheter is left in place in the renal pelvis. This catheter stays in place for approximately 48 hours and allows subsequent nephrostograms to be carried out to check stent patency.

Ureteric balloon angioplasty

This procedure is largely reserved for benign strictures. It is very effective for relatively fresh post-traumatic strictures, e.g. post-accidental ligature, with a 90% success rate (Lang, 1986) in these cases. It is much less useful for chronic strictures, especially when ischaemia and fibrosis have developed.

The stricture is traversed using the techniques described above for ureteric stents following an antegrade puncture. A balloon angioplasty catheter, which is slightly larger in diameter than the underlying ureter, is inflated in the stenosed area and a large diameter ureteric stent is left in place for approximately four weeks post-procedure.

Renal calculus extraction

Indications

This procedure, together with extracorporeal shockwave lithotripsy (ESWL) has virtually eliminated open surgical nephrolithotomy. Over the last five years, with the more widespread availability of ESWL, percutaneous stone extraction (PSE) has significantly decreased in frequency. However, it remains an important procedure since a substantial proportion of patients with renal calculus disease are unsuitable for ESWL. The current major indications for PSE are as follows:

1   renal calculi larger than 3 cm in diameter and staghorn calculi. Staghorn calculi are best treated by a combination of percutaneous debulking plus ESWL for the residual calculus load
2   cystine stones which usually do not respond to ESWL
3   stones in obstructed collecting systems or in calyceal diverticula.

Pre-procedure patient evaluation

All patients having PSE should have had either an IVU with oblique films of the stone-bearing kidney, or a well carried out retrograde study of the affected side, to assess the position of the calculus and to help in planning the puncture site. In complicated cases, particularly when the kidney is malrotated or unusually situated, computerized tomography may give further useful information for puncture planning.

Technique

Most PSE cases are performed as one-step procedures under general anaesthetic. Two-step procedures, where the track dilation is carried out 48 hours or more prior to the nephroscopic manipulation, are as successful, but have the disadvantage of a much longer hospital stay. The technique described below is as used in a one-step procedure, but is very similar in the two-step procedure.

A retrograde ureteric catheter is placed in the side to be punctured, and the collecting system is distended with a mixture of dilute contrast medium and methylene blue dye, to allow easy visualization of the system. The methylene blue dye allows immediate appreciation of when the collecting system has been entered, since any aspirated urine will be blue. The choice of the puncture site is often crucial to the success of the procedure, particularly if one is dealing with calyceal stones. The following are general guidelines on the selection of puncture sites.

1   Stones lying in the renal pelvis can usually be approached by lower or middle calyceal punctures.
2   Upper pole calculi can usually be approached by a lower pole puncture if there is a normal renal pelvis that the nephroscope may pass across. If there is an upper pole calyceal stem stenosis, a direct puncture of the stone bearing upper pole calyx may have to be carried out and this puncture may be above the twelfth rib.
3   Middle group calyceal and lower pole calyceal stones should be approached by a puncture of the affected calyx, ideally along the medial aspect of the stone.
4   Staghorn calculi may be extremely difficult to tackle, particularly if they occupy the whole of the collecting system. Usually, a lower pole puncture is performed into a calyx, which will allow access to as much of the calculus bulk as possible.

The puncture technique is as described in the nephrostomy section and, ideally, a heavy-duty guidewire is placed in the lower ureter or, less satis factorily, in the renal pelvis to allow confident track dilation. The track is subsequently dilated up to 28–30 French with large balloon catheters, Teflon or concentric metallic dilators. A large Teflon sheath is then left *in situ* along the dilated track, which allows easy access to the kidney and tamponades the track created. A rigid or fibre-optic nephroscope is then passed into the collecting system. The calculi are either removed with grabbing forceps if they are small enough to pass up the track, or they are lithotripsied *in situ* using the shock wave lithotripsy probe or the ultrasonic lithotripsy probe. A large bore nephrostomy drain is left in position at the end of the study for approximately 24–48 hours.

Biliary intervention

Percutaneous transhepatic cholangiography (PTC)

Indications

1   As a prelude to drainage or stenting procedures.
2   To demonstrate common bile duct anatomy and pathology when these areas are not clearly seen on ultrasound, or when results of investigations conflict.
3   To demonstrate congenital abnormalities of the biliary tree.

Contraindications

Bleeding diathesis.

Procedure

Prior to the procedure, the patient is appropriately sedated, and given prophylactic antibiotics if a biliary tree obstruction is suspected. All of the procedures below are carried out using fluoroscopy, although it is also possible to carry out biliary tree punctures under ultrasonic control.

The patient is placed in the supine position and a 21 or 22 gauge Chiba needle is used for the puncture. The position and direction of the puncture are chosen using the following criteria:

1   the puncture should be just anterior to the mid axillary line
2   the position of the puncture is at the junction of the upper two thirds and the lower one third of the liver, using screening to help outline the liver position.

The needle is passed into the liver after copious local anaesthesia in a slightly cephalad direction, parallel to the table top up to the midline (Figure 4.4). It is then slowly withdrawn and contrast is injected as the needle is pulled back. When a bile duct is entered, contrast rapidly forms well-defined branching structures which are not flowing, unlike vascular structures where contrast rapidly flows away from the needle tip, either to the liver periphery or in a cephalad direction. Once the biliary tree is entered, contrast is injected to fill the whole system and appropriate films are obtained to demonstrate it. Multiple passes through the liver may be required to puncture a non-obstructive system, and there is little risk of significant complications using this small diameter needle.

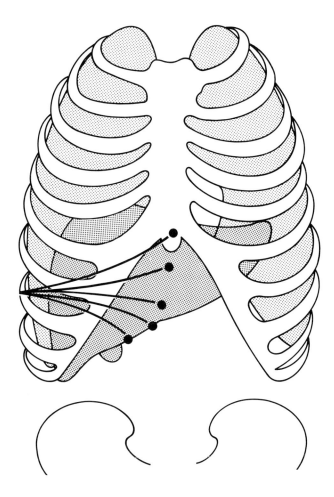

Figure 4.4: The position and direction of fine needle puncture in a transhepatic cholangiogram.

Complications

Significant haemorrhage is very rare with Chiba needles, and puncture of adjacent organs is again of little significance with the above small needle technique. Intraperitoneal contrast injection may, however, cause moderately severe abdominal pain.

Biliary drainage and stent insertion

Indications

1   Palliation of biliary tract obstruction due to malignancy.
2   Placement of intraductal wires for local radiotherapy (Nunnerley and Karani, 1990).

Technique

The basic techniques described in the PTC section above are used to puncture the biliary ducts. After the initial puncture, the appearances and configuration of the ducts are assessed to decide which is the most appropriate duct for access to the stricture/obstruction. Lateral films may often be necessary to help make this decision.

Either a one-step system with an initial 21 gauge puncture (*see* nephrostomy section for details, page 69) or an 18 gauge sheathed needle is used to puncture the selected duct. A guidewire is then passed into the biliary tree and a combination of different guidewire and catheter configurations are used to manoeuvre the catheter across the strictured segment and into the duodenum. A heavy-duty guidewire is then used, and a drainage catheter is advanced across the stenosis into the duodenum. A Ring biliary drainage catheter allows internal drainage due to its multiple side holes and external access. When an internal stent is to be placed (preferred method for patient comfort), initial dilation of the track is carried out at this stage. This is usually performed with a 12 French dilator when standard plastic stents are used, and can be an extremely painful process. Therefore, this portion of the procedure should be covered by extra sedation and analgesia. The stent is advanced along the heavy-duty guidewire until it lies in a good position, straddling the obstruction and allowing drainage from the unaffected biliary tree above into the normal ducts or duodenum below (Figure 4.5 and 4.6). The exact position depends on the type of stent used, but all stent portions should be within the biliary tree peripherally, and the stent will often protrude into the duodenum if necessary. A drainage catheter is left in place for about 48 hours to prevent bile leakage around the track, and to allow subsequent check cholangiograms. Contrast injection at the time of the stent placement should confirm that both the left and right bile ducts are drained by the stent. If this is not the case, a further stent may have to be inserted into the non-drained portion of the biliary tree. If this is the left side of the biliary tree, a subxiphisternal approach for puncture and stenting should be used.

Combined approach to stenting

The use of relatively large catheters and dilators transhepatically causes a significant increase in the complication rates for biliary stenting procedures in comparison with simple PTCs. Biliary leaks and bleeding are a particular problem. Endoscopically-guided biliary tree stenting allows the operator to place a stent without a transhepatic puncture and the overall complication rate of using this approach is substantially lower than with the transhepatic approach (Speen *et al.*, 1987). However, the longer tortuous path to the ampulla, and the nature of the procedure, often make this approach problematic, particularly when there has been previous surgery. As a result, combined procedures have been developed with substantial success. In this procedure, an initial PTC is carried out, followed by a standard duct catheterization as described above. The catheter is manoeuvred into the duodenum across the strictured segment, so that

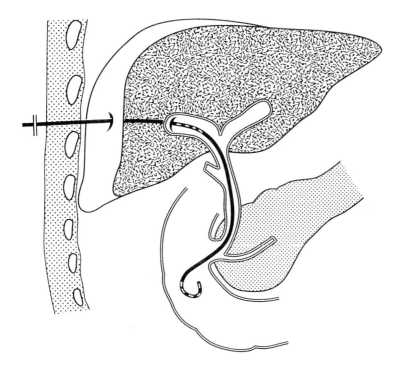

Figure 4.5: The position of an internal biliary stent with side holes in the biliary tree and further side holes distally in the duodenum which allow internal drainage. This sort of catheter also allows external access to the biliary tree.

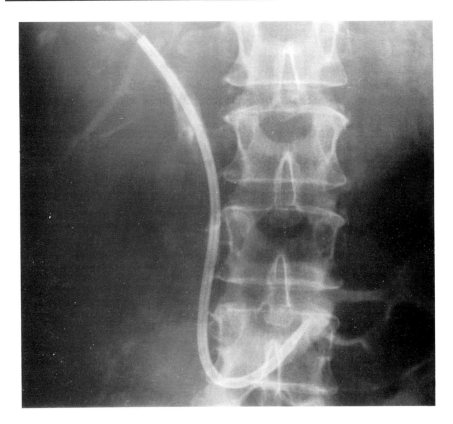

Figure 4.6: An internal biliary stent placed with distal end in the duodenum and proximal end within the biliary tree.

it can be snared by an endoscopic basket and brought out through the endoscope. The wire is then anchored at both ends and a plastic stent is pushed across the stricture via the endoscope. The guidewire is sheathed by the catheter at the skin puncture site to prevent 'cheese wiring' of the tissues. The ability to control and anchor both ends of the guidewire allows the vast majority of lesions to be stented successfully using this combined approach.

Metallic stents versus plastic stents

The main disadvantage of plastic stents is that they tend to block within three to six months, and that large bore dilators, up to 12 French, are required to place them. Metallic stents, such as the Wall stent (Medinvent), may be placed through 7 French (Figures 4.7 and 4.8). The use of this much smaller size track significantly reduces complications. Metallic stents do not block due to bacterial encrustation like plastic stents, but tumours may grow through the mesh of the stent to cause restenosis. Initial experience with the metallic stents, particularly the Wall stent type, is very promising, and results from larger series are currently awaited.

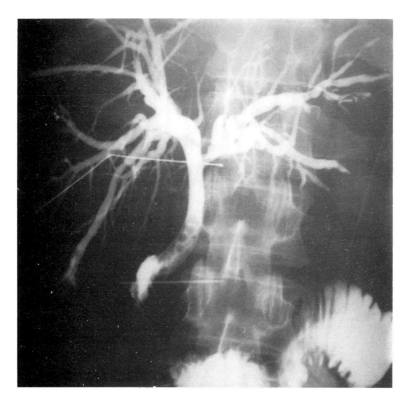

Figure 4.7: A metallic stent has been placed across the strictured biliary segment with good drainage.

Gall bladder intervention

1 **Drainage for calculous and acalculous cholecystitis.** The distended gall bladder is punctured directly via the transhepatic or transperitoneal route, and a catheter is placed in it via a guidewire. Imaging and guidance of the puncture is usually ultrasonic, but oral cholecystographic contrast can be used with fluoroscopy if the gall bladder is functioning.

2 **Percutaneous cholecystolithotomy.** A track is dilated into the gall bladder using techniques similar to those for renal stone extraction. The track is dilated up to 28 French, a rigid nephroscope is passed into the gall bladder and the stones are removed or lithotripsied *in situ*. If the procedure fails, the patient should proceed to immediate cholecystectomy (Malone, 1990).

3 **Stone dissolution.** A transhepatic catheter of small diameter is placed into the gall bladder using the above methods. The volume of the gall bladder is ascertained by gentle injection of contrast. An equal volume of methyltertbutylether (MTBE) solution is injected and aspirated 4–6 times a minute continuously until all gallstones are dissolved. Only non-calcific cholesterol stones can be dissolved. MTBE can accomplish this dissolution using an average five hours infusion per day (Malone, 1990). MTBE, however, has substantial disadvantages. It is very difficult to handle, being

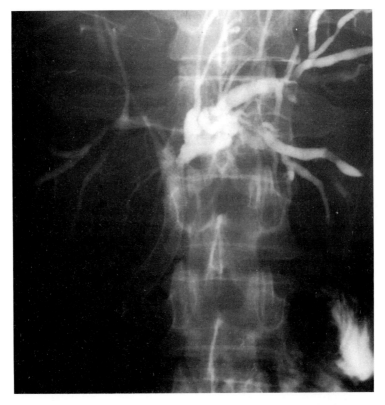

Figure 4.8: The metallic stent is seen more easily without contrast and it has expanded to its full diameter. However two stents have been used in an overlapping fashion to make sure that the narrowed area is covered.

potentially explosive, anaesthetic and haemolytic, as well as causing renal failure if it is left for any length of time in the gall bladder from where it can be reabsorbed.

Angio-intervention

Broadly speaking the principles of angio-interventional work can be divided into the following categories.

1   Methods of increasing flow
    • percutaneous transluminal angioplasty (PTA)
    • fibrinolysis
    • atherectomy and related devices
    • laser-assisted PTA
2   Methods for decreasing flow
    • embolization
3   Removal of foreign bodies from the vascular system.

Percutaneous transluminal angioplasty (PTA)

PTA has assumed an important role in the treatment of vascular disease since the introduction of the Gruntzig double lumen balloon dilation catheter in 1976. The ease of use, relative safety and success of this technique have led to it being applied in most accessible arterial sites in the body, as well as numerous extravascular sites. It is most successful in dealing with atheromatous stenoses and those due to fibromuscular hyperplasia, but it has been used with success in stenoses of other pathological origins.

Indications

1 Accessible vascular stenoses.
2 Short vascular occlusions.

Sites of use

1 Peripheral vascular disease from aorta to iliacs to femoral vessels and down to the proximal peroneal and tibial vessels.
2 Renal arteries including native and transplant arteries.
3 Mesenteric arteries.
4 Cardiac valvular disease. These are usually very selective cases.
5 Graft stenoses.
6 Coronary arteries.
7 Upper limb arteries.
8 Carotid arteries. This is a very controversial area and there are not many practitioners in this field, although it does have its enthusiasts.
9 Venous stenoses, such as portal veins, dialysis AV fistulae, etc.

See Figures 4.9, 4.10, 4.11 and 4.12.

Technique

A variety of catheters, wires and balloon catheters have been developed to allow PTA of a wide range of vessels. The general principle is that a guidewire is first manoeuvred across the stenosed or occluded segment, followed by a catheter. This catheter causes some predilation and allows the placement of a more heavy-duty guidewire if necessary. The catheter is then withdrawn over the guidewire and an appropriate PTA catheter is advanced over the guidewire into the area of abnormality. The balloon is then inflated in the stenosed area, causing dilation of that segment (Figure 4.13). The diameter of the balloon is generally chosen so that slight over-dilation of the vessel, in comparison with more normal parts of that vessel, is carried out. The length and number of inflations vary substantially between operators and with the site being dilated, e.g. peripheral arterial stenoses are often treated with 2–3 dilations with inflations of between 45–60 seconds. Heparin is usually given just before dilation and vasodilators may be used in conjunction with this to decrease the amount of distal spasm.

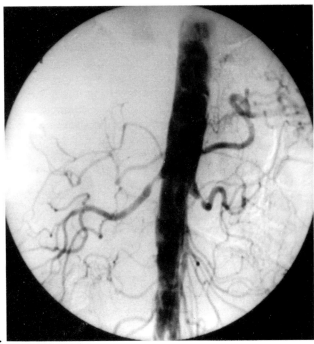

Figure 4.9: Bilateral renal artery stenoses.

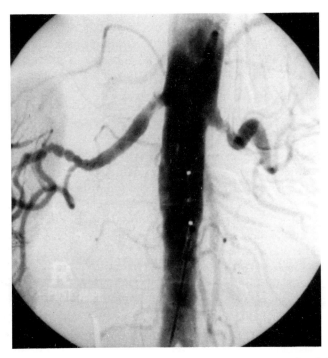

Figure 4.10: Significant improvement in both renal artery stenoses after bilateral renal angioplasty.

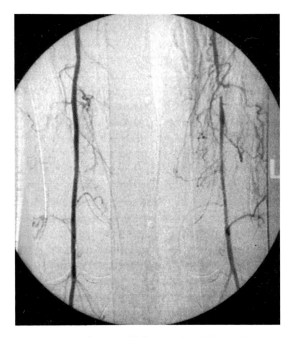

Figure 4.11: Localized short occlusion of left superficial femoral artery.

The above are very general guidelines for PTA, and variations in all aspects of the described technique are common. The technique is carried out using fluoroscopy coupled with digital subtraction angiography (DSA) or cut film.

The mechanism of action of PTA and the requirements of different anatomical areas are beyond the scope of this chapter.

Local fibrinolysis

The technique described below is that of low dose local thrombolysis (first described by Dotter *et al.*, in 1964).

Indications

1 Relatively recent arterial occlusion and graft occlusion due to thrombosis.
2 A venous thrombotic occlusion especially in the axillary and subclavian regions. There is controversy surrounding the value of more peripheral thrombolysis.

Technique

The site of occlusion/thrombus is determined by initial good quality angiography. History is important, because recent occlusions respond much

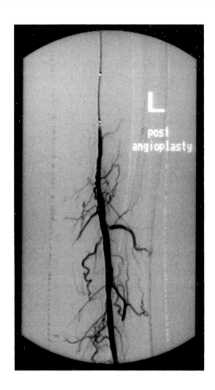

Figure 4.12: Appearance post-angioplasty of this area with no residual occlusion or stenosis visible.

better to thrombolysis than well established occlusions, and the risk from haemorrhage should always be balanced against the potential benefits to the patient. The main risk of this local procedure is haemorrhage, usually at vessel puncture sites. Other complications include significant more distal bleeding (although rare, it has been described, Totty *et al.*, 1982), allergic reactions to streptokinase and distal emboli as the clot undergoes fragmentation.

A catheter with multiple side holes is placed into the area of the clot and infusion of the thrombolytic agent, e.g. streptokinase 5000–10 000 u/hr, is started. Subsequent check arteriograms are carried out at regular intervals and as thrombolysis proceeds, the catheter is advanced further into the previously thrombosed area, until complete lysis has occurred (Figure 4.14, 4.15 and 4.16). The time period over which thrombolysis is carried out varies between practitioners, but many put an upper limit of 72 hours for success or failure of thrombolysis. Urokinase or tissue plasminogen activator (TPA) may be used instead of streptokinase with similar good effects. The lysis of clot in this situation usually reveals an underlying stenosis. This has to be dealt with subsequently, either by further PTA or surgery, otherwise it is likely that the thrombus will recur.

Miscellaneous

1   **Atherectomy and related devices.** There are several new devices currently marketed which remove or destroy atheroma in a mechanical

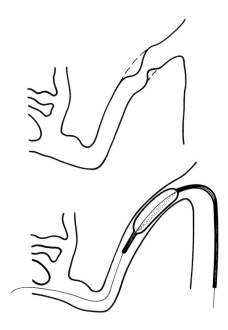

Figure 4.13: Stenosis in a renal artery is cannulated by a guidewire and catheter combination followed by the balloon catheter which is inflated within the stenosed segment causing dilation.

    fashion. The indications for the use of these new machines are not yet clear, nor has their usefulness in comparison with PTA been established.

2 **Lasers.** This is potentially a huge topic with many different types of laser commercially available. They are usually used as an adjunct to angioplasty to allow the operator to cross badly stenosed or occluded areas and subsequently carry out PTA. Once again, there is a fair amount of literature concerning the use of lasers (*see* Chapter 9), but no trial has reported a significant advantage of lasers alone as opposed to conventional PTA techniques (Strandness *et al.*, 1989), and further, more conclusive results are awaited.

Embolization

There are almost as many techniques available for embolization as there are potential applications. Many of the applications are controversial and practices vary widely between institutions. Only the general principles of this technique are described here.

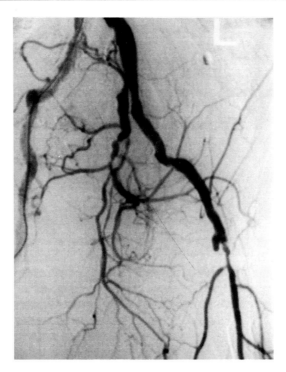

Figure 4.14: Small stump of an occluded femoropopliteal graft is visible arising from the common femoral artery. There is a stenosis of the left proximal profunda.

Indications

1   Uncontrolled haemorrhage sites:
    • gastrointestinal, such as bleeding duodenal ulcers, etc
    • trauma causing bleeding, such as pelvic fractures or following biopsy or surgical procedures
    • haemorrhage from tumours or inflammatory sites, such as bronchiectatic arteries.
2   Tumour/organ/ablation, e.g. prenephrectomy.
3   Arteriovenous malformations.
4   Aneurysms, e.g. caroticocavernous fistulae or pseudo aneurysms at other sites.
5   Miscellaneous conditions, e.g. varicocele embolization.

Materials

A large variety of embolic agents have been used over the years and new materials are continuously being developed.
1   Gelfoam – this is a reabsorbable particulate embolic agent which is now not available in the UK.
2   'Ivalon sponge' – either as a particulate powder or in large pledgets.
3   Dura mater.

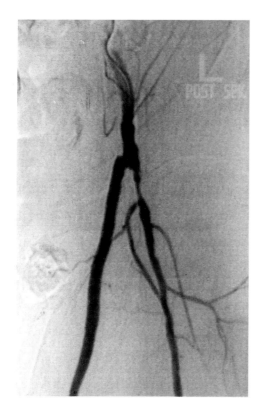

Figure 4.15 (above) and 4.16: After 24 hours of localized streptokinase infusion, the graft is now patent from the origin down to the popliteal artery.

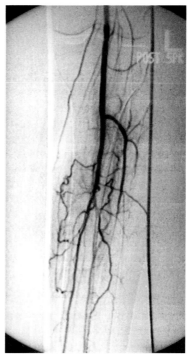

4   Coils – such as the Gianturco variety. Coils are probably the most popular and easiest to use embolic devices. They are very versatile and are available in a wide variety of sizes.
5   Absolute alcohol.
6   Miscellaneous proprietary liquid sclerosing agents.
7   Cyanoacrylate.
8   Detachable balloons.

Technique

The essential principle of embolization is to deliver the embolic agent into the vessel of choice with minimal or no spillage. When dealing with a bleeding vessel, one can usually arrest haemorrhage by placing embolic material anywhere along the vessel supplying the bleeding point, provided that there are no large distal collaterals which refill the bleeding vessel beyond the occlusion. When dealing with an arteriovenous malfunction (AVM) however, the situation is much more complex. If the feeding vessel is blocked proximally, collaterals continue to feed the AVM and therefore, if successful embolization of such a lesion is to be achieved, all feeding arteries should be blocked as close to the centre of the AVM as possible and, ideally, embolic material should be placed in the AVM nidus itself.

Coils and their variants are easy and safe embolic agents to use. They have an effect akin to surgical ligatures in that they cause a localized blockage of a vessel. They are not, however, ideal for use when embolization of tumours or peripheral lesions is required, since collateral flow will often continue to feed the lesion beyond the occluded main artery. In these situations, particulate matter should be used in conjunction with the coils. Liquid embolic agents require great care and expertise in their use, since the danger of reflux or the passage of the agent through the collaterals to reach other normal areas is very real. They should not be used by the occasional practitioner.

Foreign body removal

A variety of grasping and basket tools are available to grip foreign bodies, such as broken off catheters, within the vascular system. The essential principle is that a catheter which will allow the passage of one of these grasping devices, is manoeuvred up to the foreign body, and the material is then grasped and pulled down into the puncture site region. It can then be removed in one piece, either through a sheath, which is the preferred method, or, if it is too large, by a localized surgical cut down at the puncture site.

Abscess drainage

Open operative drainage of abscesses may carry a mortality of up to 43% (Ariel and Karazrian, 1977), compared to figures of about 6% (Martin et al., 1983) for percutaneous drainage procedures. Consequently, it is not surprising that percutaneous drainage of abscess cavities has become widely accepted as the first line of management in the majority of cases in areas such as the abdomen.

Imaging

Fluid collections are usually best visualized by ultrasound or computerized tomography. Other modalities such as radio-isotopes, may suggest an abscess, but further imaging is always required if drainage is intended to allow access route planning.

Ultrasound is a very cost-effective, quick method for imaging abscesses, and in many cases, drainage can be carried out immediately using ultrasound guidance for the placement of the catheter. If the pathway to the abscess is obscured by bowel gas, or the collection is in close proximity to the bowel, or is not well visualized, computerized tomography is usually used to plan the puncture site and carry out the drainage. Computerized tomography is more time consuming and more expensive, but it does allow the bowel to be visualized accurately, and puncture routes to be planned, in such a way as to avoid putting large drainage catheters through loops of bowel and other viscera.

Indications

1 Most abdominal abscesses can be successfully drained percutaneously.
2 Empyema drainage via the percutaneous route is a rather more controversial topic, but there have been reports of significant successes in this area, particularly in association with the use of urokinase to break down septae within the collections.

Contraindications

1 Bleeding diatheses.
2 Fungal infections do not respond well to percutaneous drainage.
3 Necrotic tumours show little response.
4 Cavitating haematomas have only a moderate response to percutaneous drainage.

Technique

Using either ultrasound or computerized tomography as described above, a safe access route to the collection is determined. A trocar and catheter system are guided into the abscess, with regular imaging to make sure that the correct line of approach is being used, and that the catheter enters the cavity. Once the catheter is in the cavity, the trocar is removed and the catheter advanced, so that it coils up within the abscess cavity. Regular aspiration is carried out to make sure that good drainage will be achieved.

There are several variations to this technique. The main alternative is to place an 18 gauge needle into the cavity under imaging control, and then advance a guidewire into the abscess over which a drainage catheter is placed. A single step technique may alternatively be used with a 21 gauge puncture, but both these last two methods may require additional fluoroscopy for optimal siting of the catheter, and this will mean that the patient will have to be moved from the CT room. The one-piece trocar system is a quicker procedure, but it does require a larger bore initial puncture and therefore accurate imaging is essential.

Once the catheter is in place, the collection should be drained dry and re-imaging carried out to assess whether the whole collection has drained via the puncture site that has just been made, or whether further punctures will be required, with further catheter placement, to achieve complete drainage. Multilocular lesions may sometimes be drained by one tube, but it is not uncommon in this situation for several punctures to be required to allow complete drainage.

References

Ariel IM and Karazrian KK (1977) *Diagnosis and treatment of abdominal abscesses.* Williams & Wilkins, Baltimore.

Coleman CC, Casteneda-Zaniga WR and Kimura Y *et al.*, (1984) A systematic approach to puncture site selection for urinary tract stone removal. *Seminars Intervent. Radiol.* 1: 70.

Dotter CT, Rosch J and Seaman AJ (1974) Selective clot lysis with low dose streptokinase. *Radiology.* 111: 31.

Lang EK Transluminal dilation of ureteropelvic junction strictures, ureteral strictures and strictures at ureteroneocystostomy sites. *Radiolog. Clin. N. Amer.* 24: 4.

Malone DE (1990) Interventional radiologic alternatives to cholecystectomy. *Radiolog. Clin. N. Amer.* 28: 1145–1156.

Martin EC, Fankuchen EI and Nuff RA (1983) Percutaneous drainage of abscesses – report 100 cases. *Clin. Radiol.* 28: 97.

Mitty NA, Train JS and Dan SJ (1986) Placement of ureteral stents by antegrade and retrograde techniques. *Radiolog. Clin. N. Amer.* 24: 4.

Nunnerley HB and Karani JB (1990) Intraductal radiation. *Radiolog. Clin. N. Amer.* 28: 1237–1240.

Salazar JE, Johnson JB and Scott R *et al.*, (1983) A simplified method for placement of internal ureteral stents. *Amer. J. Roentgenol.* 140: 611–612.

Speen AG, Cotton PB and Russel RC *et al.*, (1987) Randomized trial of endoscopic versus percutaneous stent insertion in malignant obstructive jaundice. *The Lancet.* 2: 57–62.

Strandness D, Barnes RW, Katzen B and Ring EJ (1989) Indiscriminate use of laser PTA. *Radiology.* **172**: 945–946.

Totty WG, Giula LA, McLennan BL, Ahmad P and Sherman L (1982) Low dose intravascular fibrinolytic therapy. *Radiology.* **143**: 59.

5

General Surgery

SARAH CHESLYN-CURTIS

Introduction

There is a trend towards less or 'minimally' invasive surgery, with an increasing number of procedures being performed using endoscopes and laparoscopes with direct visual, fluoroscopic or ultrasound guidance, either alone or in combination. The major advantage to the patient of minimal access techniques is that it reduces disruption to their pattern of life. The operation can be performed less painfully, through small incisions, without the legacy of a large unsightly scar, and with a much reduced incidence of wound-related complications such as infection, incisional hernia and chronic pain which is experienced by 20% of patients with post-cholecystectomy symptoms (Bates *et al.*, 1984). Also, despite the 'major' nature of the operation, hospital stay is reduced and recovery is rapid, enabling the patient to go back to work and play strenuous sports within 1–2 weeks. Less invasive surgery is viewed favourably by the public if it has these advantages and an outcome which is similar to the conventional operation.

There has been a lot of interest in the last 5–10 years in developing less invasive techniques, particularly for the management of gallstone disease. These techniques have included extracorporeal lithotripsy, oral and contact dissolution therapy, percutaneous cholecystolithotomy and minicholecystectomy, but it is the introduction of laparoscopic cholecystectomy that has caught the imagination of the world. Laparoscopic surgery has become an effective and useful tool for the gynaecologist, and there is no reason why it should not be employed for operations performed by general surgeons. Techniques for these operations are being developed and, apart from cholecystectomy, include appendicectomy, oversewing of perforated peptic ulcers, vagotomy, gastro-oesophageal anti-reflux procedures, oesophagectomy, bowel resection and herniorrhaphy.

Gall bladder and bile ducts

Laparoscopic cholecystectomy

The first laparoscopic cholecystectomy reported was performed in March 1987 by Mouret in Lyon, France. This was followed by Dubois in March 1988, and Reddick and Perissat later that year. Since then there have been many surgeons interested in obtaining the instruments and learning the technique.

Technique

The procedure is performed under general anaesthesia. Patients are placed in either the supine position, with the operating surgeon standing on the left side, or in the Lloyd-Davies position, with the operating surgeon standing between the patient's legs (Figure 5.1). A nasogastric tube is used intraoperatively to decompress the stomach, but only 55% of European surgeons perform urinary catheterization to empty the bladder before the procedure (Cuschieri *et al.*, 1991).

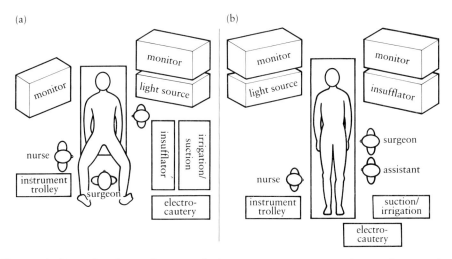

Figure 5.1: Operating theatre layout with the operating surgeon standing (a) between the patient's legs, or (b) on the left side.

As in diagnostic laparoscopy, a pneumoperitoneum is created, by inserting a Verres needle through a small infra-umbilical incision, aimed towards the pelvis. The abdomen is insufflated with 3–5 litres of CO_2 and the intra-abdominal pressure is maintained at about 14 mmHg during the operation. A 10 mm trocar is inserted through the infra-umbilical incision pointing towards the right upper quadrant, and the peritoneal cavity inspected with a video-laparoscope. Three other trocars and cannulae are sited as shown in Figure 5.2. The second 10 mm cannula, positioned in the midline between the xiphoid process and umbilicus, is used for dissecting instruments. Ratcheted grasping forceps are passed through the 5 mm cannula in the anterior axillary

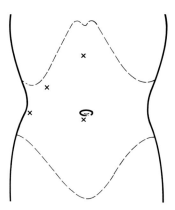

Figure 5.2: Trocar insertion sites for laparoscopic cholecystectomy. Two 10 mm diameter trocars are used in the midline and two 5 mm trocars are used at the anterior axillary and midclavicular sites.

line to retract the fundus of the gall bladder, pushing it with the liver towards the patient's right shoulder. A second pair of grasping forceps are applied to Hartmann's pouch via the trocar in the midclavicular line. These manoeuvres expose the gall bladder, subhepatic space and porta hepatis.

Dissection of Calot's triangle

The peritoneum over Calot's triangle is divided with the diathermy hook, and fibroareolar tissue cleared. The cystic duct is then exposed, cleaned circumferentially and traced on to the gall bladder. The cystic artery is similarly dissected. The Hartmann's pouch forceps can be manipulated to expose both anterior and posterior surfaces of Calot's triangle so that the dissection can proceed from both sides. Once the anatomy in Calot's triangle has been clearly identified, the cystic duct is ligated with titanium or biodegradable polydioxanone (Ethicon) clips, and divided with hooked scissors. The cystic artery can be dealt with similarly, but many surgeons regard it as safer to divide the branches of the cystic artery on the gall bladder wall with diathermy alone or clips, rather than the main trunk.

Cholangiography

A peroperative cholangiogram can be performed before ligating the cystic duct. Some surgeons believe that this should be done routinely, others selectively and still others, not at all. The importance of cholangiography is to confirm that the anatomy has been correctly identified before proceeding with the dissection. The time of greatest risk for bile duct injury is during the learning curve for the operation, when cholangiography is often not attempted because it adds another difficult stage to the operation. Most surgeons perform cholangiography selectively when there is difficulty in identifying the anatomy, or there is suspicion of a stone in the bile duct.

The cystic duct is clipped at the neck of the gall bladder and a small nick made in the duct. A cholangiocatheter is introduced into the cystic duct, using either specially designed forceps (Storz) which grasp the cystic duct, or simply through a 14 French Abbocath placed through the abdominal wall in the right hypochondrium. The cholangiocatheter is secured in the cystic duct with a clip. A cholangiogram is obtained in the normal way, using an image intensifier with the ability to produce hard copies. The catheter is removed and the cystic duct clipped.

Dissection of gall bladder

The next stage is to dissect the gall bladder from the liver bed by dividing its peritoneal attachments and fibroareolar tissue. The dissection is best performed by taking small bites of tissue with the diathermy hook and ensuring complete haemostasis throughout. Once detached, the gall bladder is removed through one of the 10 mm cannulae, usually the infra-umbilical which is in the thinnest part of the abdominal wall.

To do this, the video-laparoscope is transferred to the subxiphoid port. The cystic duct is grasped through the infra-umbilical cannula and pulled into it. As the cannula is removed, the cystic duct and neck of gall bladder appear on the surface of the abdominal wall. To facilitate extraction, the gall bladder is opened, the bile aspirated with a sucker, and the stones are crushed and removed with grasping forceps. If the stones cannot be removed, the umbilical incision may need to be enlarged to extract the gall bladder. The Laparolith (Baxter Healthcare Ltd, California), an instrument similar to the Rotalith (*see* page 103), has been devised rapidly to reduce gallstones to a sludge to aid gall bladder extraction.

Laser energy or diathermy

When laparoscopic cholecystectomy was first introduced, the publicity gave the impression that laser energy was necessary, and it was called laparoscopic laser cholecystectomy. Diathermy or laser energy can be used for the dissection. Diathermy is a better coagulator, and it appears that the dissection takes longer with laser energy. Of more importance is that every operating theatre is equipped with diathermy apparatus. Laser units cost about £25–50 000. It is interesting to note, that surgeons in seven out of 12 centres who participated in a multicentre study, started out using laser and changed to diathermy (Southern Surgeons Club, 1991).

Selection and contraindications

Treatment with laparoscopic cholecystectomy is probably indicated only in patients with symptomatic gallstones. The technical feasibility or difficulty of the laparoscopic operation can be predicted from an ultrasound examination, which includes assessment of gall bladder emptying by measuring its volume before and after a fatty meal.

A thick-walled gall bladder with a small fasting volume which fails to contract after a fatty meal suggests that there have been previous episodes of inflammation. These thick-walled, shrunken, fibrosed gall bladders which are often surrounded by adhesions and have short cystic ducts, are more difficult to dissect even at open operation. Findings such as these are a relative contraindication to laparoscopic cholecystectomy, and warn the surgeon of the likely technical difficulty to be encountered and that extra time will be required for the operation.

Contraindications to laparoscopic cholecystectomy have gradually diminished with greater experience of the technique. There are probably no absolute contraindications. Relative contraindications include acute gallstone disease, previous upper abdominal surgery, pregnancy, advanced liver disease, bleeding disorders and patients who are high risk for general anaesthesia. Obesity is not a contraindication in women as their fat is largely stored in the abdominal wall and does not interfere with the operation, whereas in men, fat is stored intra-abdominally which often creates major technical difficulties.

Results

Several early series of laparoscopic cholecystectomy have been reported, the largest by the Southern Surgeons Club (1991) of 1518 cases performed by 59 surgeons in 20 different centres. Conversion to the open operation was necessary in less than 5%, for reasons including uncontrolled bleeding from the cystic artery, technical difficulties due to complicated gall bladder disease or to anatomical anomalies, bile duct injury, adhesions and bowel injury.

The procedure at present takes longer to perform, but operating times are reducing as experience increases. The average operating time for 20 expert European surgeons varied between 30–90 minutes (Cuschieri et al., 1991), although most series give operating times with means of 90 minutes or more, ranging from 20 to over 300 minutes. The main advantage of the laparoscopic technique is the short recovery period. Patients are able to eat, drink and become mobile as soon as they have recovered from the anaesthetic, and experience minimal pain, thus removing the need for opiate analgesia. The 1518 patients reported by the Southern Surgeons Club, (1991) had a mean hospital stay of only 1.2 days and, in Reddick and Olsen's series (1990), 37 of 83 patients (45%) were treated as out-patients.

The convalescent period is extremely short, and patients are often able to return to normal activities within a few days. In a survey of 104 French and 84 American patients two weeks after laparoscopic cholecystectomy, discomfort had resolved in 73–93% of patients (Vitale et al., 1991). In the same period, 89–94% of patients had returned to normal activity and 63% of employed Americans had returned to work, contrasting with only 25% of the French. An early return to work is possible, but will not be a reality until it is accepted that major surgery no longer requires a prolonged convalescent period.

The difficult gall bladder

Laparoscopic cholecystectomy has been accepted as a major advance in the management of uncomplicated symptomatic gallstone disease. Those experienced at the technique are now offering the operation to patients with acute cholecystitis, common duct stones and those who have had previous surgery.

The operation is more difficult when the gall bladder is acutely inflamed, and in one study, five out of 15 patients were converted to the open operation (Flowers *et al.*, 1991). Adhesions following previous surgery add to the difficulty of the operation, making access hazardous and exposure of the gall bladder difficult. Dubois *et al.*, (1990), who have published an experience of 330 operations, find that adhesions are still a problem.

Bile duct stones can be removed by preoperative or postoperative endoscopic retrograde cholangiopancreatographic examination (ERCP) with endoscopic sphincterotomy, or by laparotomy and exploration of the common bile duct. Duct stones have been successfully removed by laparoscopic choledochoscopy or choledochotomy (Petelin, 1991), but this may not be justified with the availability and ease of endoscopic techniques.

Complications

All of the complications described for diagnostic laparoscopy may occur during laparoscopic cholecystectomy and, in addition, there are those specifically associated with cholecystectomy. The morbidity associated with laparoscopic cholecystectomy is not accurately known, but is reported to be between 1.6% and 11% (Cuschieri *et al.*, 1991; Schirmer *et al.*, 1991). There have also been fatalities. Complications include bleeding, biliary leak, bile duct injury, retained ductal stones, perihepatic collections and infection.

Bile duct injury is a serious complication occurring in 0.1–0.4% of open cholecystectomies (Raute and Schaupp, 1988; Habib *et al.*, 1990). The potential for such injury may be greater with the laparoscopic approach, and a 0.5% incidence has been reported (Southern Surgeons Club, 1991). Despite the many advantages of the technique, its use may not be justified if it proves to be less safe than the open operation.

Minicholecystectomy

Although technically demanding, cholecystectomy can be safely performed through 4–6 cm transverse incisions (Dubois and Berthelot, 1982). One method uses a stabilized ring retractor (Codman) which comes with a variety of fixed and malleable blades, and provides accurate fixed retraction with excellent exposure, despite the small incision.

The surgeon's hand does not enter the abdomen at any stage and the operation can be performed without an assistant. The gall bladder is dissected retrogradely, using diathermy scissors or hook, to ensure haemostasis throughout. A peroperative cholangiogram is performed, securing the cholangiocatheter with a metal clip. The cystic duct and artery are also clipped, and the wound closed without drainage.

No modification of the incision is required for the more difficult gall bladder, for exploration of the bile duct or for choledochoduodenostomy. The cosmetic result is excellent, especially when the incision is made in a skin crease and closed with an absorbable subcuticular skin suture.

Results

Over 80% of patients are discharged by the third postoperative day, although a mean hospital stay of 1.5 days has been reported (Goco and Chambers, 1983). Patients require less analgesia than following standard cholecystectomy and are able to return to work after a mean 18.6 days (Russell and Shankar, 1987).

Percutaneous gall bladder techniques

Over the past decade, direct percutaneous access to the gall bladder has opened new avenues for minimally invasive therapeutic procedures. These include percutaneous cholecystostomy in acute cholecystitis, mechanical stone extraction by percutaneous cholecystolithotomy or rotary lithotripsy, and contact dissolution of stones with solvents. The main criticisms of these techniques are the risk of stone recurrence and that a diseased gall bladder is left *in situ*.

Percutaneous cholecystostomy

Direct percutaneous access to the gall bladder is being increasingly used for the treatment of acute cholecystitis, empyema and even the perforated gall bladder with localized abscess formation, particularly in elderly and high risk patients. Drainage of the gall bladder under these conditions, as with any localized septic focus, produces immediate relief of symptoms with resolution of fever and leucocytosis.

The procedure is performed with local anaesthesia and carries minimal morbidity and mortality. In the elderly, emergency cholecystectomy carries a mortality rate of 10–14% (Huber et al., 1983; Addison and Finan, 1988), and 5% after surgical cholecystostomy (Winkler et al., 1989). When the acute phase has resolved, the stones can be extracted by percutaneous methods without the need for cholecystectomy.

Percutaneous cholecystolithotomy

Percutaneous puncture of the gall bladder is usually transhepatic as it avoids bowel injury and leakage of bile. Kellet et al., (1988) described percutaneous cholecystolithotomy, adapting it from percutaneous nephrolithotomy, using the transperitoneal approach to the gall bladder, which allows larger cannulae to be introduced (28–30 French) for easier stone extraction. Cheslyn-Curtis et al., (1992) have successfully performed transperitoneal, fundal punctures of the gall bladder, with dilatation of a track, in 100 of 113 patients without complication.

Technique

The procedure is performed under general anaesthesia or local anaes-thesia with intravenous sedation, and takes 25–90 minutes. A percutaneous cholecystogram is performed, and then the fundus of the gall bladder is punctured with a Kellett needle, using a combination of ultrasound and fluoroscopic guidance. A guidewire is placed in the gall bladder for the entire procedure as a safety measure. The track is dilated to 28–30 French using Teflon and telescoping metal dilators, before inserting a Teflon sheath (Figure 5.3). The gall bladder is inspected with a rigid cholecystoscope, and stones up to 10 mm in diameter are flushed out or removed with forceps. Stones too large to pass through the Teflon sheath are fragmented by intracorporeal electrohydraulic laser or ultrasound lithotripsy and removed piecemeal (Figure 5.4).

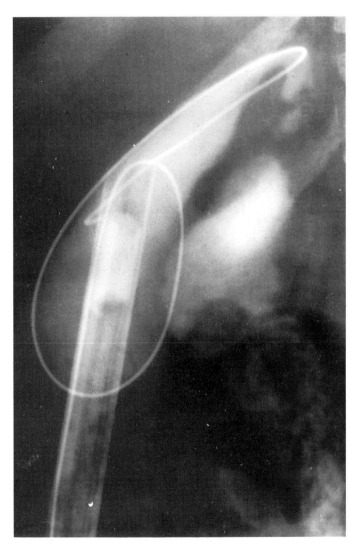

Figure 5.3: Cholecystogram showing a guidewire coiled in the gall bladder lumen and the 30 French Teflon sheath through which the stones are removed. Contrast is also seen in the duodenum.

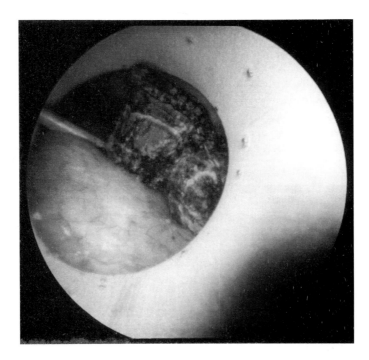

Figure 5.4: View down the Amplatz sheath of a solitary 2 cm diameter stone lying on the gall bladder mucosa. The stone has been fragmented by electrohydraulic lithotripsy to facilitate extraction. The guidewire is also visible.

The gall bladder is carefully inspected and, following radiological confirmation that all the stones and fragments have been removed, a Foley catheter is introduced through the Teflon sheath and placed on free drainage. Patients are discharged from hospital after 24–48 hours, and are able to return to normal activities as soon as the Foley catheter is removed 10 days later, although many return to work before this.

Selection and contraindications

Patients are selected by ultrasound scanning of the gall bladder before and after a fatty meal. Information is obtained on the number and size of stones and gall bladder position, wall thickness and its ability to empty. Almost 80% of patients with symptomatic gallstones of any number, size or composition, are suitable for treatment. The only patients to be rejected are those with thick-walled contracted gall bladders, which are diseased and difficult to puncture and dilate a track. Patients with acute complications, and those with non-function due to a stone impacted in Hartmann's pouch, are also suitable for treatment, but the gall bladder is decompressed percutaneously for 7–10 days before stone extraction, to allow the acute phase to resolve or the stone to disimpact.

Results

In the largest study (Cheslyn Curtis *et al.*, 1992) the procedure was successful in 100 of 113 patients, failures being due to failed puncture and dilatation, or to residual cystic duct stones. Among those treated were 14 patients with acute gall bladder disease and 30 who were regarded as high risk and unfit for open cholecystectomy. The 15 complications were mainly of a minor nature and intervention was only needed to drain one subhepatic bile collection percutaneously.

Outcome was assessed in 92 patients, followed up for a mean 14 months (range 6–37), of whom 90% were asymptomatic or had minimal discomfort. There have been nine stone recurrences (9.8%), five recurring within six months of treatment. These are believed to be due to residual fragments, as they were suspected on the post-procedure contrast study, but not confirmed by additional radiological examination. 93% of gall bladders are functioning, including 80% of those treated with acute gall bladder disease.

Ultrasound guided minicholecystostomy with radiological stone removal (Gibney *et al.*, 1987), and laparoscopic cholecystolithotomy (Perissat *et al.*, 1989) are more invasive than percutaneous cholecystolithotomy, but can be used if expertise to puncture the gall bladder percutaneously is not available.

Percutaneous rotary lithotripsy

Technique

This method is performed under local anaesthesia and uses the Rotalith (Baxter Healthcare Ltd, California), which consists of a rotating metal arm (impeller) held within a rigid basket. It is introduced into the gall bladder in compressed form through a 10 French percutaneous catheter. The Rotalith rotates at over 30 000 revolutions per minute and generates a vortex sucking the stones into the basket (Figure 5.5). The impeller reduces the stones to a sludge which is flushed out at the end of the procedure.

Results

Selection is similar to percutaneous cholecystolithotomy, but has been restricted to non-acute gallstone disease. It has been successfully undertaken in nine out of 10 patients, but long-term outcome is unknown (Gillams *et al.*, 1991).

Contact dissolution therapy

Technique

A 5 French transhepatic catheter is passed into the gall bladder under local anaesthesia and intravenous sedation. Thistle *et al.*, (1989) continuously infused and aspirated methyl tert butyl ether (MTBE) by hand for an average of five hours per day, over 2–3 days. Leuschner *et al.*, (1991) report a mean

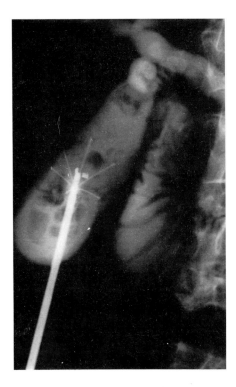

Figure 5.5: Cholecystogram of the Rotalith, (a) (above) within a gall bladder containing stones and (b) (right) after the stones have been reduced to sludge and flushed out. Contrast is also seen in the bile duct and duodenum.

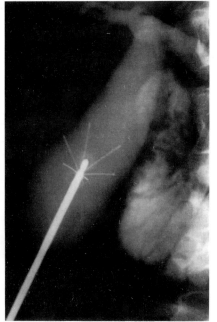

dissolution time for solitary stones of four hours, and for multiple stones of 10 hours. A microprocessor-assisted solvent transfer system has now been developed to regulate the infusion and aspiration of MTBE at high flow rates, and to control gall bladder pressure preventing solvent escape into the duodenum (Zakko and Hofmann, 1990).

Selection

MTBE is only effective against cholesterol gallstones. Leuschner *et al.*, (1991) carefully selected 120 out of 612 patients (20%) for MTBE therapy.

Results

In the original study (Thistle *et al.*, 1989), MTBE produced complete or more than 95% stone dissolution in 72 out of 75 (96%) patients. Leuschner *et al.*, (1991) obtained successful puncture of the gall bladder and stone dissolution in 113 out of 120 (97%) patients. There are several side-effects with this therapy including nausea, vomiting, burning pain, transient sedation due to systemic absorption of the solvent, intravascular haemolysis, duodenal erosions, haematobilia and destruction of certain catheter materials. The treatment requires considerable care and skill and, because of the potential for complications, is unlikely to become a standard method except in a few specialist centres.

Summary

Laparoscopic cholecystectomy has rapidly become the procedure of choice for the management of symptomatic gall bladder stones. Minicholecystectomy should be used in patients unsuitable for the laparoscopic technique, and for those requiring conversion to the open operation. A small group of patients, perhaps 5%, will continue to be unfit for operative treatment, and it is in these patients that one of the percutaneous techniques is invaluable in removing their stones and symptoms.

Other general surgical procedures

With the rapidity and enthusiasm with which laparoscopic cholecystectomy has been introduced, there is now a lot of interest in developing laparoscopic techniques for other general surgical operations. Most of the techniques that follow are performed by a few laparoscopic 'enthusiasts' and should be regarded as at a developmental stage.

Oesophageal surgery

Anti-reflux procedures

Oesophageal reflux disease is common and mainly treated with H_2-receptor antagonists, alginates or, more recently, omeprazole, a proton-pump inhibitor. Anti-reflux procedures are indicated when there is a failure or non-compliance in medical therapy, or if complications arise. The most common operation performed is a total or partial fundoplication and this has been performed laparoscopically. An alternative anti-reflux procedure, the ligamentum teres cardiopexy, acts by lengthening the intra-abdominal segment of oesophageal sphincter (Narbona Arnau *et al.*, 1980). Nathanson *et al.*, (1991) have adapted this procedure to be performed laparoscopically.

Technique

Five cannulae are sited as shown in Figure 5.6. A fan-like retractor, used to lift the left lobe of the liver, is passed through the small paraxiphisternal cannula and opened out. The two large cannulae at the umbilical level are used for the telescopes (0° and 30°) and clip applicator, but can also be used for grasping forceps and scissors. Two other small cannulae are used for dissecting instruments, grasping forceps and needle holders.

The operation is performed in three stages. Firstly, the ligamentum teres (falciform ligament) is mobilized off the anterior abdominal wall, from the upper part of the anterior surface of the liver down to the umbilicus, preserving its blood supply from the liver and detaching it from the umbilicus.

Secondly, the abdominal oesophagus is mobilized. The peritoneum over the oesophagus is grasped and divided with scissors. The right margin of the oesophagus is exposed using dissection with pledget and sucker until the posterior wall is reached. The left margin of the oesophagus is similarly mobilized and then the phreno-oesophageal membrane is dissected upwards off the anterior oesophageal wall. Curved long grasping forceps, introduced through a flexible silicone cannula sited in the left upper quadrant, are used to pass a silicone sling around the oesophagus. Both ends of the sling are made to

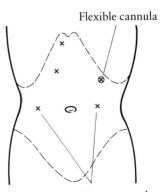

Flexible cannula

11 mm cannulae

Figure 5.6: Trocar insertion sites for ligamentum teres cardiopexy.

emerge through a stab incision, and external traction is applied to retract the oesophagus anteriorly, allowing the posterior oesophageal mobilization to be completed.

The third stage in the operation is to perform the cardiopexy. The curved grasping forceps are used to grip the end of the previously mobilized ligamentum teres, and to pass it from right to left behind the mobilized oesophagus. The end of the ligament is pulled down along the anterior wall of the stomach. The degree of traction is adjusted using oesophageal manometry, and has been shown to affect the length of intra-abdominal oesophagus.

The ligamentum teres sling is sutured to the left side of the oesophagus, and then the gastric fundus is sutured to the oesophagus above the sling. The rest of the sling is attached to the anterior wall of the stomach, roughly parallel to the lesser curvature. Suturing is performed using 3/0 silk sutures and a two needle holder technique with internal knotting, a technique which requires considerable training.

Results

Nathanson et al., (1991) have reported laparoscopic ligamentum teres cardiopexy in five patients with oesophageal reflux disease including two with hiatus hernia. The procedure time was long at 2.5–5 hours, but all patients were discharged within five days. All patients were relieved of their reflux symptoms and none complained of dysphagia or gas bloat symptoms, but follow-up was short (1-6 months).

Cardiomyotomy

This operation is performed for achalasia and oesophageal motility disorders, such as diffuse oesophageal spasm and nutcracker oesophagus. Laparoscopic techniques have been developed to perform the myotomy by both the thoracic and abdominal approaches.

Technique

Using the abdominal approach (Shimi et al., 1991), the peritoneum over the oesophagus is divided to expose the hiatal crura. The right and left margins of the oesophagus are mobilized from the crura and anteriorly, the phreno-oesophageal membrane is teased up until the mediastinum is reached. About 5 cm of oesophagus is exposed, but care is taken to preserve anchoring bands of the phreno-oesophageal membrane and the posterior vagus nerve. The anterior vagus nerve is identified, and a vertical myotomy performed lateral to it along the oesophagus on to the stomach wall.

Results

Cuschieri (personal communication) has successfully performed six cardiomy-otomies for achalasia, complicated by perforation of the oesophagus in one patient.

Gastric surgery

Peptic ulcer surgery

Until the 1970s, peptic ulcer disease was largely managed by operative intervention such as partial gastrectomy or different types of vagotomy. The success of effective medical treatment with H_2-receptor antagonists has resulted in a major decline in the role of surgery. Operative intervention is now largely confined to patients who are unresponsive to, or fail to comply with, medical treatment, or who develop complications of the disease such as haemorrhage, perforation or pyloric stenosis.

Endoscopic therapy

Using endoscopic methods of arresting haemorrhage, such as diathermy (heater probe) or injection of adrenaline around a bleeding ulcer, an operation can be avoided in some patients. However, there is no evidence that the use of endoscopy in gastrointestinal haemorrhage has resulted in a reduction in mortality (Steele, 1989). Pyloric stenosis, which would formerly have been treated by vagotomy and gastroenterostomy or gastric resection, can also be managed endoscopically by pneumatic dilatation with a balloon catheter.

Laparoscopic repair of perforated peptic ulcer

The conventional operation for managing a perforated duodenal ulcer is laparotomy with oversewing of the perforation with an omental patch and peritoneal toilet. A perforated gastric ulcer can be managed similarly, provided that a biopsy is performed to ensure that it is benign. These perforations can now be managed laparoscopically (Mouret *et al.*, 1990; Nathanson *et al.*, 1990).

Technique

Laparoscopy is performed under general anaesthesia and the diagnosis confirmed by the demonstration of turbid fluid, mainly in the subhepatic pouch, right paracolic gutter and pelvis, associated with a perforation in the duodenum or stomach. Acute duodenal perforations are usually anterior and easily identified through the laparoscope.

Trocar and cannulae may be sited in the right subcostal region, for an instrument to retract the liver off the duodenum, and in the left and right upper quadrants for suturing and grasping instruments. Peritoneal toilet is performed, to clean the contaminated peritoneal cavity, by systematically irrigating with saline and aspirating the turbid fluid using the combined irrigator/aspirator. The perforation is closed using an omental patch, which is fixed by two or three sutures with internal or external knotting. A tissue glue (Tiseel, collagen/fibrinogen spray) can be sprayed over the operative site.

An alternative technique described for closure of a duodenal perforation is a combined endoscopic and laparoscopic approach (Mouret *et al.*, 1990). Grasping forceps are passed through the operating channel of the endoscope and out through the duodenal opening. The grasping forceps are used to pull a segment of omentum over the duodenal opening and then the omentum is secured to the duodenum by laparoscopic sutures.

Vagotomy

The operation of choice for patients with ulcer disease unresponsive to medical management, is highly selective vagotomy which preserves antropyloric innervation and motility. Laparoscopic vagotomy has been described using three methods: anterior lesser curve seromyotomy and posterior truncal vagotomy (Taylor *et al.*, 1982), posterior truncal vagotomy combined with selective anterior vagotomy (Hill and Barker, 1978) and truncal vagotomy combined with pneumatic dilatation of the pylorus (Mouiel and Katkhouda, 1991). Taylor *et al.*, (1990) showed that with their technique, a similar degree of vagal denervation could be obtained, with a lower incidence of dumping and diarrhoea than truncal vagotomy. However, recurrent ulceration occurred in 6.5% of patients, which was more frequent than the 2.9% for truncal vagotomy.

Technique: posterior truncal vagotomy and anterior seromyotomy

A pneumoperitoneum is created via an umbilical puncture and a 0° video-laparoscope inserted through a 10 mm umbilical cannula. Four other trocar and cannulae are inserted (Figure 5.7); a 5 mm trocar to the right of the xiphoid process for the liver retractor and the combined irrigator/aspirator; two other 5 mm trocars subcostally in the right and left midclavicular lines for atraumatic grasping forceps; and a 10 mm trocar 6 cm to the left of the umbilicus, used as an operating channel for dissecting scissors, diathermy hook and the clip applier.

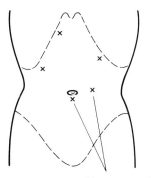

Figure 5.7: Trocar insertion sites for posterior truncal vagotomy and anterior seromyotomy.

10 mm cannula

The operation begins by dissecting the avascular portion of the lesser omentum and clipping and dividing the left gastric vein. Identification of the oesophagus is aided by the light of an endoscope introduced alongside the nasogastric tube. The overlying peritoneum is incised, and careful dissection using the diathermy hook, frees the left side of the right crus. With two grasping forceps separating the oesophagus and right crus, the posterior vagus nerve is identified as a thick white filament. The nerve is divided between two clips and a specimen sent for histological examination.

The anterior lesser curve seromyotomy is started at the cardia and extended in a curved fashion, at a distance of 1.5 cm from the lesser curve, to 6 cm from the pylorus (at the Crow's foot). The diathermy hook is used to incise the gastric wall, while two grasping forceps retract the edges of the seromyotomy. The exposed mucosa is visually checked for any perforation, and methylene blue can be injected into the stomach for the same purpose.

Any perforation is closed with 4-0 monofilament nylon using two needle holders and internal knotting, a technique which requires considerable training. The edges of the seromyotomy are approximated with sutures to aid haemostasis, and fibrin sealant may also be used. The cannulae are extracted and the skin wounds sutured.

Results

Katkhouda and Mouiel, (1991) have reported the procedure in 10 patients with a mean age of 32 and long histories of chronic duodenal ulceration (mean duration 3.8 years and mean 2.8 recurrences). The mean duration of the procedure was 60 minutes (range 55–110 min). There were no complications. All patients were discharged from hospital within five days and able to return to work 10 days postoperatively. Gastric acid studies, performed before and one month postoperatively, showed a mean reduction in basal acid output of $79 \pm 1.32\%$ and in maximal acid output of $83 \pm 1.23\%$. All patients were asymptomatic two months postoperatively and the ulcers had completely healed in nine patients.

Technique: posterior truncal vagotomy and anterior selective vagotomy

This laparoscopic procedure has been described by Bailey et al., (in press), based on the open operation reported by Hill and Barker (1978), where branches of the anterior nerve of Latarjet are individually divided as they enter the stomach. Five trocar and cannulae are sited as above. The left lobe of the liver is mobilized by dividing the left triangular ligament, and is retracted with the fan-like retractor. A 48 French oesophageal bougie is passed and used to keep the stomach on tension. The lesser omentum is opened and the posterior vagus is identified and divided between titanium clips. The anterior vagus is identified on the front of the oesophagus and put on tension with a probe.

The serosa is carefully opened along the lesser curve of the stomach, to display individual branches of the anterior nerve of Latarjet as they enter the stomach. The laparoscopic magnification often enables the nerve to be dissected and divided separately from the adjacent blood vessels. The branches of the nerve of Latarjet, innervating the gastric antrum, are easily identified and preserved. The oesophagogastric junction is carefully dissected to divide vagal branches innervating the cardia.

Technique: truncal vagotomy (Mouiel and Khathouda, 1991)

Five trocar and cannulae are used and sited as above. The left lobe of liver is retracted with the fan-like retractor. The lesser omentum is opened towards the oesophageal hiatus and the peritoneum over the oesophagus divided with the diathermy hook. The posterior vagus nerve is located and divided between clips sending a segment for histological examination. The anterior vagus is snared with the hook dissector and similarly divided between clips. The entire circumference of the oesophagus is then examined and other vagal branches are divided. To avoid problems with gastric emptying, pneumatic dilatation of the pylorus is performed, using a 16 mm balloon at 45 psi pressure. This partially ruptures the oblique and circular muscles of the pylorus and results in a widely patent channel.

Summary

There has been a major decline in the number of patients undergoing elective duodenal ulcer surgery, largely as a result of successful medical treatment with H_2-receptor antagonists, but also due to the unwanted side-effects of truncal vagotomy and the recurrence rate after highly selective vagotomy. Nevertheless, on stopping treatment with H_2-receptor antagonists, ulcer recurrence rates approach 90% at one year. With the minimally invasive method of laparoscopic vagotomy, many more patients may benefit from operative intervention rather than continue with long-term medication to prevent ulcer recurrence.

Percutaneous gastrostomy

This technique can be used in patients with diseases of the pharynx and oesophagus who need a gastrostomy, provided that an endoscope can be passed into the stomach. Different methods have been described including the 'pull' technique in which the feeding catheter is railroaded down via the mouth, and the 'introducer' technique in which a percutaneous tract into the stomach is dilated before introducing the feeding catheter (Ponsky and Gauderer, 1989; Miller et al., 1989).

Technique

Using the introducer technique, endoscopy is performed under intravenous sedation with local anaesthesia and antibiotic cover. The stomach is inflated with air and a small incision made in the left upper quadrant, adjacent to the light from the endoscope, which is visualized on the anterior abdominal wall. The stomach is punctured percutaneously with a long 18 gauge needle through which a guidewire is threaded. A special dilator and sheath are threaded over the wire into the stomach. The inner dilator is replaced with a gastrostomy tube, the balloon inflated and the sheath peeled off. Percutaneous gastrostomy is widely used and has few complications (Miller *et al.*, 1989). It can be used for the majority of patients formerly treated by surgical gastrostomy.

Diagnostic laparoscopy

Until the introduction of laparoscopic cholecystectomy, general surgeons showed very little interest in diagnostic laparoscopy, although it had been performed for nearly 90 years (Kelling, 1923). It is useful in the investigation of patients with malignancy, to determine the extent of spread, to assess the stage of the disease, to assess operability and, with developments in operative laparoscopy, to perform laparoscopic bypass surgery. Second-look laparoscopy has been successfully used in ovarian cancer patients, treated with a combination of surgery and intraperitoneal chemotherapy, to assess the significance of new symptoms.

It is also useful for staging lymphoma and for diagnosing the cause of PUO (pyrexia of unknown origin), such as abdominal tuberculosis or lymphoma. During laparoscopy, biopsies of various organs can be performed under direct vision, with the advantages that a biopsy can be taken from the correct area. Sites such as the parietal peritoneum, omentum or mesentery, which are not easily accessible to radiologically guided percutaneous biopsy, can be sampled, and bleeding at the biopsy site can be directly controlled with a coagulating probe.

Emergency laparoscopy

Diagnostic laparoscopy may be more accurate than peritoneal lavage in assessing the need for laparotomy in patients with blunt or penetrating abdominal trauma. The incidence of unnecessary laparotomies following positive peritoneal lavage is 15–20% (Berci and Sackier, 1991). In a series of 150 diagnostic laparoscopies for trauma (Berci and Sackier, 1991), 38 out of 64 patients (59%), in whom intraperitoneal blood was found, did not require exploration, as the findings were of minimal to moderate haemorrhage, with no identifiable injury or only minor lacerations. One of these patients had a sealed sigmoid colonic perforation and underwent a subsequent laparotomy. The findings in the 28 who were explored were seven liver lacerations, 11 splenic injuries, four organ perforations and six arterial haemorrhages.

The use of laparoscopy for the diagnosis of acute abdominal pain was described in 1975 (Sugerbaker *et al.*, 1975), and a number of studies have since shown that it is useful in determining an accurate diagnosis of right iliac fossa and pelvic pain. In patients with acute abdominal pain, in whom there is uncertainty about the need for operation, both diagnostic and therapeutic errors can be significantly reduced from 19% to zero, by selectively performing laparoscopy (Paterson-Brown *et al.*, 1986).

An argument can be made for performing laparoscopy in all women with suspected appendicitis, irrespective of the certainty of diagnosis, because of the high error rate in this group. Laparoscopy is a safe procedure, which is relatively simple to learn, with a complication rate of about 3% and a mortality rate of 8 per 100 000 (Chamberlain and Carron Brown, 1978), whereas the reported complication rate following the removal of a normal appendix is 13–17% (Chang *et al.*, 1973; Deutsch *et al.*, 1983).

Appendicectomy

Appendicectomy for acute appendicitis is one of the most common operations performed by general surgeons. It is performed through a small incision, classically over McBurney's point, with a good cosmetic result, a short hospital stay (about 3–4 days) and minimal morbidity. Removal of a normal appendix, using a laparoscopic technique, was first reported in 1983 by Semm, but it was not until 1987, that laparoscopic appendicectomy for acute appendicitis was described (Schreiber, 1987).

Technique

The patient is placed supine or in the Lloyd-Davies position, with a moderate head down and left lateral tilt. A pneumoperitoneum is created and the video-laparoscope introduced through a 10 mm cannula at the umbilicus. A 5 mm trocar is inserted in either the left iliac fossa or just suprapubically, for the dissecting instruments. The abdomen is thoroughly inspected with the help of an atraumatic rod, and the diagnosis of appendicitis confirmed or refuted.

For appendicectomy, the appendix is gripped with grasping forceps through a third 5 mm cannula sited over McBurney's point in the right iliac fossa. The vessels in the mesoappendix are dissected out and divided either with the diathermy hook or between metal clips with scissors. The newly developed EndoGIA stapler (Autosuture), which is 30 mm long with three rows of haemostatic staples and a cutting blade, may also be suitable for this purpose. The dissection is continued until the appendix has been freed down to its base, which is ligated with a pre-knotted O-catgut Roeder's loop. The base of the appendix is cut across with the diathermy hook, 6–7 mm distal to the ligature.

The stump can be invaginated by placing a purse-string suture as in the open operation, using a straight needle and two laparoscopic needle-holders, but is technically difficult and time-consuming. As recent evidence (Engstrom and Fenyo, 1985) has shown that there is no advantage in invaginating the appendix stump over simple ligation, it seems unnecessary to do so during the laparoscopic operation. The appendix is extracted through the umbilical cannula, necessitating removal of the laparoscope and resiting of a 5 mm scope through the suprapubic/left iliac fossa cannula.

If the appendix is very fat or swollen, the 10 mm cannula can be replaced by a 15–20 mm appendiceal extraction sheath, so that the appendix is removed without contaminating the abdominal wall. Patients usually recover rapidly and can resume normal activities within 48 hours.

Results

Several series have reported the feasibility and safety with which laparoscopic appendicectomy can be performed. In a recent series (Gotz *et al.*, 1990), only 12 out of 388 laparoscopic appendicectomies were converted to the open operation. 74% of patients had histologically proven acute appendicitis of which eight were gangrenous, 43 phlegmonous and five perforated. The remainder showed subacute or chronic appendicitis (14%) or were normal (12%). The average procedure time was 15–20 minutes. Two patients developed abscesses which were drained at laparotomy, and 14 umbilical wound infections were treated with antibiotics.

This series has shown that laparoscopic appendicectomy can be performed safely with a low complication rate in all stages of appendicitis. The laparoscopic approach is particularly useful for the diagnosis of non-specific lower abdominal pain in young women, as 20% or more will be due to a gynaecological problem (Paterson Brown *et al.*, 1990). For those with appendicitis, appendicectomy can be performed at the time of laparoscopy without the need for conversion to the open operation, and adds 10–15 minutes to the procedure.

Summary

Although open appendicectomy can be performed through a 2–4 cm incision, the laparoscopic approach seems to have the benefit of more accurate diagnosis as well as the advantages common to other laparoscopic operations: greater cosmesis, less postoperative pain and shorter recovery period.

Hernia repair

Extraperitoneal inguinal herniorrhaphy repairing the posterior wall of the inguinal canal, first proposed by Bassini in 1884, has undergone many modifications but, as evident from the large literature on suturing techniques, the use of different suture materials and different hernia repair techniques, no single technique is entirely satisfactory.

The most important criterion used to measure the success of herniorrhaphy is the incidence of recurrence. Closure of the neck of the sac, narrowing of the internal ring, combined with repair of the posterior wall are, important in the prevention of recurrence. In a large collected review (Condon and Nyhus, 1989) of inguinal herniae repaired by the Bassini method and its various modifications, recurrence rates were 0–7% for indirect hernias, 1–10% for direct hernias and 5–35% for recurrent hernias.

In addition to recurrence, injury to the spermatic cord or postoperative epididymo-orchitis can occur, and chronic pain due to neuromata may develop. The conventional operation is painful, and for those whose occupation involves heavy lifting, it requires several weeks away from work.

Laparoscopic herniorrhaphy is performed transabdominally using prosthetic mesh. Prosthetic mesh is usually used for repairing recurrent or unusually large hernias, with the aim of providing a tension-free repair, but Lichtenstein et al., (1989) use prosthetic material for their standard hernia repair, and have reported 1000 consecutive cases, followed up for 1–5 years, without a single recurrence or prosthetic infection. Other surgeons investigating preperitoneal prosthetic repair of groin hernias in first-time operations have reported large series with low recurrence rates of 1.4% (Stoppa and Warlaumont, 1989) and 1.7% (Nyhus et al., 1988).

Techniques and results

Several techniques have been described for laparoscopic inguinal herniorrhaphy, but none is entirely satisfactory. Usually a 30° or 45° angled laparoscope is inserted at the umbilicus, and two other trocar and cannulae (5 and 10 mm) in the iliac fossae for dissecting instruments. Popp (1990) reported the first repair of a direct inguinal hernia at the time of laparoscopic myomectomy.

In the method described by Schultz (1990), the hernia sac is incised along its superior margin and, with a combination of laser dissection of the preperitoneal tissues and downward traction on the sac, it is easily removed. Polypropylene mesh, in the form of a roll tied by a dissolvable suture, is placed directly through the musculofascial defect and additional rolls are used to fill the defect completely. Finally, two to three 25 × 50 mm pieces of mesh are placed over the defect and the peritoneum is closed over them with endoclips.

Twenty male patients have been treated by this method, mostly as day cases, with follow-up ranging from 3–11 months. There has been one recurrent hernia at two weeks, because the direct component of a pantaloon hernia had been missed at operation. Patients were able to return to unrestricted activity within a mean 3.3 days, and to employment in under four days.

Corbitt et al., (1991) used a similar technique by placing a single 50 mm × 130 mm piece of polypropylene, rolled into a plug, through the internal ring into the inguinal canal, covering the internal ring with a 50 mm square mesh and closing the peritoneum with the EndoGIA (Autosuture). This procedure is not now used because of a 20% recurrence rate.

Another variation is to use aquadissection of the preperitoneal space (Popp, 1991). The hernia sac is visualized endoscopically, and an injection needle is introduced through the skin until its tip is visualized endoscopically under the peritoneum of the sac. Aquadissection is performed by instilling 100–300 ml saline. The sac is inverted into the peritoneal cavity, and the water pillow in the area surrounding the hernia defect is dissected out. A Vicryl mesh patch is introduced and spread out in the dissected preperitoneal space. Fixation of the patch is not thought to be necessary as it is trapped in the preperitoneal space.

A different approach has been demonstrated by Katkhouda (personal communication). The laparoscope is passed from the umbilical site preperitoneally, without entering the peritoneal cavity, and a pneumopreperitoneum is created. A large mesh patch is placed over the internal ring and posterior wall of the inguinal canal and stapled in place, leaving the hernia sac in situ.

Summary

There is no adequately evaluated technique for laparoscopic herniorrhaphy to allow its widespread use at present, and most surgeons remain sceptical about its advantages. It is difficult to believe that by simply placing a plug in the inguinal canal, recurrence of a hernia will be prevented. The advantages of the laparoscopic approach should be reduced postoperative pain, enabling an earlier return to full activity, and prevention of local groin complications such as chronic pain due to neuromata and testicular atrophy due to ischaemic orchitis.

Discussion

The development of minimal access surgical techniques marks an advance in the specialty of general surgery. These techniques are unlikely to replace open operations completely, but will become a part of surgical practice, and patients will demand their use. The term 'minimal access' is perhaps inappropriate, as it implies that these procedures are easier and simpler to perform and the operative risks are minimal. This is not true. This type of surgery tends to involve greater technical expertise meaning that some procedures are only suitable for performance by a limited number of surgeons.

Many advances have been made in minimal access surgery, but further developments are needed to improve instrument design, lighting and imaging techniques. The development of three-dimensional imaging for laparoscopic surgery will be an advance over two-dimensional imaging, which at present poses real problems with hand-eye co-ordination and the appreciation of depth of visual field.

There is no doubt that minimal access surgery is less traumatic to the patient with the advantages of minimal postoperative pain, rapid recovery and avoidance of chronic wound problems. The reasons for this are not entirely understood, but very small wounds almost abolish the trauma of access, and operating in a largely closed environment with delicate instruments avoids exposure of the tissues, with cooling and drying of the viscera, and tissue damage due to retraction, instrument trauma and handling. Psychological factors influence the patient's response, but obviously if little pain is experienced, their ordeal is very much reduced.

The future of these techniques requires critical evaluation of their benefits and problems. For example, the safety and efficacy of laparoscopic cholecystectomy has not been properly evaluated, but many believe it is not ethical to run a randomized controlled clinical trial (Neugebauer *et al.*, 1991). Others advocate monitoring the technique through a national audit as is being undertaken by the Association of Surgeons of Great Britain together with the Society of Minimally Invasive General Surgeons, or the National Laparoscopic Cholecystectomy Registry in the USA. The purpose of audit is to collect clinical data relevant to the laparoscopic procedure, which should provide surgeons with realistic information concerning the appropriate and safe use of the technique. Other minimal access techniques need similar scrutiny.

Most surgeons believe that future advances in endoscopic gastrointestinal surgery should remain the surgeons' domain, unlike diagnostic and therapeutic ERCP which, 20 years ago, were taken over by gastroenterologists, largely due to the indifference of the surgeons at the time towards new technology. There is likely to be a continued trend towards a reduction in hospitalization, with more daycase surgery, to which minimal access techniques are ideally suited.

References

Addison NV and Finan PJ (1988). Urgent and early cholecystectomy for acute gall bladder disease. *Br. J. Surg.* **75**: 141–143.

Bailey RW, Flowers JL and Graham SM (In press) Combined laparoscopic cholecystectomy and selective vagotomy. *Surg. Laparosc. Endosc.*

Bates T, Mercer JC and Harrison M (1984) Symptomatic gallstone disease: before and after cholecystectomy. *Gut.* **24**: A579–580.

Berci G and Sackier JM (1991) Emergency laparoscopy. *Am. J. Surg.* **161**: 332–335.

Chamberlain GVP and Carron Brown JA (1978) *Report of the working party of the confidential enquiry into gynaecological laparoscopy.* Royal College of Obstetricians and Gynaecologists, London.

Chang FC, Hogle HH and Welling DR (1973) The fate of the negative appendix. *Am. J. Surg.* **126**: 752–754.

Cheslyn-Curtis S, Gillams A and Russell RCG *et al.*, (In press) Selection, management and early outcome of 113 patients with symptomatic gallstones treated by percutaneous cholecystolithotomy. *Gut.* **33**: 1253–1259.

Condon RE and Nyhus LM (1989) Complications of groin hernias. In: Nyhus LM and Condon RE (eds) *Hernia.* JB Lippincott, Philadelphia, pp 253–269.

Corbitt JD (1991) Laparoscopic herniorrhaphy. *Surg. Laparosc. Endosc.* **1**: 23–25.

Cuschieri A, Dubois F and Mouiel J *et al.*, (1991). The European experience with laparoscopic cholecystectomy. *Am. J. Surg.* **161**: 385–387.

Cuschieri A (personal communication).

Deutsch AA, Shani N and Reiss R (1983) Are some appendicectomies unnecessary? *J. R. Coll. Surg. Edin.* **28**: 35–40.

Dubois F and Berthelot G (1982) Cholecystectomie par minilaparotomie. *Nouv. Presse. Med.* **11**: 1139–1141.

Dubois F, Berthelot G and Levard H (1990) Cholecystectomie sous coelioscopie, 330 cas. *Chirurgie.* **116**: 248–250.

Engstrom L and Fenyo G (1985) Appendicectomy: An assessment of stump invagination. A prospective trial. *Br. J. Surg.* **72**: 971–972.

Flowers JL, Bailey RW, Scovill WA and Zucker KA (1991) The Baltimore experience with laparoscopic management of acute cholecystitis. *Am. J. Surg.* **161**: 388–392.

Gibney RG, Fache JS and Becker CD *et al.*, (1987). Combined surgical and radiological intervention for complicated cholelithiasis in high risk patients. *Radiology.* **165**: 715–719.

Gillams A, Lake S, Cheslyn-Curtis S, Lees WR, Hatfield ARW and Russell RCG (1991) The treatment of symptomatic cholecystolithiasis under local anaesthesia using the percutaneous rotary lithotrite. *Gut.* **32**: A568.

Goco IR and Chambers LG (1983) 'Mini-cholecystectomy' and operative cholangiography. A means of cost containment. *Am. Surg.* **49**:143–145.

Gotz F, Pier A and Bacher C (1990) Modified laparoscopic appendectomy in surgery: a report on 388 operations. *Surg. Endosc.* **4**: 6–9.

Habib NA, Foo CF, Cox S, El-Masry R, Salem R, Todd V, Sung D and Benjamin IS (1990) Complications of cholecystectomy in district general hospitals. *Br. J. Clin. Pract.* **66**: 189–192.

Hill GL and Barker CJ (1978) Anterior highly selective vagotomy with posterior truncal vagoomy: A simple technique for denervating the parietal cell mass. *Br. J. Surg.* **65**: 702–705.

Huber DF, Martin EW and Cooperman M (1983) Cholecystectomy in elderly patients. *Am. J. Surg.* **146**: 719–721.

Katkhouda N and Mouiel J (1991) A new technique of surgical treatment of chronic duodenal ulcer without laparotomy by videocoelioscopy. *Am. J. Surg.* **161**: 361–364.

Katkhouda N (personal communication).

Kellett MJ, Wickham JEA and Russell RCG (1988) Percutaneous cholecystolithotomy. *Br. Med. J. Clin. Res.* **296**: 453–455.

Kelling G (1923) Zur coelioskopie. *Arch. Klin. Chir.* **126**: 226–229.

Leuschner U, Hellstern A and Schmidt K *et al.*, (1991) Gallstone dissolution with methyltertbutylether in 120 patients–efficacy and safety. *Dig. Dis. Sci.* **36**: 193–199.

Lichtenstein IL, Shulman AG, Amid PK and Montllor MM (1989) The tension-free hernioplasty. *Am. J. Surg.* **157**: 188–193.

Miller RE, Castelmain B, Lacqua FJ and Kotler DP (1989) Percutaneous endoscopic gastrostomy. Results in 316 patients and review of literature. *Surg. Endosc.* **3**: 186–190.

Mouiel J and Katkhouda N (1991) Laparoscopic truncal and selective vagotomy. In: Zucker KA (ed) *Surgical laparoscopy*. Quality Medical Publishing, St Louis, pp 263–279.

Mouret P, Francois Y and Vignal J *et al.*, (1990) Laparoscopic treatment of perforated peptic ulcer. *Br. J. Surg.* **77**: 1006.

Narbona-Arnau B, Olavarietta L and Lloris J *et al.*, (1980). Reflujo gastroesofagico hernia hiatal. Rehabilitacion quirurgica del musculo esofagico mediante pexia con el ligamento redondo. Resultados (1143 operados en 15 anos). *Bol. Soc. Val. Digest.* **1**: 21–28.

Nathanson LK, Easter DW and Cuschieri A (1990) Laparoscopic repair/peritoneal toilet of perforated duodenal ulcer. *Surg. Endosc.* **4**: 232–233.

Nathanson LK, Shimi S and Cuschieri A (1991) Laparoscopic ligamentum teres (round ligament) cardiopexy *Br. J. Surg.* **78**: 947–951.

Neugebauer E, Troidl H, Spangenberger W, Dietrich A, Lefering R and The Cholecystectomy Study Group (1991) Conventional versus laparoscopic cholecystectomy and the randomized controlled trial. *Br. J. Surg.* **78**: 150–154.

Nyhus LM, Pollak R, Bombeck TC and Donahue PE (1988) The preperitoneal approach and prosthetic buttress repair for recurrent hernia. *Ann. Surg.* **208**: 733–737.

Paterson-Brown S, Eckersley JRT, Sim AJW and Dudley HAF (1986) Laparoscopy as an adjunct to decision making in the acute abdomen. *Br. J. Surg.* **73**: 1022–1024.

Paterson-Brown S and Vipond MN (1990) Modern aids to clinical decision-making in the acute abdomen. *Br. J. Surg.* **77**: 13–18.

Perissat J, Collet D and Belliard R (1990) Gallstones: laparoscopic treatment – cholecystectomy, cholecystostomy and lithotripsy. *Surg. Endosc.* **4**: 1–5.

Petelin JB (1991) Laparoscopic approach to common duct pathology. *Surg. Lap. End.* **1**: 33–41.

Ponsky JL and Gauderer MWL (1989). Percutaneous endoscopic gastrostomy: indication, technique and results. *World J. Surg.* **13**: 165–170.

Popp LW (1990) Endoscopic patch repair of inguinal hernia in a female patient. *Surg. Endosc.* **4**: 10–12.

Popp LW (1991) Improvement in endoscopic hernioplasty: Transcutaneous aquadissection of the musculofascial defect and preperitoneal endoscopic patch repair. *J. Laparoendosc. Surg.* **1**: 83–90.

Raute M and Schaupp W (1988) Iatrogenic damage of the bile ducts caused by cholecystectomy. *Langenbeck's Arch. Chir.* 373: 345–354.

Reddick EJ and Olsen DO (1990) Out-patient laparoscopic laser cholecystectomy. *Am. J. Surg.* 160: 485–487.

Russell RCG and Shankar S (1987) The stabilized ring retractor: a technique for cholecystectomy. *Br. J. Surg.* 74: 826.

Schirmer BD, Edge SB, Dix J, Hyser MJ, Hanks JB and Jones RS (1991) Laparoscopic cholecystectomy. Treatment of choice for symptomatic cholelithiasis. *Ann. Surg.* 213: 665–676.

Schrieber J (1987) Early experience with laparoscopic appendectomy in women. *Surg. Endosc.* 1: 211–216.

Schultz LS, Graber JN, Pietrafitta JJ and Hickok DF (1990) Laser laparoscopic herniorrhaphy. *J. Laparoendosc. Surg.* 1: 41–45.

Semm K (1983) Endoscopic appendectomy. *Endoscopy.* 15: 59–64.

Shimi S, Nathanson LK and Cuschieri A (1991) Laparoscopic cardiomyotomy for achalasia. *J. R. Coll. Surg. Edin.* 36: 152–154.

Southern Surgeons Club (1991) A prospective analysis of 1518 laparoscopic cholecystectomies. *New Eng. J. Med.* 324: 1073–1078.

Steele RJC (1989) Endoscopic haemostasis for non-variceal upper gastrointestinal haemorrhage. *Br. J. Surg.* 76: 219–225.

Stoppa RE and Warlaumont CR (1989) The preperitoneal approach and prosthetic repair of groin hernia. In: Nyhus LM and Condon RE (eds) *Hernia.* JB Lippincott, Philadelphia, pp 199–225.

Sugarbaker PH, Bloom BS and Sanders JH *et al.*, (1975) Preoperative laparoscopy in diagnosis of acute abdominal pain. *The Lancet.* i: 442–445.

Taylor TV, Gunn AA and Macleod DAD (1982) Anterior lesser curve seromyotomy and posterior truncal vagotomy in the treatment of chronic duodenal ulcer. *The Lancet.* ii: 846–848.

Taylor TV, Lythgoe JP and McFarland JB *et al.*, (1990). Anterior lesser curve seromyotomy and posterior truncal vagotomy versus truncal vagotomy and pyloroplasty in the treatment of chronic duodenal ulcer disease. *Br. J. Surg.* 77: 1007–1009.

Thistle JL, May GR and Bender CE *et al.*, (1989). Dissolution of cholesterol gallbladder stones by methyltertbutyl ether administered by percutaneous transhepatic catheter. *New Eng. J. Med.* 320: 633–639.

Vitale GC, Collet D, Larson GN, Cheadle WG, Miller FB and Perissat J (1991) Interruption of professional and home activity after laparoscopic cholecystectomy among French and American patients. *Am. J. Surg.* 161: 396–398.

Winkler E, Kaplan O, Gutman M, Skornick Y and Rozin RR (1989) Role of cholecystectomy in the management of critically ill patients suffering from acute cholecystititis. *Br. J. Surg.* 76: 693–695.

Zakko SF and Hofmann AF (1990) Microprocessor-assisted solvent-transfer system for gallstone dissolution. In vitro and in vivo validation. *Gastroenterology.* 99: 1807–1813.

6

Orthopaedics

DAVID HUNT

The concept of minimal access in orthopaedic surgery is not entirely new. With the development of the cystoscope, it was realized that the same instrument could be used to look inside joints. Tagaki in Japan is credited with being the first to use a cystoscope to look inside a knee joint, in 1918. This was the beginning of arthroscopy. However, arthroscopy is not the only minimal access technique in orthopaedic surgery. The principle of minimal invasion, with the advantages of reduced morbidity and shorter hospital stay, has been followed in other areas of orthopaedics, particularly in spinal surgery and hand surgery. Although microsurgical techniques do not strictly qualify as minimal access, other areas of hand surgery, such as carpal tunnel release are proving amenable to endoscopic and thus minimal access techniques.

A history of arthroscopy

At the same time as Tagaki, Bircher in Switzerland was using an early laparoscope. He published the results of 20 'arthro-endoscopic' examinations of the knee in 1921. These early instruments were large – more than 7 mm in diameter. Finer instruments were soon developed specifically for arthroscopy. They were then tried in other joints. Burman *et al.*, in 1933 reported the use of a 4 mm arthroscope to examine the knee, ankle, shoulder and elbow. There was a lot of scepticism initially, critics referring to the arthroscope as a 'gonoscope' and suggesting it was impossible to get a good view inside a joint without opening it fully.

However, arthroscopy flourished, with attempts at surgical procedures being carried out almost as soon as it was possible to get a view. Geist in 1926 described synovial biopsy being performed.

Most of the development was carried out by Tagaki and his successor, Masaki Watanabe. In 1957, Watanabe published an atlas of arthroscopy, the first specialist monograph on the subject. Watanabe made two other major contributions. The first was his continued development of the arthroscope, culminating in the number 21, in 1960, which had a small tungsten bulb fixed at the tip giving an excellent view. This instrument was taken up by surgeons around the world, and was not improved upon for many years (*see* Figure 6.1).

Watanabe's second contribution was the first description of an arthroscopically performed meniscectomy, when he removed part of the posterior horn of the medial mensicus in 1962. This was seized upon by Dr Robert Jackson from Toronto, who described the removal of loose bodies and later the removal of a complete bucket handle tear of the medial meniscus in 1970.

There followed an explosion in the development of arthroscopic instrumentation and techniques which has continued unabated. In 1980, Dandy wrote that *'after such an explosion of enthusiasm there must follow a trough of disappointment and disillusion'*. It appears he was wrong. The

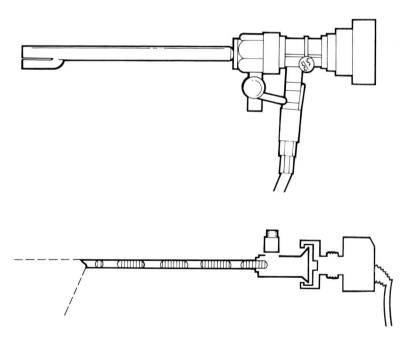

Figure 6.1: The Watanabe 21 arthroscope and a modern arthroscope with microchip camera attached.

complication rate has been gratifyingly low and the success rate high. More and more complex procedures are being undertaken in many joints. Arthroscopic surgery is very much a standard technique used by all orthopaedic surgeons.

Instruments and equipment

The development of the rod lens system and the fibre-optic light source meant that the size of the arthroscope could be reduced and the view obtained very much improved. The sterilizable micro-chip camera made arthroscopy into a sterile procedure, and facilitated instrument manipulation. Modern arthroscopes have a variety of lenses giving wide angles of vision, or offset ends to give a 180° field (*see* Figure 6.2).

The range of instruments available for arthroscopic procedures is now vast. They vary from simple hooks and knives, through special punches to power tools and laser probes. It is now not only possible to achieve a high level of diagnostic accuracy with the arthroscope, but also to undertake a great many operative procedures from simple removal of loose bodies to torn menisci and even ligament reconstruction.

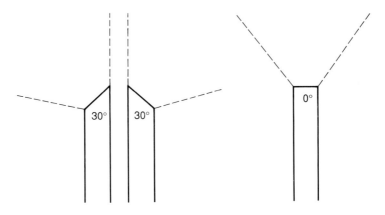

Figure 6.2: 30° offset field showing how 180° can be visualized.

Principles of arthroscopy

Arthroscopy is principally a diagnostic tool. It is important that training surgeons spend a lot of time looking inside a joint before attempting any procedures. Similarly, the importance of the history and examination of a joint cannot be over stressed. While arthroscopy is a useful tool, it is essentially only an investigation, and as such should only endorse or refute a clinical diagnosis.

The taking of an accurate history and careful clinical examination will indicate which part of a joint to examine and probe most carefully. For example, the history of locking and pain posterolaterally in the knee, will suggest careful inspection of the posterolateral gutter and milking the popliteus tendon, which can deliver the cartilaginous loose body, not visible on X-ray, into the joint. This may well have been missed on routine arthroscopy. With the advent of magnetic resonance imaging (MRI), the role of arthroscopy as a diagnostic technique is not so important. It should now be reserved for cases where a precise diagnosis can be made clinically and a definite procedure planned. If there is doubt, a MRI scan should be performed if it is available.

Arthroscopy of the knee

Not only is the knee the joint most likely to sustain an intra-articular injury, but it is also the joint which is most amenable to arthroscopic examination. It is with arthroscopic surgery of the knee, that minimal access techniques have had the most impact on orthopaedic surgery.

Pre-operative preparation

Arthroscopic surgery is better performed under general anaesthesia using a tourniquet. The relaxation obtained under general anaesthetic allows a full examination of the joint, which can give as much information as the arthroscopy, and is an essential part of the assessment of the knee. Local anaesthesia, either by local infiltration or by epidural anaesthetic, is possible and adequate for simple diagnostic arthroscopy or very short procedures such as synovial biopsy.

Examination under anaesthesia

With the patient asleep, and before the tourniquet is applied, the limb is examined. The range of movement is established. If the knee was locked, it is unlocked if possible, and the full range of flexion tested. The ligaments are tested individually. The collaterals are examined in extension and flexion. The posterior cruciate ligament is examined with the knee flexed to 90° by the posterior draw test. Finally, the anterior cruciate ligament is tested by Lachmann's test, which involves rocking the tibia in an anteroposterior direction on the fixed femur (*see* Figure 6.3).

This is a test which takes some practice to master; examining knees under anaesthetic is the best way to achieve this. Rotary instability, which accompanies anterior cruciate instability, can also be tested for by the 'pivot shift' or 'jerk' test, which relies on the fact that damage to the anterior cruciate ligament allows the tibia to internally rotate excessively on the femur. In extension, the tibia is forced into internal rotation. The knee is then gently flexed, at approximately 20° of flexion, the tibia relocates on the femur with a clunk or 'jerk', which will not be present if the anterior cruciate ligament is intact (*see* Figure 6.4).

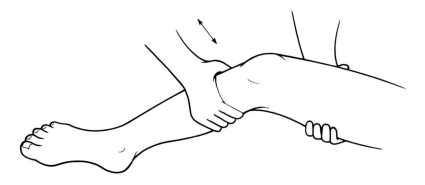

Figure 6.3: Lachmann's test for anterior cruciate ligament damage.

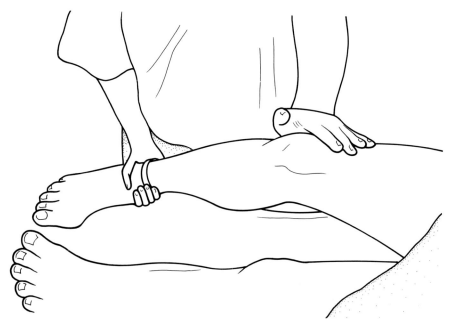

Figure 6.4: Examination of the knee for instability (the pivot shift test).

Procedure

After the examination under anaesthetic, the tourniquet is inflated. A leg holder which immobilizes the thigh and allows manipulation of the lower leg may be used. The leg is prepared and draped. Special disposable knee drapes, which have a rubber seal around the knee, are an asset as they allow manipulation of the leg without disturbing the drapes.

The arthroscope is inserted through a simple stab incision which can be made at a number of sites. The anterolateral portal is the usual choice (*see*

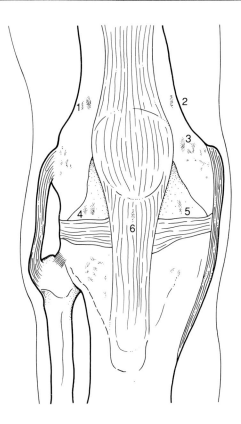

Figure 6.5: Entry portals in common use. Number 4 is the most common.

Figure 6.5). An irrigation cannula is inserted into the suprapatella pouch on the lateral side, to give a good through-flow of irrigation fluid. Normal saline is the irrigation fluid of choice. The light and camera are attached.

The knee is now inspected in a routine fashion. The anatomy of the normal knee must be well-known before arthroscopy is performed. The suprapatella pouch is inspected first, examining for loose bodies and evidence of abnormal synovial folds or inflammation. The under surface of the patella (see Figure 6.6) is inspected next, by rotating the telescope through 180° looking particularly for areas of damaged articular cartilage.

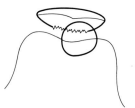

Figure 6.6: The undersurface of the patella.

The lateral gutter is visualized to look for loose bodies. The telescope is then returned to the suprapatella pouch and swept down the medial side to demonstrate the medial synovial shelf. This brings the telescope into the medial compartment. The knee is flexed and a valgus strain applied to open up the medial compartment and allow inspection of the medial meniscus (*see* Figure 6.7). A probe is now inserted through a medial portal and the meniscus probed, as it is inspected to visualize the under surface and to examine for tears.

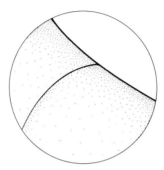

Figure 6.7: The normal medial meniscus.

The telescope passes into the intercondylar notch. By pressing medially on the patella tendon, and slightly extending the knee, the telescope can be advanced medial to the anterior cruciate ligament into the back of the knee, demonstrating the back of the medial meniscus. Next it is withdrawn and the contents of the intercondylar notch are examined. The normal anterior cruciate ligament appears as a smooth pale white column of tissue with a diaphenous film of synovial tissue covering it (*see* Figure 6.8). Any split in the film suggests damage to the underlying fibres, although the ligament itself may appear intact.

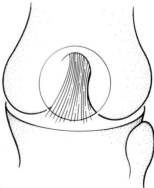

Figure 6.8: The normal anterior cruciate ligament.

It is not possible to visualize the posterior cruciate ligament well. However, by passing the telescope through to the back of the knee on the lateral side of the anterior ligament, and turning the telescope through 90° to look medially, part of the posterior cruciate ligament can be seen.

This leaves only the lateral compartment. The knee is flexed to 90°, and the foot placed on the operating table allowing the knee to drop out laterally, opening the lateral compartment. The whole of the lateral meniscus can be seen and probed (*see* Figure 6.9). At the back of the lateral compartment, the popliteus tendon is seen passing upwards and outwards.

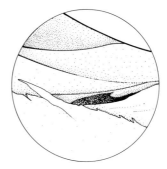

Figure 6.9: The normal lateral meniscus.

Principles of arthroscopic surgery

Arthroscopic procedures in any joint are based on the technique of triangulation. *See* Figure 6.10. This is the ability to bring the tips of the two instruments together in a closed space without visual contact. This is true of most endoscopic techniques. At first it seems difficult, but it is surprising how quickly surgical trainees master it. By getting into the habit of using a probe, it is a small step to manipulating an instrument under direct vision.

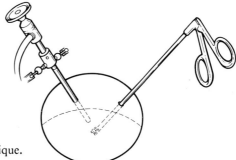

Figure 6.10: The triangulation technique.

Pathology of the knee and arthroscopic techniques

Loose bodies

One of the most straightforward arthroscopic surgical manoeuvres is removal of loose bodies. Loose bony or cartilaginous fragments may separate from the articular cartilage or from the menisci. They may be fragments of osteochondritis disseccans, the result of trauma or osteophytes associated with osteoarthritis. The loose body is identified, and a grasping forcep is introduced through a separate portal near the loose body.

The number of places where a portal can be sited is almost infinitessimal. It is a good guide to observe the light of the telescope through the skin, and indent the skin while observing through the telescope. A needle can be introduced to check, and then a small stab incision is made. It can be surprisingly difficult to get hold of even the smallest of loose bodies.

Articular cartilage defects

Loose bodies may arise from defects in articular cartilage. Pain is also commonly associated with defects in articular cartilage. This may be the softening of articular cartilage seen in adolescents, so-called chondromalacia of the patella or osteochondritis disseccans. It may result from a blow to the articular surface.

At arthroscopy, such an area should be trimmed down to subchondral bone and the floor smoothed with a power-driven burr. Better healing of such a defect has been shown to follow this treatment than trimming alone or drilling the base (Kim *et al.*, 1991). Attempts to fill large defects with material such as carbon fibre or transplanted meniscal tissue by arthroscopic techniques, is at present experimental, but looks promising for the future (Shahgaldi *et al.*, 1991).

Synovial plica

The medial synovial shelf in particular can become traumatized as it is stretched over the medial femoral condyle in flexion and extension of the knee. It then causes pain. It is a simple manoeuvre to remove a segment of it arthroscopically.

Menisci

Arthroscopy has demonstrated that the range of meniscal pathology is much greater than is generally appreciated. There is the well-known bucket handle tear, but there are also radial tears, horizontal cleavage tears, parrot beak tears, degenerate tears and the problems of the congenital discoid meniscus. All of these are amenable to arthroscopic treatment. It is unusual now to perform an arthrotomy to treat a meniscal lesion.

Bucket handle tear

Although more common in the medial meniscus, bucket handle tears can occur in either meniscus and the principles of removal are similar. The lesion is identified arthroscopically and the bucket handle fragment delivered into the intercondylar notch, by passing a hook under the fragment and pulling it forward.

Removal of the bucket handle fragment

The precise technique for removal of the bucket handle fragment is always a matter of personal preference. The following description is a standard technique and the author's preferred method (*see* Figure 6.11).

Through a medial portal, sited near the front end of the tear, a straight-bladed knife is introduced, and the anterior attachment of the fragment cut smoothly where it joins the rim of intact meniscus. The arthroscope is now removed and reintroduced through an anteromedial portal. Through the anterolateral portal, a pair of grasping forceps are now inserted. The anterior end of the cut fragment is seized and traction applied pulling the attached posterior horn forward into the intercondylar notch. A pair of arthroscopic scissors can now be introduced, again through the most medial portal, across the front of the femoral condyle to the back of the fragment, which is eased between the blades of the scissors. With traction still applied to the fragment through the grasping forceps, the blades of the scissors are closed, cutting the posterior end. The freed fragment is then delivered through the anterolateral portal. The rim of meniscus is inspected and trimmed as necessary.

With the lateral meniscus, access to the anterior part of the meniscus is more difficult. The same three portals are used. The medial portal described above gives surprisingly good access to the front. It is better to cut the anterior end of a bucket handle of this meniscus from the medial side and from the front, rather than a separate portal placed over the front end of the tear.

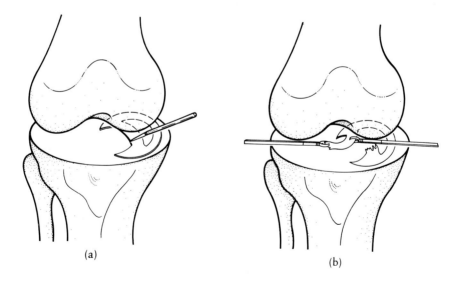

(a) (b)

Figure 6.11: Removing a bucket handle tear of the medial meniscus. (a) Division of the anterior end. (b) Division of the posterior end.

Radial tears, cleavage tears and parrot beak or flap tears

These tears are removed by trimming the torn part of the meniscus back to normal meniscal rim, using either a punch basket forcep or a powered meniscal shaver. For a fragmented degenerate tear of the posterior horn, usually of the medial meniscus, the fine probe of the pulsed laser beam can be very useful, allowing access to the area most difficult to reach, particularly in the early osteoarthritic knee. Treatment of the discoid meniscus when it is symptomatic, by arthroscopic techniques, is contentious. When the meniscus is stable, partial arthroscopic meniscectomy is effective. If the posterior horn of the meniscus is detached, arthroscopic treatment may not be possible, and the whole meniscus should be removed using an open technique.

Meniscal repair

When there is a detachment of the meniscus from the capsule at its outer edge, or there is a limited peripheral tear which cannot be dislocated into the intercondylar notch, it is possible to repair the meniscus rather than remove it. This can now be done arthroscopically (*see* Figure 6.12). The periphery of the meniscus is roughened to promote healing to the capsule. This is best done with a power tool.

An absorbable suture with a needle at both ends, is now introduced down a double lumen tube, in which the two lumens communicate allowing the tube to be withdrawn leaving the suture behind. The needles are passed through the meniscus and out through the capsule of the knee. A small skin incision is made at the exit point of the sutures. Great care must be taken, as the exit point is often well to the back of the knee. The ends of the sutures are tied, tethering the torn meniscus to the capsule.

Meniscal transplantation

The long-term results of open complete meniscectomy are well known. Complete meniscectomy results in significant osteoarthritic change in the knee in more than 80% of patients within 20 years. Hence the development of minimal access techniques. In young patients with complete absence of the meniscus, there is a place for allografting a meniscus. Early results of this are encouraging, but the technique is not established (Garrett, 1991).

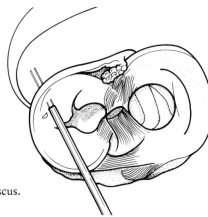

Figure 6.12: Repairing a meniscus.

Arthroscopic treatment of the osteoarthritic knee

Treatment of the early osteoarthritic knee by arthroscopic irrigation, removal of loose bodies and trimming of osteophytes and articular cartilaginous flaps has been shown consistently over the past decade to produce significant improvement in up to 80% of patients, and the benefit may last five years (Bert, 1989).

Arthroscopic ligament reconstruction

Over the past 20 years, there has been increased awareness of the importance of general fitness and sporting activity to health. Higher standards of sports, and an increase in professionalism, have meant that it is no longer acceptable to patients to give up sports when a significant ligament injury is sustained. The demand for rapid and effective rehabilitation has led to the development of minimal access techniques of ligament reconstruction, particularly the anterior cruciate ligament. Although it is now satisfactory to treat collateral ligament injuries conservatively, cruciate ligament injuries require surgical treatment when damaged sufficiently to cause instability.

Modern instrumentation has enabled cruciate ligament reconstruction to be performed arthroscopically. This reduces the morbidity associated with an open arthrotomy, protecting the vulnerable articular cartilage from dessication and subsequent damage.

There are many different techniques, but the most commonly performed technique for anterior cruciate ligament reconstruction uses autogenous patella tendon, taken as a free graft at the time of reconstruction, with a bone plug at either end from the lower pole of the patella and the upper tibia. This is threaded through a tunnel drilled in the upper tibia to come out in the knee at the site of insertion of the anterior cruciate ligament. It is inserted into a similar tunnel, made in the lateral femoral condyle at the normal insertion of the ligament. The graft is tensioned to prevent instability, and held with a wide-threaded interferential screw holding the bone blocks (see Figure 6.13a–d).

Arthroscopy of the shoulder

After the knee, the shoulder is the joint most commonly arthroscoped. An explosion is occurring in shoulder arthroscopy similar to the explosion over the past 10 years in knee arthroscopy. As a result, a far more accurate knowledge of the pathology of shoulder conditions has been acquired, with modification of the surgical procedures to treat the conditions, many of which are now being done utilizing the arthroscope and the principles of minimal access.

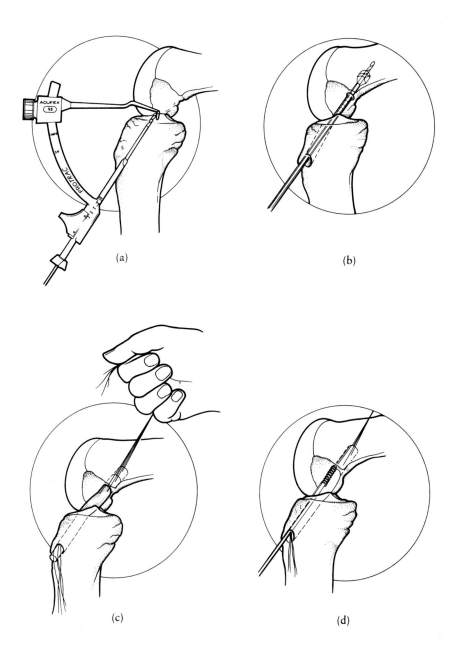

(a)

(b)

(c)

(d)

Figure 6.13: Anterior cruciate reconstruction using a bone-patellar tendon-bone graft inserted under arthroscopic control. (a) Siting the tibial drill hole. (b) Drilling the femoral tunnel. (c) Threading the graft through. (d) Placing the interferential screw in the femur.

Procedure

As in all joints, the procedure begins with examination under anaesthesia. For this reason, general anaesthesia is preferred. It is the only option in shoulder arthroscopy.

The shoulder is examined for a full range of movement and for instability in any direction. One of the major contributions of arthroscopy has been the realization that shoulder instability can be inferior, posterior or even multidirectional in addition to the more common anterior, and surgical treatment of the instability is directed towards repair in this particular area.

The examiner holds the patient's elbow in one hand and with the other, grasps the upper humerus just below the shoulder joint and attempts to displace the head of the humerus anteriorly, posteriorly and inferiorly. The affected shoulder is compared with the normal. It may be possible to dislocate the shoulder completely.

Arthroscopy

The patient is placed on the side with the affected shoulder uppermost (*see* Figure 6.14). The whole arm is prepared to allow easy manipulation. A

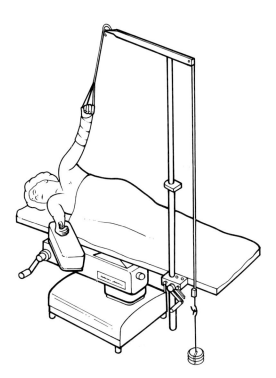

Figure 6.14: The set-up for shoulder arthroscopy.

stockinette can be used to cover the lower arm and suspended from a drip stand as an arm holder. The shoulder is distended with 40 ml of saline. The arthroscope is introduced through a posterior approach. A stab incision is made 2.5 cm below, and medial to the lip of the acromion, where a 'soft spot' can be palpated (*see* Figure 6.15).

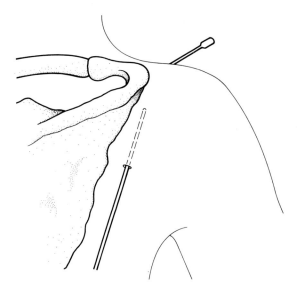

Figure 6.15: Posteriorly introducing the arthroscope in a right shoulder.

The arthroscope is introduced and passed over the humeral head. Under direct vision, where the light of the arthroscope can be seen anteriorly, just below the biceps tendon, an anterior stab incision is made for the introduction of instruments. An irrigation cannula can be introduced laterally below the tip of the acromion.

When the joint is entered, the humeral head is immediately identified, and once orientated, the glenoid cavity can be found. The labrum can then be visualized and probed, to demonstrate a detachment or 'Bankart lesion'. Passing over the top of the humeral head from the top of the glenoid, the biceps tendon is seen. Passing over this, and turning the arthroscope through 180°, the undersurface of the supraspinatus tendon and the rotator cuff can be identified and probed for defects. When a defect is present, the undersurface of the acromion will be seen. Finally, passing down the anterior capsule, the glenohumeral ligaments and the subscapularis tendons are seen (*see* Figures 6.16 and 6.17).

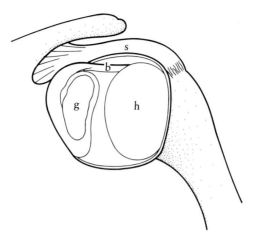

Figure 6.16: Normal appearances. S: supraspinatus tendon. B: biceps. G: glenoid. H: head of humerus.

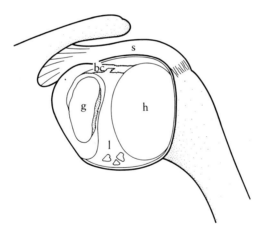

Figure 6.17: Pathological appearances. B: damaged biceps tendon. G: Bankart lesion. L: loose bodies in the infraglenoid.

Pathology and arthroscopic treatment

Frozen shoulder

Cases of frozen shoulder syndrome which do not respond to physiotherapy or even manipulation under anaesthesia, can respond to arthroscopic washout and breakdown of adhesions leading to a more rapid recovery.

Impingement syndrome and rotator cuff tears

It is in this condition, that arthroscopic techniques have had most benefit. A difficult condition to diagnose, classify and treat by conventional methods, the arthroscope has not only facilitated accurate diagnosis, but has enabled simple minimal access and effective treatment to be carried out.

The impingement syndrome is the most common cause of pain at the front of the shoulder (Neer, 1972). The rotator cuff comprises the tendons of subscapularis, supraspinatus and infraspinatus, stretching over the head of the humerus to their insertions on the greater tuberosity (*see* Figure 6.18). They pass through the narrow gap between the head of the humerus and the undersurface of the acromion. As the shoulder abducts, they impinge on the acromion, which can result in inflammation, swelling and eventually a tear in the cuff, with loss of the ability to abduct the arm.

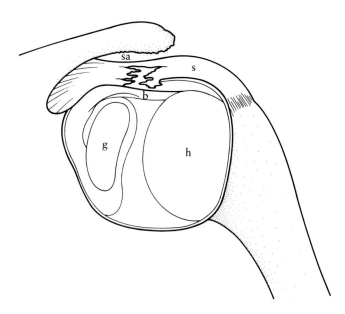

Figure 6.18: A partial rotator cuff tear in supraspinatus (s), providing communication with the subacromial space.

In the early stages, this condition responds to conservative treatment such as physiotherapy and anti-inflammatory agents. When chronic fibrosis is present, physiotherapy has limited use. When there is a complete tear, standard treatment is by open repair of the cuff, and this is still the treatment of choice in the younger athletic patient.

In the older patient, the results of repair are disappointing. An option which is proving more satisfactory is arthroscopic acromioplasty (Altcher *et al.*, 1990). Trimming and removal of damaged cuff with shaving of the undersurface of the acromion relieves the impingement, allowing free movement of the cuff. It is conventionally done by an open technique, by a deltoid splitting incision, with or without splitting the acromion. Interference with the deltoid mechanism causes significant disability and, if the muscle is not closed meticulously, recovery time is unacceptably long and the results disappointing. By achieving the same decompression arthroscopically, the postoperative morbidity is avoided, and the procedure is rapidly beneficial.

The shoulder is examined under general anaesthetic. It is essential to exclude any co-existing instability of the shoulder. If the rotator cuff damage is secondary to instability, the shoulder must be stabilized. Arthroscopic examination will also reveal any damage to the capsule or labrum suggesting instability.

The arthroscope is introduced posteriorly, and an anterior portal is made. Full inspection of the joint is carried out, with a probe inserted through the anterior portal. If there is a complete tear of the cuff, the subacromial space may be inspected. If not, the arthroscope is withdrawn from the posterior cannula, and a blunt trocar inserted. The cannula and trocar are withdrawn from the joint, and swept upwards and forwards to enter the subacromial space. The tip of the trocar can be palpated as this is being done. A cannula is similarly introduced through the anterior portal, into the space which can now be distended and inspected, by removing the trocar and replacing it with the telescope. The undersurface of the acromion is inspected from below and the rotator cuff from above.

It is important to establish a good inflow and outflow of irrigation fluid before removal of soft tissue and bone is started. The cannula in the anterior portal is used as an exit portal for fluid. A pressure pump is normally required.

Next a lateral portal is made 2 cm below the most lateral point of the acromion. This is used for the introduction of instruments. All damaged soft tissue is removed with punches and rongeurs. The undersurface of the acromion is shaved using a powered burr (see Figure 6.19). The complete anterior edge of the acromion is removed with the coraco-acromial ligament. From the anterior edge of the acromion, the bone is shaved to a depth of almost 1 cm, extending posteriorly and gradually sloping to provide a smooth, wedge-shaped undersurface, over a distance of approximately 2 cm. Posteriorly, the arm is supported in a sling and exercises start immediately. Approximately 90% of patients can expect to return to work within a week and the procedure is carried out as a day case.

Tears of the glenoid labrum

A torn labrum is readily identified arthroscopically. In the absence of instability, removal of the tear arthroscopically is straightforward and, when it is the cause of symptoms such as clicking and pain with use, as in throwers and swimmers, produces very satisfactory relief.

Shoulder instability

The precise cause of instability and the site of the defect can be accurately assessed arthroscopically. It is an important diagnostic tool. It is also technically possible to repair the instability by the percutaneous insertion

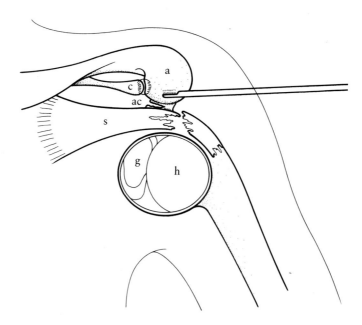

Figure 6.19: Subacromial decompression. Showing the undersurface of the acromion (a). The coraco-acromial ligament, partly divided (ac) and a power burr clearing the undersurface of the acromion.

of staples or screws under arthroscopic control. The results of this are as yet unpredictable, but it is another area of minimal access surgery which holds promise for the future.

Arthroscopy of other joints

Arthroscopy has now been applied to many other joints including the ankle, hip, wrist and elbow. In these joints, the main value of arthroscopy is diagnostic, but removal of loose bodies, small fragments of cartilage and debridement and washing out of osteoarthritic joints can all be done, and arthroscopy has a place in the treatment of these conditions.

Other orthopaedic applications of minimal access techniques

Although the principles of minimal access are being tested in other areas of orthopaedic surgery, for example endoscopic release of the carpal tunnel for compression of the median nerve, the other major area in which minimal access has led to reduced morbidity, length of hospital stay and rapid rehabilitation is in the field of spinal surgery.

Microdiscectomy and percutaneous discectomy

Microdiscectomy

Over the past 10 years this technique has been developed to remove the sequestrated disc in patients who have not had previous disc surgery. It is a technique which is at present confined to the lumbar spine. It avoids the need for a laminectomy or removal of bone from the posterior laminae, and avoids damaging the facet joints. The extradural soft tissues are preserved, but adequate disc removal is possible. Blood loss is minimal, the patient is mobilized early and the hospital stay is reduced by two-thirds. The majority of patients are back at work within six weeks compared with over two months by standard laminectomy. Criticisms of the technique are that location of the correct level can be difficult. An image intensifier is mandatory. Secondly, the procedure is of no use in spinal stenosis. Recently, multiple level microdiscectomies have been performed when multiple levels are affected.

Technique

The patient is positioned prone (*see* Figure 6.20). The correct level is identified, using a marker and screening the spine on a lateral view with an image intensifier. A small skin incision is made in the midline, between the spines of the vertebra adjacent to the prolapsed disc (approximately 1 inch long). The interspinous ligament is incised in the midline, and the paravertebral muscles mobilized sub-periosteally from the spine and the lamina. A finger is used to identify the interlaminar space and the microlumbar retractor is inserted down to the ligamentum flavum. An operating microscope with a 400 mm lens is brought in, and under magnification the ligamentum flavum is excised, using a fine blade followed by Kerrison rongeurs. Using a fine nerve hook, the dura is mobilized and the nerve root identified. The nerve root is retracted and the sequestrated disc is exposed. It is removed using microdisc forceps. Only exposed disc material is removed. Limited removal of residual disc material is possible, but complete discectomy is not necessary. The wound is closed by a conventional technique. The patient is mobilized on the first postoperataive day and usually discharged by the third day.

Percutaneous discectomy

For the patient with a prolapsing disc instead of a full sequestrated disc, the options for treatment have been chymopapain injection to produce lysis of the disc, or microdiscectomy. Chymopapain injection has largely fallen into disrepute, because of the incidence of anaphylactic reaction to it. As an alternative, and as a less invasive procedure than microdiscectomy, percutaneous discectomy has been developed. It is technically difficult, but the results are encouraging (Schaffer and Parviz Kambin, 1991).

Technique

It is performed under local anaesthetic. An image intensifier is used to identify the correct level, and a trocar is introduced 9 cm from the midline on the

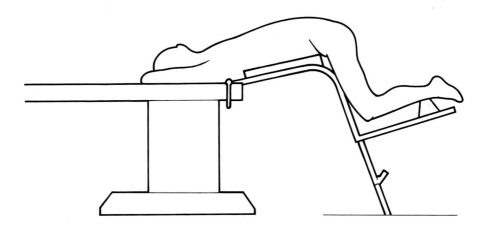

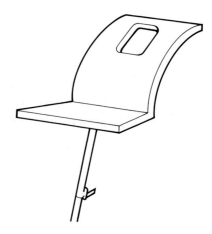

Figure 6.20: Microdiscectomy positioning.

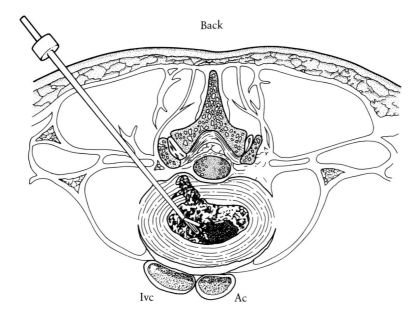

Back

Ivc   Ac

Figure 6.21: Percutaneous discectomy technique.

affected side, and advanced under image intensifier control to the disc space, checking that the patient feels no root pain. The trocar stops at the annulus fibrosus, and a 4.9 mm cannula is inserted over the trocar, which is withdrawn. A cutting instrument is inserted, and a window cut in the annulus. The disc material is then removed using suction punches. Recently, aspiration probes and laser probes have been developed to remove the disc (*see* Figure 6.21).

Summary

Minimal access techniques in orthopaedic surgery have developed extensively over the past decade. There is little doubt that the surface has only been scratched. The potential for ever more sophisticated procedures to be undertaken endoscopically or percutaneously is large, particularly in the fields of treatment of intra-articular fractures, ligament reconstruction and surface replacement of damaged articular cartilage, either traumatic or arthritic.

References

Altcher DW *et al.*, (1990) Arthroscopic acromioplasty. *J. Bone and Jt. Surg.* **72A:** 1198–1207.

Bert JM and Mashra K (1989) The arthroscopic treatment of unicompartmental gonarthrosis. *Arthroscopy.* **5**: 25–32.

Bircher E (1921) Die Arthroendoskopie. *Zentralbl. Chir.* **48**: 1460–1461.

Burman MS, Finkelstein H and Mayer L (1934) Arthroscopy of the knee joint. *J. Bone and Jt. Surg.* **16**: 255–268.

Bunker TD and Wallace WA (1991) *Shoulder arthroscopy.* Martin Dunitz, London.

Dandy DJ (1978) Early results of closed partial meniscectomy. *Br. Med. J.* **1**: 1099–1100.

Dandy DJ (1981) *Arthroscopic surgery in the knee.* Churchill Livingstone, London.

Elsmont FJ and Currier B (1989) Surgical management of lumbar intevertebral disc disease. *J. Bone and Jt. Surg.* **71A**: 1266–1271.

Garrett JC and Stevenson RN (1991) Meniscal transplantation in the human knee. *Arthroscopy.* **7**: 57–62.

Geist ES (1926) Arthroscopy: preliminary report. *The Lancet.* **46**: 306–307.

Jackson RW and Abe J (1972) The role of arthroscopy in the management of disorders of the knee. *J. Bone and Jt. Surg.* **54B**: 310–322.

Kim HKW, Moran ME and Salter RB (1991) The potential for regeneration of articular cartilage in defects created by chondral shaving and sub chondral abrasion. *J. Bone and Jt. Surg.* **73A**: 1301–1315.

Neer CS (1972) Anterior acromioplasty for the chronic impingement syndrome in the shoulder. *J. Bone and Jt. Surg.* **54A**: 41–50.

Schaffer JL and Kambin P (1991) Percutaneous posterolateral lumbar discectomy versus decompression with a 6.9 mm cannula. *J. Bone and Jt. Surg.* **73A**: 822–831.

Shahgaldi BF *et al.,* (1991) Repair of cartilage lesions using biological implants. *J. Bone and Jt. Surg.* **73B**: 57–64.

Tagaki K (1933) Practical experience using Tagaki's arthroscope. *J. Jap. Orthopaed. Assoc.* **8**: 132.

Watanabe M, Takeda S and Ikenchs H (1957) *Atlas of arthroscopy.* Igaku Shoin Ltd, Tokyo.

7

Colorectal Surgery

MICHAEL HERSHMAN

Introduction

Minimal access colorectal surgery may be endoluminal or laparoscopic. Endoluminal approaches include colonoscopy and transanal endoscopic microsurgery. Colonoscopy has progressed over the past 15 years, from a technique performed by a few pioneers, to one of the most widely used diagnostic and therapeutic tools of both gastroenterologists and surgeons. Transanal endoscopic microsurgery is a technique for local excision of benign sessile neoplasms and small carcinomas of the upper rectum, which would previously have required open surgery. Although originally described in 1984, it has only recently achieved popularity.

The introduction of therapeutic laparoscopy into general surgery in the last five years has dramatically changed the management of common intra-abdominal conditions. Preliminary applications of laparoscopy to colorectal surgery are currently emerging. The mobility of the colon, its ample mesentery, and long pedicle blood supply make it eminently suitable for laparoscopic surgery. This, together with the high incidence of colonic disorders, will almost certainly lead to widespread application of these techniques.

Colonoscopy

Colonoscopy is often an alternative to barium enema for examining the colon. Most physicians prefer colonoscopy, because direct visualization does not depend on a radiologist's interpretative skills, and therapeutic intervention is possible. However, colonoscopy is a highly skilled procedure, and there is a steep learning curve for the first 100 examinations (Parry and Williams, 1991). A skilled colonoscopist should be able to examine the left colon fully in almost every patient, and to reach the caecum in over 90% of cases (Williams, 1987).

Indications

The indications for colonoscopy are outlined in Table 7.1. Strictures and carcinomas are easily recognized and biopsied. Polyps are very common, particularly small 2–3 mm sessile metaplastic ones. Polyps greater than 1 cm in diameter are more likely to be malignant, and should always be excised or biopsied.

Diagnostic	Therapeutic
Tumours (benign or malignant) • follow up • screening Inflammatory bowel disease • assess extent and nature • follow-up • surveillance Stricture on barium enema Bleeding source Ischaemic colitis Pseudomembranous colitis Terminal ileum visualization	Tumour • polypectomy • fulguration • intubate obstruction Decompress • pseudo-obstruction • volvulus Dilate strictures Arrest bleeding Remove foreign bodies

Table 7.1: Indications for colonoscopy.

The extent and severity of inflammatory bowel disease is well assessed by colonoscopy. In ulcerative colitis, there is uniform rectal mucosal inflammation which spreads proximally continuously. There may be frank bleeding, but the ulcers are usually too small to identify. In Crohn's disease, similar inflammation is seen, but with discrete ulcers and relatively normal mucosal areas between inflammatory patches.

Colonoscopy for diverticular disease may be very difficult, because the colon is tortuous with prominent vascular folds. In addition, diverticula may be large enough to simulate the bowel lumen. Angiodysplasia is recognized as small leashes of vessels with venous lakes.

Contraindications to colonoscopy include severe pain during the examination, severe acute inflammatory bowel disease, toxic megacolon and acute diverticular disease (Galandiuk, 1992).

Technique

Bowel preparation is crucial, and the aim is to produce fluid diarrhoea at the time of colonoscopy. Many techniques of bowel preparation are described, but two sachets of Picolax (magnesium oxide, citric acid and sodium picosulphate) given during the 24 hours prior to colonoscopy are as effective as any. Local enemas may be used for severe constipation, or in an emergency for colonic bleeding. Patients with inflammatory bowel disease may require no preparation.

The patient is placed in the left lateral position with knees drawn up and buttocks on the edge of the bed. An intravenous analgesic and sedative is then administered, with dose reduction in patients who are elderly or have respiratory problems. The colonoscope is introduced after rectal examination. Several lengths are available, but the 140 cm and 180 cm scopes which have a single biopsy and suction channel are most useful. Shorter instruments of 60 or 100 cm are more manoeuvreable, and may be used to inspect the left colon.

The colonoscope is advanced by following the bowel lumen, using a combination of the directional controls, withdrawal and torsion. If the lumen is not seen, gentle insufflation is performed. The sigmoid colon is tortuous and often difficult to traverse, particularly when sigmoid loops or diverticular disease are present. The sigmoid can usually be straightened out after the descending colon has been reached. This is done by gently withdrawing the scope, making the sigmoid concertina over it, and can be confirmed by using an image intensifier (Cotton and Williams, 1991). The descending colon is usually straight and traversed with ease. The splenic flexure is variable, but the purplish appearance of the spleen is a useful landmark. The transverse colon is recognized by its triangular shape, and the ascending colon is short and usually easily passed. The caecum has a cul-de-sac appearance often with prominent folds. It is often possible to enter the terminal ileum (Cotton and Williams, 1991). The colonoscope is withdrawn gently, the colonic mucosa is inspected and any necessary intervention performed.

Polypectomy is the most common intervention performed. Small polyps are removed by hot biopsy. The technique is to grasp the polyp apex with insulated forceps and create a pseudopedicle. A blended diathermy current is then applied for 2–3 seconds, causing whitening of the visible part of the polyp but not the bowel wall. This enables complete excision and enough tissue for histology. When large polyps are present, the colonoscopist must decide whether they should be removed surgically or if snare removal can be performed safely. It should be appreciated that the smaller the area of tissue between the polypectomy snare (or hot biopsy forceps), the greater the tissue heating. Thus, if the snare is too loose, there may be insufficient tissue heating for adequate cutting. Conversely, if it is too tight, the stalk may be severed, with minimal haemostasis (Cotton and Williams, 1991).

When difficult midsigmoid polyps are present, it may be possible to snare the polyp and intussuscept it into the rectum for surgical removal. Another possibility is stalk injection with adrenaline (or sclerosant/adrenaline mixtures). This should not be performed if the stalk is less than 1cm, because of the risk of bowel wall necrosis.

Other therapeutic colonoscopic techniques include colonoscopic balloon dilatation of malignant obstruction and colonoscopic Nd:YAG laser palliation (Table 7.1) (Galandiuk, 1992). Intraoperative colonoscopy can identify the source of lower gastrointestinal bleeding or localize tumours for laparoscopic excision.

An intriguing new technique is fistuloscopy, in which an endoscope is

inserted into a fistula (Nakagawa *et al.*, 1990). Fistuloscopy has been performed for colocutaneous and other gastrointestinal fistulae, and the authors
claim that irrigation can be performed, infectious sources removed, histology
obtained and some fistulae closed with fibrin glue (Nakagawa *et al.*, 1990).

Complications

Colonoscopy is a safe procedure, with no mortality in over 4500 procedures
(Reiertson *et al.*, 1987). The complication rate is 0.14% for diagnostic
colonoscopy and 2% for therapeutic colonoscopy. Major complications
include perforation and bleeding. Large perforations require laparotomy,
but small perforations without local peritonism may be treated conservatively
(Hall *et al.*, 1991). The incidence of bleeding after polypectomy is 0.72–2.5%
and it may occur up to two weeks after the procedure (Webb, 1991). Bleeding
may require resnaring, diathermy or surgery. A transmural burn may also
occur during polypectomy and causes localized peritoneal signs.
    Complications can be prevented by rigorous bowel preparation, avoiding
mannitol which can cause an explosive large bowel gas mixture, meticulous
diathermy technique, as well as recognition and acceptance of personal
limitations.

Laparoscopic colonic surgery

The colon is easily visualized at laparoscopy except for the splenic flexure, which is often obscured by bowel and omentum. Laparoscopy for
colorectal disorders may be diagnostic or therapeutic. Indications for diagnostic laparoscopy include both acute and chronic abdominal pain. It is
particularly helpful in a young female patient with right iliac fossa pain,
in determining whether the aetiology is gynaecological or gastrointestinal.
In penetrating abdominal trauma, a peritoneal breach can be demonstrated
by indenting the puncture site. If traumatic injury has occurred, the feasibilty
of laparoscopic repair can be assessed.
    In oncology, diagnostic laparoscopy can assess the nature and extent of
the disease and the efficacy of treatment. In addition, biopsies of liver or
abdominal masses may be taken. Other indications for diagnostic laparoscopy
include assessment of abdominal masses, PUO, and intra-abdominal abscesses
which can be drained. Laparoscopy may be useful in conjunction with other
intraoperative investigations, such as colonoscopy and angiography, for
identifying obscure bleeding sites or localizing small tumours for laparoscopic
excision.
    The introduction of therapeutic laparoscopy has dramatically changed the
management of many common intra-abdominal disorders. The advantages
of laparoscopic over conventional surgery include reduced hospitalization
and recovery times, reduction of complications, and consequently quicker
return to normal functional activity. For laparoscopic colonic surgery to be
successful, it must have the above advantages and also prove to be as safe
and effective as open surgery. In particular, sound anastomoses without

faecal contamination must be fashioned and where indicated, *adequate* cancer clearance operations must be performed.

The following is an outline of colorectal procedures currently being performed or assessed.

Adhesiolysis

Laparoscopic adhesiolysis has been performed electively and for emergency intestinal obstruction. Adhesions should be divided close to the peritoneum, as the diathermy current usually runs to the narrowest part of the adhesive band (Sackier, 1992).

Appendicectomy

Laparoscopy is very valuable for patients with right iliac fossa pain, especially young females. Appendicectomy should be performed if there is acute appendicitis, visible faecoliths, a normal appendix with no other pathology, or recurrent right iliac fossa pain.

The technique involves placing additional ports in the right iliac fossa (10 mm) and in the left iliac fossa (5 mm). The appendix is mobilized and drawn into the right iliac fossa port with a grasper. The mesoappendix is divided by diathermy, laparoscopic stapler or between ties or clips. The appendix base is then stapled or doubly ligated usually with endoloops. It is then removed through the right iliac fossa port (Semm, 1983).

Caecal procedures

Laparoscopically guided caecostomy has been performed for poor risk patients with intestinal obstruction or with pseudo-obstruction (Ponsky *et al.*, 1986). Caecopexy for poor risk patients with caecal volvulus has also been performed.

Right hemicolectomy

Several different techniques have been described (Schlinkert, 1991; Cooperman and Zucker, 1991; Jacobs *et al.*, 1991). Generally, the patient is placed supine with legs in stirrups. The surgeon and camera operator stand on the patient's left and the first assistant is positioned between the patient's legs (Cooperman and Zucker, 1991). The scrub nurse usually stands on the patient's left, although some prefer the right (Jacobs *et al.*, 1991).

The abdomen is insufflated with carbon dioxide and a 10–11 mm port and cannula are inserted at the umbilicus. A full laparoscopy is performed, to assess the presence of metastases. Three other ports are usually placed as shown (Figure 7.1). Some prefer the right iliac fossa port to be placed in the right hypochondrium (Jacobs *et al.*, 1991). They are all 10–11 mm cannulae so that endobabcocks and staplers can be passed and the video camera moved. Recently, 5 mm bowel graspers have become available, which allow some cannulae to be reduced to 5 mm (Jacobs *et al.*, 1991). An additional 5 mm port in the epigastric region is sometimes helpful.

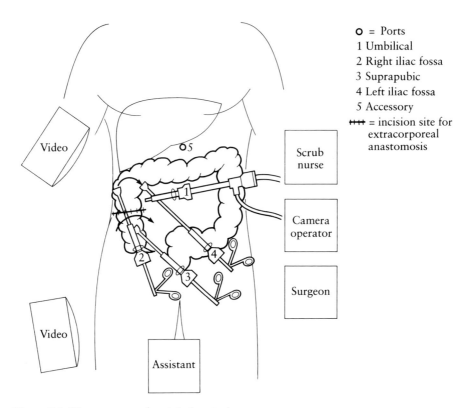

o = Ports
1 Umbilical
2 Right iliac fossa
3 Suprapubic
4 Left iliac fossa
5 Accessory
+++ = incision site for
    extracorporeal
    anastomosis

Figure 7.1: Theatre set-up for right hemicolectomy.

The caecum and ascending colon are grasped and rotated towards the midline. The avascular plane lateral to the ascending colon is incised using laser or diathermy, and the hepatic flexure mobilized. The mesentery is divided between clips or using a stapler. If the bowel is to be anastomosed extracorporeally, a small abdominal incision is made over the lesion. When a right hypochondrial port is used, the incision can incorporate it. The bowel ends are exteriorized, resected and anastomosed. Alternatively, a 30 or 40 mm port and sheath may be used and this has the advantage of maintaining pneumoperitoneum. An extracorporeally hand-sewn or stapled anastomosis is performed, the bowel replaced and the incision closed.

Intracorporeal anastomoses have been performed by dividing the bowel and either hand sewing, stapling or a combination of the two. The initial results are encouraging. One author reports a hospital stay of 3–5 days and a mean operating time of 155 minutes (Jacobs *et al.*, 1991).

Left hemicolectomy

The theatre set-up for the left hemicolectomy is the mirror image of that for right hemicolectomy, except that a Trendelenberg position with lateral tilt is adopted to position the small bowel. Similarly, several techniques and port sites are described (Cooperman and Zucker, 1991; Jacobs *et al.*, 1991; Fowler and White, 1991). The usual positions are as shown in Figure 7.2. The left iliac fossa port is placed on a proposed line of a grid iron incision if an extracorporeal anastomosis is to be performed.

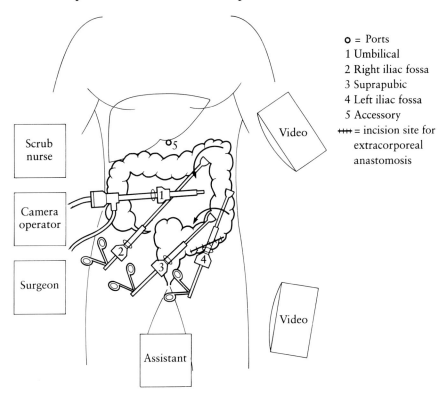

Figure 7.2: Theatre set-up for left hemicolectomy.

The left colon is rotated towards the right, and mobilized along its avascular plane. The splenic flexure is generally more difficult to mobilize than the hepatic flexure. The mesentery is divided with a stapler or clips. When an intracorporeal anastomosis is performed, the colon can be removed transanally, or via a small abdominal incision. An end to end stapling device is passed through the anus and the anastomosis performed (Figure 7.3) (Fowler and White, 1991). The anvil is placed in the abdomen if the rectal stump has been closed, and is attached to the endoanal stapler when the rectum has been divided and left open. Purse string sutures are either hand-sewn or secured with pretied Roeder knots.

In a recent study (Jacobs *et al.*, 1991), laparoscopic left hemicolectomy was performed for adenomas, carcinomas, diverticulitis and an endometrioma, with a hospital stay of 3–8 days, and a mean operating time of 170 minutes.

Rectal procedures

Laparoscopic anterior resection may be made easier by slinging the sigmoid colon to the anterior abdominal wall in order to aid posterior rectal dissection (Buess, personal communication). In females, the uterus position can be manipulated transvaginally as an aid to anterior rectal dissection. Recently, laparoscopic-assisted abdominoperineal excision of the rectum has been performed laparoscopically, and the colon removed via the perineal incision.

Laparoscopic rectopexy has been performed by mobilizing the posterior rectal wall from the sacrum, and suturing in a synthetic mesh.

Loop colostomy

This operation is performed for patients with irresectable distal colonic carcinoma, irradiated anal carcinoma or for patients who have undergone complicated fistulae or incontinence operations. Clearly an abdominal incision is best avoided in these cases. The operation is performed by inserting two additional trocars in the upper and lower abdomen. The sigmoid colon is mobilized and a sling passed through a mesenteric window (Lange *et al.*, 1991). The colostomy site is fashioned and the bowel brought to the surface, via the lower abdominal trocar. It is matured after the completion of the laparoscopy.

Complications

Laparoscopy is a safe procedure, and a study by the Royal College of Obstetricians and Gynaecologists reported a mortality of 8 in 100 000 with a complication rate of 3% (Chamberlain and Carron Brown, 1978). This study was based on laparoscopy in fit young women. These rates will undoubtedly become higher with more laparoscopists, newer techniques and older and sicker patients.

In addition to the general complications of laparoscopy and pneumoperitoneum, a particular complication of colorectal surgery is bowel perforation, usually due to a trocar. Perforation usually occurs when distended bowel or adhesions are present. Preoperatively localizing adhesions by ultrasonic mapping, using spontaneous and evoked visceral slide, may help avoid this injury (Sigel *et al.*, 1991). It is sometimes possible to repair a full thickness bowel injury by laparoscopic suturing (Reich *et al.*, 1991). Another technique is to convert the injury into a colostomy using a balloon catheter (Birns, 1989). Subsequent radiological studies to exclude further peritoneal leakage can then be performed.

The future

Laparoscopic colonic surgery is still in its infancy. Only time will tell whether laparoscopic colonic surgery can be as safe as open surgery, and whether adequate cancer clearance operations can be performed. Encouragingly, preliminary studies have shown that the extent of bowel and lymph node resection at laparoscopic colectomy was similar to that normally obtained by open surgery (Jacobs *et al.*, 1991).

Advances will come with improved instrument design. Although instrument designers have rapidly produced laparoscopic staplers, retractors, graspers and clamps, many techniques, for example suturing, remain time-consuming and frustrating. Continued and improved instrument design is urgently needed. New techniques for creating purse strings, vessel ligation, and anastomoses including fibrinogen glue and laser welding, are currently being developed. Further improvements will come with better optics; a three-dimensional optic system is already being developed (Buess, personal communication).

Transanal endoscopic microsurgery

Local excision is the treatment of choice for rectal adenomas and selected rectal carcinomas. Transanal resection avoids the mortality and morbidity of conventional abdominal surgery. This is especially important in the elderly and those at high operative risk. Transanal excision of lesions in the lower rectum has been performed for many years using standard abdominal instruments via a proctoscope. However, transanal excision of upper rectal lesions has proved impossible, due to lack of instruments for operating and providing exposure above 8 cm. Previously, these lesions have been removed by either the abdominal approach (low anterior resection), presacral approach (Kraske, 1885) or by incising and splitting the anal sphincter (York Mason, 1970).

The transanal endoscopic microsurgery system was reported by Professor Gerhard Buess in 1984 (Buess *et al.*, 1984). It provides an alternative for removing lesions in the upper rectum.

Instruments

The key instrument is an operating proctoscope which is 20 cm long and 4 cm in diameter. It is introduced into the rectum using an obturator, and a glass window plate is applied at the viewing end. The proctoscope is then positioned and fixed using an adjustable clamp (Martin arm). The glass window plate is replaced by a face plate, through which the operating binocular scope is passed. The scope enables close-up three-dimensional vision with six times magnification. The face plate also has four airtight ports through which instruments are inserted (Figure 7.3). The instruments used are long and include a needle holder, electric knife, scissors, forceps, sucker and a special clip applicator, which attaches a silver clip to the suture in place of a knot.

An 'endosurgical unit' is connected to the proctoscope. This provides a constant rectal pressure state (15 mmHg) by continuous infusion of CO_2, which may flow at up to 6 litres/minute. The sucker is designed to suck at

1 Operating proctoscope   2 Stereo telescope   3 Assistant's optics
4 Needle holder   5 Grasping forceps   6 Suction
7 Adjustable clamp (Martin arm)

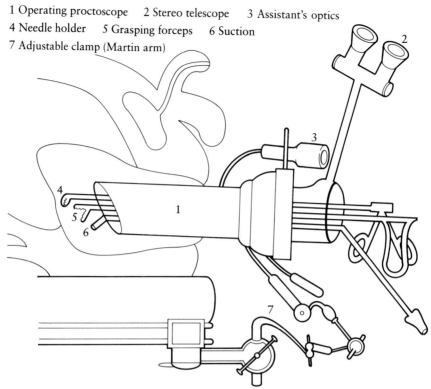

Figure 7.3: Operating proctoscope and optics.

less than 15 mmHg, so that the rectal wall does not collapse when suction is performed. The endosurgical unit also has a pump for irrigation.

Technique

Patients must undergo full bowel preparation and consent for possible laparotomy. General anaesthesia is usually performed, although occasionally regional anaesthesia is used. The patient is positioned on the operating table so that the tumour is below the end of the proctoscope. Thus, the patient may require a prone, lithotomy or lateral position and the operating table is adjusted accordingly. The Martin arm is fixed and CO_2 insufflation is commenced (Figure 7.4).

The operation begins by marking out the resection margins using the high frequency electric knife. They should include at least a 1 cm normal tissue cuff. A submucosal excision is performed if the tumour is benign, and a full thickness excision if it is suspicious or frankly malignant (Buess et al., 1988). The surgeon must utilize predominantly fingers and wrists as the instruments are used in parallel (Kipfmuller et al., 1988). Haemostasis is carefully maintained as dissection continues. Both the forceps and suction can be connected to the diathermy. It is necessary to readjust the proctoscope position more frequently by releasing the Martin arm.

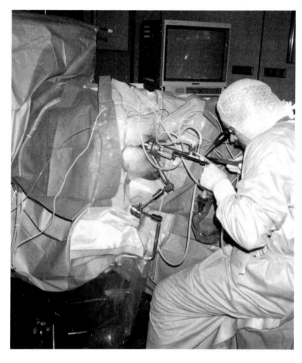

Figure 7.4: Transanal endoscopic microsurgery.

The wound is closed with a 6 cm length of monofilament suture, with a silver clip attached to one end. The suture is tightened and a further silver clip applied to the other end. Several sutures may be required to close a large wound. The resected specimen is pinned flat prior to histological examination.

Indications and results

Using this technique, benign lesions that are confined to the mucosa may be excised by submucosal dissection, whereas superficial cancers are excised by full thickness excision. Only cancers that are small, mobile, well or moderately differentiated and confined to the mucosa or submucosa should be selected. Tumours that invade the muscularis propria should undergo more radical surgery. On table ultrasound may be useful to confirm the clinical impression of degree of spread. If the tumour has been removed locally, and is subsequently found to have lymphatic invasion, or penetration of the muscularis propria, then a more radical surgical procedure should be performed.

Buess *et al.*, have now operated on more than 300 patients. The mortality is 0.5% and the complication rate is 9%. 51 patients had stage T1 carcinoma and only one developed a local recurrence. Transient incontinence occurred in 10% of patients but was permanent in only one patient. The mean site of lesions excised was 17 cm from the anal margin and their mean hospital stay was eight days (Buess *et al.*, 1988; Buess *et al.*, 1991; Buess *et al.*, 1992). A series of 27 patients from another centre reports a mean operating time of 130 minutes and a mean hospital stay of one day (Smith, 1992).

Future developments include transanal endoscopic rectopexy and combined laparoscopic and transanal endoscopic colonic excision; these are currently being assessed (Buess, personal communication).

References

Birns MT (1989) Inadvertent instrumental perforation of the colon during laparoscopy: non surgical repair. *Gastrointest. Endosc.* 35: 54–56.

Buess G *et al.*, (1984) Endoscopic operative procedure for the removal of rectal polyps. *Coloproc.* 6: 254 –260.

Buess G *et al.*, (1988) Technique of transanal endoscopic microsurgery. *Surg. Endosc.* 2: 71–75.

Buess G *et al.*, (1988) Clinical results of transanal endoscopic microsurgery. *Surg. Endosc.* 2: 245–250.

Buess G *et al.*, (1991) Minimal invasive surgery in the local treatment of rectal cancer. *Int. J. Colorect. Dis.* 6: 77–81.

Buess G *et al.*, (1992) Technique and results of transanal endoscopic microsurgery in early rectal cancer. *Am. J. Surg.* 163: 63–70.

Buess G (Personal communication).

Chamberlain GVP and Carron Brown JA (1978) *Report of the working party of the confidential inquiry into gynaecological laparoscopy.* Royal College of Obstetricians and Gynaecologists, London.

Cooperman AM and Zucker KA (1991) Laparoscopic guided intestinal surgery. In: *Surgical laparoscopy* Ed. Zucker KA *et al.*, Quality Medical Publishing Inc, St. Louis.

Cotton PB and Williams CB (1991) *Practical gastrointestinal endoscopy* 3rd ed. Blackwell Scientific Publications, Oxford.

Fowler DL and White SA (1991) Laparoscopy-assisted sigmoid resection. *Surg. Laparosc. Endosc.* 3: 183–188.

Galandiuk S (1992) Colonoscopy to the cecum. *Seminars in Colon and Rectal Surgery.* 3: 18–23.

Hall C *et al.*, (1991) Colon perforation during colonoscopy: surgical versus conservative management. *Br. J. Surg.* 78: 542–544.

Jacobs M *et al.*, (1991) Minimally invasive colon resection (laparoscopy colectomy). *Surg. Laparosc. Endosc.* 3: 144–150.

Kipfmuller K *et al.*, (1988) Training program for transanal endoscopic microsurgery. *Surg. Endosc.* **2**: 24–27.

Kraske P (1885) Zur exstirpation hochsitzender mastdarmkrebse. *Verh. Dtsch. Ges. Chir.* **14**: 464–474.

Lange V *et al.*, (1991) Laparoscopic creation of a loop colostomy. *J. Laparosc. Surg.* **5**: 307–312.

Mason AY (1970) Surgical access to the rectum – a trans-sphincteric exposure. *Proc. Roy. Soc. Med.* **63**: 91–94.

Nakagawa K *et al.*, (1990) Endoscopic examination for fistula. *Endosc.* **22**: 208–210.

Parry BR and Williams SM (1991) Competency and the colonoscopist: a learning curve. *Aust. N. Z. J. Surg.* **61**: 419–422.

Ponsky JL *et al.*, (1986) Percutaneous endoscopic cecostomy: a new approach to a nonobstructive colonic dilatation. *Gastrointest. Endosc.* **32**: 108–111.

Reich H *et al.*, (1991) Laparoscopic repair of full-thickness bowel injury. *J. Laparoendosc. Surg.* **2**: 119–121.

Reiertsen O *et al.*, (1987) Complications of fiberoptic gastrointestinal endoscopy – Five years' experience in a central hospital. *Endosc.* **19**: 1–6.

Sackier JM (1992) Laparoscopy. Applications to colorectal surgery. *Seminars in Colon and Rectal Surgery.* **3**: 2–8.

Schlinkert RT (1991) Laparoscopic-assisted right hemicolectomy. *Dis. Colon. Rectum.* **34**: 1030–1031.

Semm K (1983) Endoscopic appendectomy. *Endosc.* **15**: 59–64.

Sigel B *et al.*, (1991) *Technique of ultrasonic detection and mapping of abdominal adhesions.* Society of American Gastrointestinal Endoscopic Surgeons Postgraduate Course, Monterey, California.

Smith LE (1992) Transanal endoscopic microsurgery. *Seminars in Colon and Rectal Surgery.* **3**: 9–12.

Webb WA (1991) Colonoscoping the 'difficult' colon. *Am. Surg.* **57**: 178–182.

Williams CB (1987) Colonoscopy. *Curr. Opin. Gastroenterol.* **3**: 36–42.

8

Gynaecology

STEPHEN GROCHMAL

Introduction

The recent upsurge of interest in using minimal access surgical procedures in the fields of general surgery, urology and neurosurgery is related to the efforts and enthusiasm of the gynaecologist who practises operative endoscopic procedures. Operative endoscopic procedures have, in the last 25 years, become the mainstay of therapy in the armamentarium of the gynaecologist. Although dating back to the early 1800s, it has been the gynaecologist who has brought the techniques of operative endoscopy to the forefront. The explosion in technology in the last two years has led to an increased interest in operative endoscopic procedures by other surgical specialties, and has enabled general surgeons to perform laparoscopic cholecystectomies or allowed urologists to begin exploring the abdominal cavity, utilizing operative endoscopy for laparoscopic lymphadenectomies. The increase in the use of both these techniques has been related to the enthusiasm and assistance of gynaecologists, working with other surgical specialties, to perfect the techniques of basic operative laparoscopy, and thus to enhance general surgeons' surgical abilities by performing manipulations that were once practised only by gynaecologists. Therefore, it is not unusual to see a gynaecologist assisting or consulting with other surgical specialists in specific applications of their surgical expertise.

This chapter intends to explore and introduce the many different alternative surgical therapies that have been introduced into gynaecology for the treatment of various disorders, both in the intraperitoneal and intrauterine cavities.

Intrauterine minimal access procedures

The first hysterosocopy was performed in 1869 by Pantaléone and, although

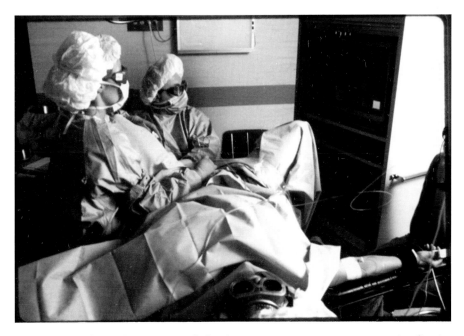

Figure 8.1: Video enhancement of the hysteroscopic image improves visualization, leading to increased precision and patient safety, as well as increased convenience for theatre staff.

well-described throughout the medical literature in the late 19th and early 20th centuries, hysterosocopy has, until recently, been utilized only as a diagnostic tool. However, because of advances in both optics and electronic ability to enhance the operative site image, hysterosocopy now occupies a useful place in the treatment of several gynaecological maladies within the uterine cavity (*see* Figure 8.1).

Treatment of menorrhagia (hypermenorrhoea)

Early in 1981, Milton Goldrath published his initial findings on the use of the Nd:YAG laser for the treatment of excessive uterine bleeding (also known as menorrhagia).

Approximately one million hysterectomies are performed throughout the world each year, 40% of which are performed for the treatment of menorrhagia which has failed to respond to the usual treatment of dilatation and curettage, hormonal suppression therapy and minor surgical procedures within the uterine cavity. Goldrath, and later Lomano (1986) and others, have described an effective alternative to conventional abdominal hysterectomy, which is treating the bleeding problem via hysteroscopy within the uterine cavity. This procedure, known as ablation of the endometrium, utilizes the deep penetrating power of the contact Nd:YAG laser and penetrates through the basalis endometrial layer in the uterine cavity, to destroy the blood vessels and regenerative endometrial tissue layer that is found to be the cause of excessive monthly bleeding. This procedure is performed using a fibre delivery laser system via an operating channel within the hysteroscope. The hysteroscopic image is enhanced by video enlargement, and the physician operates via a video monitor. A major factor that allows the physician to use this laser energy safely is the ability to distend the uterine cavity sufficiently enough so as to be able to see during the operative procedure. Recently Zimmer & Co (Figure 8.2) have introduced a hysteroscopic pump designed specifically to distend the uterine cavity at a safe intrauterine pressure of no greater than 80–90 mmHg, and allow a continuous inflow and outflow of the distension medium – normal saline. This adequate distension of the uterine cavity is critical to the outcome of the surgical procedure (Garry, 1992). However, this distension can lead to a complication known as 'fluid overload' syndrome. Since the electronic pump, maintaining a constant intrauterine pressure, will not increase over 90 mmHg, this greatly decreases the risk of fluid overload particularly if the procedure is prolonged.

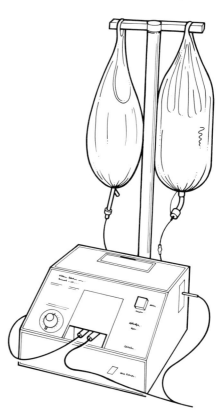

Figure 8.2: The hysteroscopic pump (CDis) consistently maintains the intrauterine pressure at 80 mmHg. (Reproduced with the kind permission of Zimmer & Co, USA.)

The effect of the laser energy is such that small furrows are created within the uterine cavity, which allow seepage of the distension medium into the uterine and ovarian venous circulatory system, and which can eventually lead to retention of the saline solution. Generally, mild diuretics and close postoperative observation will allow these patients to recover relatively quickly from the suspected fluid overload syndrome. In some instances, pulmonary oedema has been reported as a complication to the procedure;

however using the constant distension irrigation system pump, this is now rare. Other complications originally reported by Goldrath and others (1981), included postoperative bleeding due to damage of the endocervical canal as well as the minor risk of uterine perforation (*see* Figure 8.3). These complications are now infrequent due to the improved techniques of visualizing the uterine cavity under magnified video imaging. Caution, however, must be practised by the gynaecologist who performs endometrial ablation, as proper knowledge of the technology of the pump mechanics as well as use of the laser energy within the cavity must be well-understood. Recently, several deaths have been reported during laser endometrial ablation because the physician was unfamiliar with the techniques and dangers that can occur when improper fibre selection or incorrect distension medium was used (Baggish and Daniell, 1989a; 1989b). The author has demonstrated that endometrial ablation with laser energy is a safe procedure if all factors are taken into consideration prior to initiating therapy (Grochmal, 1988).

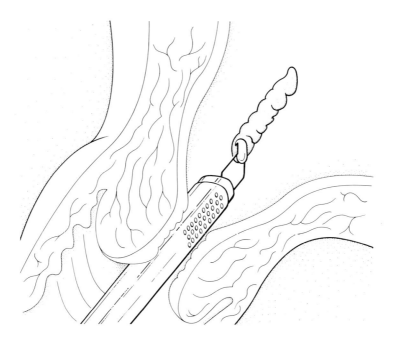

Figure 8.3: Recognition of the internal cervical os is critical, as most operative procedures (resection/ablation) are terminated 1 cm above or at the level of the os.

The outcome for patients undergoing this type of surgery is quite satisfactory. Generally, the procedure can be done under general anaesthesia or local paracervical block with iv sedation. The latter approach has a quicker recovery time and allows for easier monitoring of the patient for signs of fluid overload. Patients usually return to work within 24–48 hours and resume their life-style within three days (Garry, Erian and Grochmal, 1991).

The postoperative results are promising. The elimination of uterine bleeding has, in some studies, been reported as high as 60% in a three-year follow-up evaluation. When taken into account, amenorrhoea in association with hypomenorrhoea or scanty 1–2 day menstrual bleeding patterns, the success rate approaches 99% (Goldrath, 1981). As this procedure eliminates most of the risks associated with hysterectomy, including significant postoperative complications and the 6–8 week recuperation time, this minimal access procedure has gained a significant amount of interest in the last five years.

Endometrial resection

Apart from the use of contact Nd:YAG laser therapy for the treatment of menorrhagia, the gynaecologist has now borrowed instrumentation from the urologist in an attempt to use electrical energy to decrease uterine bleeding. This procedure, known as endometrial resection, uses the resectosocope (Figure 8.4) to remove or shave away layers of endometrial tissue. This procedure received FDA approval in November 1989 and within the last two years has gained increased popularity worldwide. The use of a small wire loop passing an electrical current through a glycine medium to distend the uterine cavity leads to a significant reduction in uterine bleeding problems (Magos, Bauman and Turnbull, 1989). The procedure, also performed under video enhancement, benefits from advanced intrauterine pump technology to distend the uterine cavity. Although the postoperative results appear as promising, and almost approach that of Nd:YAG laser endometrial ablation, there are some significantly greater risks associated with the operative procedure of which the gynaecologist must be aware. Because of the wire loop and its manipulation within the uterine cavity, the risk of uterine perforation is somewhat greater in this type of procedure. Also, due to the greater depths of penetration by the electrical current from the wire loop technique, the risk of postoperative haemorrhage and perhaps the need to convert to hysterectomy due to an inability to stop postoperative haemorrhage successfully is somewhat higher than laser endometrial ablation (Vancaillie, 1989).

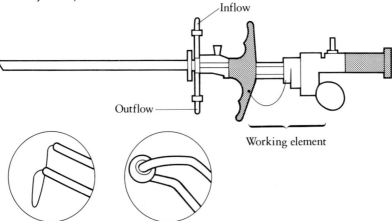

Figure 8.4: The resectoscope. (Reproduced with the kind permission of Circon/Acmi, USA.)

Rollerball (*see* Figure 8.5)

A similar procedure, using the same principles of electrical current applied to the uterine tissue, is known as rollerball. First described three years ago (Townsend *et al.*, 1990), it has also gained popularity in that its depth of penetration, although somewhat less than that achieved with the resectoscope, leads to a significant decrease in heavy uterine bleeding and satisfactory hypomenorrhoea levels (Vancaillie, 1989). The rollerball leaves a much wider tract of tissue coagulation but does not remove any tissue. This coagulation penetrates to a depth of approximately 1–3 mm (depending upon the amount of current applied) which may lead to a decrease, if not almost total elimination, of uterine endometrium (Vancaillie, 1989). Since both endometrial resection and rollerball application require an electrolyte-rich fluid medium, glycine is the distension medium of choice. Since glycine has an ability to lead to a hyponatraemic state, fluid overload risks must also be monitored (Istre *et al.*, 1992).

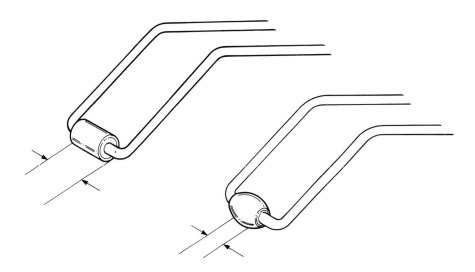

Figure 8.5: Various configurations to the electrode can alter the tissue effect and rapidity of the procedure.

Treatment of intracavitary fibroid tumours and uterine septum

As already mentioned, different energy modalities can be used to create an atrophic or sclerotic effect on the endometrium of the uterine cavity. This same principle can be applied to the treatment of other intrauterine maladies. Frequently associated with a diagnosis of menorrhagia (hypermenorrhoea), is the presence of fibroid tumours within the uterine cavity (Loffer, 1990).

Essentially, this condition has been problematic for a minimal access approach because of the difficulty in removing the tumours in small fragments. The use of the resectoscope and the wire loop for shaving off fragments of large leiomyoma within the uterine cavity can be done quickly and effectively as an out-patient under iv sedation (Corson and Brooks, 1991). As in the case of endometrial ablation or resection, pre-treatment of the patient for 3–4 weeks prior to surgery, using an antioestrogen suppression medication such as Danol (danazol) or the newer gonadotrophin-releasing hormone (GnRH) analogues such as Lupron (leuprolide acetate) or buserelin (nasal spray) enhances the effectiveness of the surgery (Grochmal, 1988). This antihormonal suppression leads to an atrophic endometrium and a brightening or whitening of the endometrial cavity due to a devascularization effect which occurs after medical therapy. Utilizing the wire loop, resection of these endometrial fibroids can be done quickly and effectively (Neuwirth and Amin, 1976). Application of laser energy, by placing the Nd:YAG laser in contact with the leiomyoma, can also be an effective approach to treatment of these tumours (Lomano, 1986). More recently, the sculptured fibres of 800 microns are enabling gynaecologists to treat the intracavitary fibroids very effectively in a 'resectoscope-like' fashion using the contact Nd:YAG laser.

Uterine septum

Treatment of uterine septum, especially in cases of repeated pregnancy loss, have now been improved due to advances in technology for hysteroscopic surgery. The use of either electrical current or contact Nd:YAG laser energy to the uterine septum allows the physician to treat this condition as a minimal access procedure. Prior to the introduction of these techniques, the treatment of intrauterine septum often required an open abdominal procedure.

The procedure itself, follows the same protocol as already described in the previous sections, and the risks and safety considerations are also similar. Postoperative outcome is greatly improved in these patients since the procedure can be performed on an out-patient basis and is less traumatic to the endometrial cavity, especially during the healing process after surgery (Grochmal, 1987). A word of caution is indicated here, in that, both these procedures, whether done with electrical or laser energy, should be done under direct laparoscopic guidance and visualization. This helps the operative surgeon have a clear view of the whole uterine fundus prior to shaving or slicing through the uterine septum. As the energy is applied to the septum, it melts away anteriorly and posteriorly and leaves a small ridge of tissue. This ridge can then be removed, either with a wire loop or ablated with a sharpened laser fibre, to create a new and larger uterine cavity. Generally, the rate of postoperative intrauterine adhesions or synechiae is significantly less with this type of approach. However, it is recommended that intrauterine stents such as a Wood's catheter or small paediatric Foley catheter be inserted into the uterine cavity for 3–4 days postoperatively to act as a stent over which the endometrium can heal and develop a new resting endometrial layer. Usually, second-look hysteroscopy is done 2–3 months after surgery to evaluate the size of the uterine cavity, and to look for any possible residual septal tissue that may still remain after the initial surgery. The rate of repeated pregnancy loss after this surgery is significantly reduced and, therefore, pregnancy rates to birth are significantly greater utilizing these advanced minimal access techniques (Grochmal, 1987).

New horizons for hysteroscopic surgery

Since 1990, a small but increasing interest has been generated by the appearance of a new miniaturized hysteroscopy system (*see* Figure 8.6). This system, known as microhysteroscopy, utilizes a 1.6 mm endoscope with an outside introducing sheath (2 mm) which can be used in the same fashion as the larger 3 and 4 mm hysteroscopes. Used as a diagnostic tool, the advantages of the microhysteroscope are several. Since it is small, it can be passed through the endocervical canal and into the uterine cavity more easily than conventional hysteroscopes. Due to its small diameter, it is not necessary to dilate the cervix prior to insertion, as the outside diameter of the scope is approximately 2 mm (Lomano and Grochmal, 1992). This makes the use of hysteroscopy more acceptable to the patient and to the physician who wishes to use this technology as a diagnostic tool. In-office (out-patient) hysteroscopy

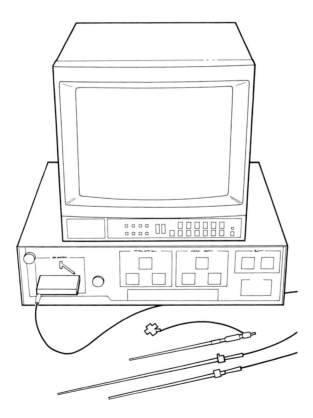

Figure 8.6: Various diameters of optical catheters can be used with this advanced miniaturized system. (Reproduced with the kind permission of Medical Dynamics Inc, USA.)

is becoming a more widely practised procedure, and will replace methods such as dilatation and curettage and blind endometrial biopsy as the procedure of choice in making diagnoses of uterine pathology.

The technology of the microhysteroscope is such that the light-carrying bundles and optical information are transmitted through a flexible cable that is part of the electronic imaging system, thus freeing the surgeon from having to manipulate a large camerahead and light cable. Because of the flexibility of the system, the hysteroscope can be shaped in order to reach difficult areas of visualization such as a retroverted or retroflexed uterus. Visualization of the tubal ostium and the initial portion of the Fallopian tubes can be done easily with this hysteroscope (Frydman *et al.*, 1987). Again, due to the small outside diameter of the hysteroscope, local infiltration of the cervix may be all that is needed to perform a diagnostic procedure. Distension of the uterine cavity is generally done with saline but, because of the small nature of the hysteroscope, the need for specialized pump systems is not essential. The visual image of the microhysteroscope is equal to that of a 3–4 mm conventional diagnostic hysteroscope. However, because of the smaller image, a good working knowledge of hysteroscopy and of the topography of the uterine cavity and its abnormalities is essential prior to using this advanced technology. The recent addition of operating channels to the outside sheath of the microhysteroscope will now enable physicians to take small hysteroscopic-directed biopsies using microinstruments through the operating channel of the system. This will truly make in-office (out-patient) hysteroscopy an essential component for every gynaecologist who is interested in treating intrauterine conditions. The system will, however, not replace conventional hysteroscopy in its specialized uses for operative procedures such as already mentioned. However, the small size of the hysteroscope and the excellent video image will make in-office consultation via hysteroscopy a practical procedure to enhance diagnostic acumen.

Laparoscopic treatment of intraperitoneal disorders

Operative laparoscopy is the usual approach that the gynaecologist uses to treat various intraperitoneal disorders in the female patient. As already described in the section on operative hysteroscopy, the recent advances and improvement in instrumentation and visualization have allowed the gynaecologist to perform most procedures via the laparoscopic approach. Laparoscopy has become a mainstay in the armamentarium of the gynaecologist for the treatment of intraperitoneal disorders. The most recent advances in the treatment of these disorders will be described. It must be remembered at all times that the techniques of haemostasis, prevention of adhesions and the general surgical principles of open abdominal surgery still prevail in treating the patient laparoscopically. The physician must be conscious that the thought process in handling difficult problems or complications that may arise during the course of operative endoscopic procedures does not differ from the thought process and techniques involved in solving problems while the peritoneal cavity is open during major abdominal procedures. This is an important concept to remember as the novice operative endoscopist may panic in a crisis situation, thus not allowing him to develop a method of treating the complication intraperitoneally. The purpose of good operative endoscopy is to perform it safely, to be able to complete the procedure as an endoscopic one, and not to have to convert to an open procedure because of a lack of understanding of the techniques, instrumentation or manoeuvres.

The gynaecologist must be fully aware of all of the instrumentation (*see* Figure 8.7a and b), electronic apparatus, suture material, haemostatic agents and other endoscopic manoeuvres that can be used to prevent an unfortunate incident converting a successful laparoscopic procedure into an open abdominal one. New safety designs for trocars, improved stability devices and enhanced cautery delivery systems have helped achieve an increased level of safety. With this in mind, the techniques that will be described can be performed safely and effectively through the endoscope with a successful outcome for the patient. The benefits to the patient are: less trauma as there are no large abdominal incisions, a reduced anaesthetic time, a shorter in-hospital stay and a more rapid recuperation phase in the postoperative period.

Endometriosis

In no other area in gynaecology has the laparoscope played such an important role than in the management of patients with endometriosis. Originally, laparoscopy was used as a diagnostic modality in evaluating patients for the presence of endometrial implants. Apart from staging the disease, the use of laparoscopy was somewhat limited because of lack of proper instrumentation and methods of safely delivering either electricity or laser energy to the operative site. In 1985, with the advent of video enhancement in endoscopy, the ability to more easily diagnose, recognize and now treat these endometrial implants became a reality. The impact of video enhancement laparoscopy is one that has opened up this field, not only to gynaecologists but also to general surgeons and urologists. The use of the video monitor and enhanced video image allows the physician to visualize the endometrial implants along the peritoneal wall, posterior aspects of the pelvic organs and in other areas of the upper abdominal cavity. The introduction of VLS has moved video enhancement on to the next plateau. Image resolution is increased to 1000 lines and the placement of the CCD chip at the distal end of the telescope eliminates heavy optical glass, thereby lightening the scope considerably. Originally, the use of the CO_2 laser (*see* Figure 8.8) was purported to be the best method, and preferred treatment modality, for endometrial implants. Apart from vaporization of small endometrial tissue sites (large areas of peritoneum were scarred), adhered portions of pelvic organs can be either vaporized and/or excised leaving behind a normal layer of tissue which can regenerate. However, CO_2 laser applications fell short of satisfactory results due to the difficulty with endoscopically manipulating them within the abdominal cavity, mostly due to the inability to maintain proper beam alignment of the laser. In 1987, the introduction of fibre delivery systems for various laser wavelengths (Nd:YAG, KTP) made the endoscopic approach for endometriosis more practical (*see* Figure 8.9). The use of fibre delivery systems

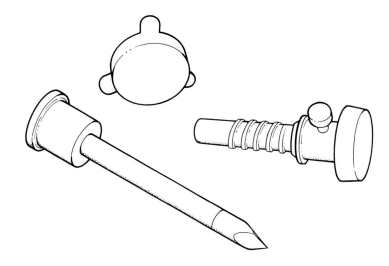

Figure 8.7a: Short trocar lengths and improved stability threads on the trocar sheaths prevent accidental removal during endoscopic procedures. (Reproduced with the kind permission of Apple Medical Corporation, USA.)

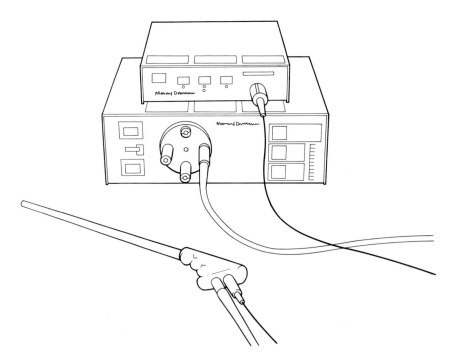

Figure 8.7b: The electronic video laparoscope (EVL) uses distal placement of the camera chip eliminating glass optics and increasing resolution to 1000 lines. Note: the eyepiece of the scope has been eliminated. (Reproduced with the kind permission of Medical Dynamics Inc, USA.)

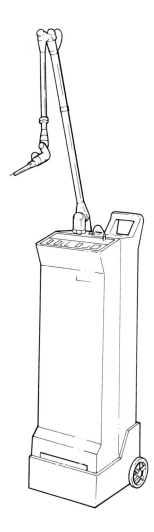

Figure 8.8: Compact size and design modifications have improved articulated arm delivery systems and portability of the CO_2 laser. (Reproduced with the kind permission of Sharplan Lasers Inc, USA.)

made transportation of the laser energy directly to the target site easier and less risky. Wavelengths such as KTP, argon and Nd:YAG can now be used endoscopically. These laser wavelengths, some of which have more affinity for dark-coloured tissue than others, aid the gynaecologist in treating endometrial implants. The fact that many of these laser wavelengths are not absorbed by water or fluid also allows the evacuation of endometriomas and excision of endometrial tissue in moist areas. Fibre delivery system lasers have also aided the reproductive endocrinologist in treating patients with endometriosis, as well as performing advanced tubal surgery, and even GIFT procedures in selective patients. Because of these developments, laser technology and further improvement in instrumentation has also coincided with the ability of the gynaecologist to improve his treatment modalities in endometriosis. New developments in instruments including multipronged forceps, atraumatic forceps and dissecting forceps designed specifically for the gynaecologist, allow the surgeon delicately to strip away and dissect tissue planes in the more advanced stages of the disease (Figure 8.10). Patients with advanced disease, such Stage III or IV, benefit from having their procedures done completely endoscopically. Using hydrodissection pumps, pressurized irrigation systems and specialized instruments which can grasp but not strangulate delicate tissues, advanced tubal surgery and more aggressive approaches in removing large portions of destroyed and scarred peritoneal tissue as well as portions of both Fallopian tubes and ovaries have now become a reality. The level of tissue damage is minimal because of these advanced instruments.

Using sculptured fibres, or sapphire probes in the fibre delivery systems of lasers, has allowed the gynaecologist to approach areas in the pelvis such as

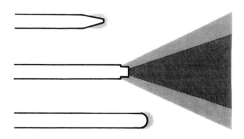

Figure 8.9: Fibre delivery systems for various wavelengths.

the ureters, small and large bowel, and bladder dome more readily. Due to the limited depth of penetration provided by the use of the sculptured fibres, areas that were once endoscopically taboo due to their location, can now be successfully treated (Figure 8.11). Despite the advances in both laser application and instrumentation, the common problems of postoperative adhesions and reformation of scar tissue can still plague the operative endoscopist. Advances in the development of material and liquid barrier methods of antiadhesion prevention are now underway and many products appear to be promising (Stovall, Edler and Ling, 1989). Of recent note, is the use of Interceed which can be applied through various ports into the abdominal cavity. This acts as a cellulose barrier and prevents the reformation of adhesions in areas where the majority of the endometriosis has been stripped away and excised. Preliminary data reported by several authors seems to indicate that the outcome in patients utilizing these advanced antiadhesive methods is promising when they are evaluated in follow-up laparoscopies.

Uterine fibroids

As previously mentioned, the hysteroscopic treatment of uterine fibroids has been improved by recent advances in technology. It is the same situation

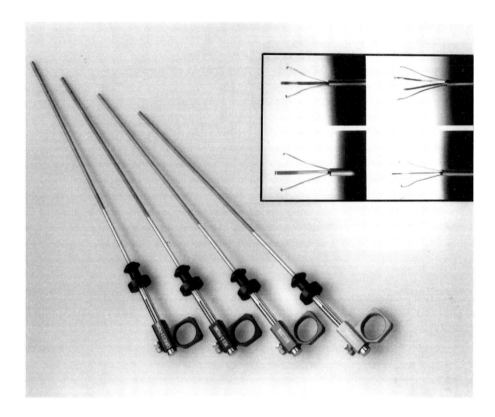

Figure 8.10: Multipronged spring-loaded forceps facilitate delicate endoscopic dissections. (Reproduced with the kind permission of Edward Weck Instruments and Linvatec, USA.)

laparoscopically. Large leiomyoma can now be removed successfully via the laparoscope (Dubuisson *et al.*, 1991). Most leiomyoma of the serosal or intramural type can be easily excised using the same techniques as used if the procedure was done conventionally through an open abdominal incision. Many physicians choose to approach leiomyoma by devascularizing them with medication prior to surgery. In Europe, buserelin is successfully used, not only to decrease vascularity of fibroid tumours but to shrink them as well. In the USA, the use of the GnRH analog Lupron (lupolide acetate) and Danol (danazol) has shown promising results in devascularizing and shrinking fibroids prior to surgery. With this in mind, excision of larger leiomyoma can be done successfully by a minimally invasive approach (Fedele *et al.*, 1990).

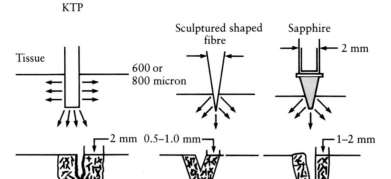

Figure 8.11: Diagram of tissue depth of penetration of KTP and Nd:YAG lasers with bare, shaped and sapphire fibres. (Reproduced with the kind permission of Sharplan Lasers Inc, USA.

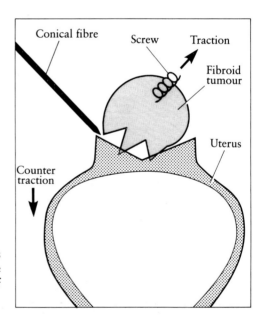

Figure 8.12: Traction of the fibroid is accomplished with a myoma screw while dissection is accomplished with the use of a contact laser fibre.

Laparoscopic myomectomy consists of utilizing some form of energy to incise the serosa in order to create an incision through the capsule of the fibroid tumour (*see* Figure 8.12). Once a small incision has been made, different alternatives and techniques can be utilized. Generally, the leiomyoma is undermined with blunt dissecting forceps. Using a twisting motion, the leiomyoma can be twisted away or 'shelled' out of its cavity in the wall of the uterus without much difficulty. Traction can be applied using a 5 or 10 mm myoma screw. Most leiomyoma have a vascular pedicle which can be either clipped or ligated using a Surgitie or endoloop (Semm, 1978). Leiomyoma can then be removed directly out of one of the larger endoscopic trocar ports. Large leiomyoma (i.e. greater than 6–8 cm) can be removed, but difficulty in extracting the specimen through the abdominal wall has been frustrating until recently. New advances in morcellators and automatic electronic tissue grinders (*see* Figure 8.13) has now made it possible to remove very large tissue masses completely endoscopically (Semm, 1987). The introduction of the endopouch, a drawstring-type plastic bag which can be inserted into the peritoneal cavity, allows fragments of fibroid tumours as they are chewed up or ground away to be collected. The entire fragmented specimen can be removed without any loss into the abdominal cavity. A simple and effective technique to remove large fibroid tissue is Semm's 'tissue extraction system'. These 15–20 mm trocars allow a serrated tip cannula to be rotated against the tissue specimen while counter traction is applied. Large cores of tissue (15–20mm) may be removed using this system (*see* Figure 8.14). The use of these techniques, benefits the patient because before laparoscopic myomectomy, conventional myomectomy meant 2–3 days postoperative stay in hospital and several weeks recovery thereafter. The need to prepare patients preoperatively with blood transfusions is unnecessary. Some endoscopic surgeons prefer to treat the operative site prior to enucleation of the leiomyoma by the injection of vasopressent. This helps in eliminating the bleeding at the operative site and has become a popular adjunct in the excision

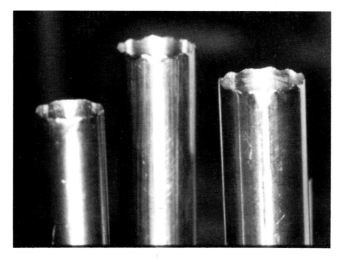

Figure 8.13: The serrated edge of extraction tube cuts a 'cone' of tissue up to 20 mm in diameter and 6 cm long. (Reproduced with the kind permission of SA Grochmal.)

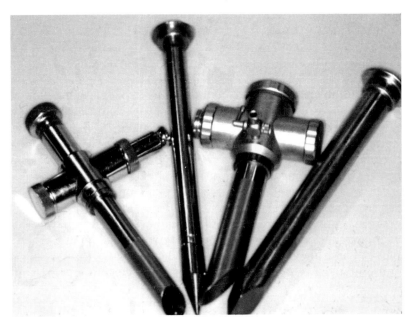

Figure 8.14: Trocars and cannulae up to 25 mm are available to facilitate tissue extracted endoscopically.

process of fibroid tumours. The use of 'dual effect' Nd:YAG laser fibre may also be used to achieve haemostasis.

Ovarian cysts

Laparoscopic treatment of ovarian cysts has raised some controversy amongst gynaecologists. The discussion in this section will address benign ovarian cysts. Even large ovarian cysts can be easily treated laparoscopically. Once an operative approach has been decided upon, and the ovarian cyst has been documented to be benign by ultrasound, chemical studies and history, the cystectomy is easily carried out (Yasilev *et al.*, 1988). Before 1986, the majority of ovarian cysts were treated by aspiration of the follicular fluid which was sent for cytology evaluation and the ovarian cyst was left behind. This caused a reaccumulation of fluid and subsequent cysts arose from the residual tissue left behind in the cyst wall. More recently, small ovarian cystotomies have been performed which allow the fluid to be removed and pressurized irrigation saline injected into the cyst wall itself. This aids in separating the cyst from the overlying ovarian stroma. Once this aspiration and irrigation technique has been completed, using an operating laparoscope, the surgeon can remove *in toto* the entire cyst wall as it is stripped away from the ovarian stroma using a grasping forcep. This method has proved very effective for acute ovarian cysts. However, more chronic ovarian cysts are difficult to enucleate and in this situation, vaporization of any residual cyst wall can be done using laser or electrocautery. Caution should always be taken when evaluating ovarian cysts, as the potential for malignancy always exists. With any suspicious appearance, a more conservative and conventional approach to the ovarian cyst should always be taken (Magge *et al.*, 1990). Recent advances in microendoscopy will allow future physicians to perform ovarioscopy via one of their laparoscopic trocar incisions.

A small optical catheter can be inserted into the ovarian cyst once it has been opened. The gynaecologist can evaluate the cyst wall, using ovarioscopy to take a small biopsy and look for excrescences etc. which may give some clue as to the best method of management of the ovarian cyst. It is optional whether to close ovarian tissue once the cyst has been removed. The ovary will usually heal within one cycle and, on second-look laparoscopies, the residual amount of adhesions or failure of the ovary to reapproximate properly has been minimal. Early data seems to indicate that on second-look laparoscopies, in infertile patients that have had multiple cystectomies, the use of cellulose barriers or other antiadhesive liquids aids the prevention or reformation of adhesions around the operative sites of the ovaries (Semm, 1987).

Adhesiolysis

Adequate treatment of pelvic pain by the gynaecologist has always been difficult. Although many surgeons feel that lysis of adhesions plays a minimal role in eliminating abdominal pain, more and more physicians are becoming convinced that the laparoscopic approach is the preferred method, and that these patients respond well to having adhesions removed. Adhesiolysis performed laparoscopically has an additional benefit in that readhesion formation appears to be much less than after the conventional open technique (not confirmed by multiple clinical studies). Adhesiolysis is preferably carried out using an operating laparoscope. The use of an operating laparoscope has several advantages in that it allows the gynaecologist to operate the camera on the eyepiece of the laparoscope and use the operating channel of the laparoscope to pass down either a laser fibre, cautery tip, suction irrigator, serrated operating scissors, or clip applier. This allows the physician to work head-on over the target site rather than from behind or sideways via secondary trocar sites. The use of the operating laparoscope for adhesiolysis is a significant improvement over the previously described endoscopic techniques for adhesiolysis.

A word of caution must be noted when considering the adhesions. The operative endoscopist should always perform as many measures as possible to make sure that initiation of the laparoscopy (i.e. insertion of the Verres needle, creation of the pneumoperitoneum and trocar insertions) is performed safely and layers of adhesions and/or intestines underlying the anterior abdominal wall are not damaged. Tests such as the Palmer needle test and the use of the new microendoscopy system will help the gynaecologist to prevent bowel perforation and damage to the underlying organs due to massive adhesions (Semm and Mettler, 1983). One of the most recent developments, which appears to be promising, is that direct visualization while inserting a Verres needle or trocar can be achieved using the optical catheter system (Curlik and Grochmal, 1993). This system of either a flexible or rigid laparoscope ranging in size from 0.4–1.6 mm and developed by Medical Dynamics in

Englewood, Colorado (*see* Figure 8.15), has made the procedure accessible to patients that would not have been treated because of the possibility of massive abdominal adhesions. With the use of the optical catheter which can be passed through the Verres needle, visualization of the abdominal cavity is possible in complicated cases.

Advances in instrumentation design and trocar development will perhaps lead the gynaecologist to a situation where laparoscopy can be performed anywhere one can place a Verres needle inside the peritoneal cavity. The use of small flexible optical catheters, which range down in size to 0.3 mm in diameter, give an adequate view of the peritoneal cavity and can actually be passed down through the channel of the Verres needle! Obviously, there are several advantages in using these more advanced techniques and operative endoscopy in a patient with a history of previous multiple abdominal operations with adhesions will become a reality within operative endoscopy.

Dyspareunia (transection of the ureterosacral ligaments and presacral neuroectomy)

Many female patients suffer from dyspareunia associated with either endometriosis, pelvic adhesions or inflammatory disease affecting the pelvic organs (Ripps and Martin, 1991). Previous evidence has shown that by transecting a portion of the ureterosacral ligaments with interruption of the nerve bundle of Frankenheimer leads to relief of the dyspareunia. Recently, a more aggressive approach, of excising the ureterosacral ligament whenever possible, leading to a more satisfactory and prolonged outcome of relief of the dyspareunia has been described (*see* Figure 8.16). This procedure can be done simply and easily via the laparoscopic approach. Preferably using a fibre delivery laser system,

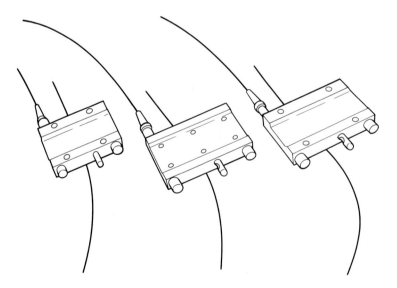

Figure 8.15: Optical catheters range in size from 0.35. 0.5 to 0.75 mm in diameter.

transection and excision of a portion of each ureterosacral ligament can be performed with a shaped fibre. However, prior to excision of any portion of the ureterosacral ligaments, proper identification of the ureters bilaterally as well as other anatomical structures in the area must be carried out. In patients with advanced stages of endometriosis, or multiple adhesions of the viscera to the pelvic sidewall, occasional use of ureterocatheters has been recommended. These illuminated catheters can be placed in the ureter so that the ureter can be palpated and retracted away from the ureterosacral ligament prior to transection or excision. Controversy still exists over the exact site along the ureterosacral ligament where the excision or the transection should be performed. However, preliminary data from several different investigators appears to indicate that no matter where the interruption of the nerve bundle occurs, relief of symptoms appears to be the same. Excision, rather than transection, is presently the preferred treatment modality. Once performed, the transected ligament does not lead, as previously thought, to significant uterine prolapse.

Laparoscopically assisted vaginal hysterectomy and total laparoscopic hysterectomy

The most advanced and aggressive procedure which is described in the current literature is that of laparoscopic removal of the uterus with or without tubes and ovaries (Magos, 1991). This approach, which appears to be a normal evolution in operative endoscopy, has several benefits.
•   For many years the traditional vaginal surgeon has been perplexed and at times frustrated in his inability to determine the precise placement of

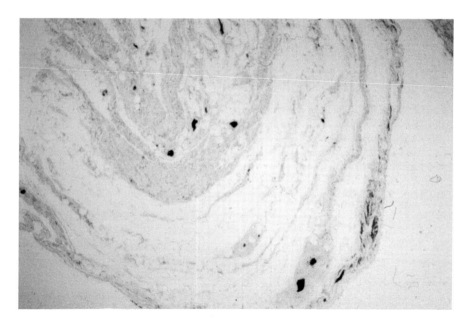

Figure 8.16: Excision of a ureterosacral ligament. (Reproduced with the kind permission of J Wright, St Peter's Hospital, Chertsey, UK.)

clamps, sutures and the division of pedicles by the vaginal approach. All of the ligaments, including the uterine artery and its corresponding pedicles, can be determined laparoscopically. Laparoscopic visualization has improved this phenomenon.

• Using the endoGIA, pedicles can be created and transected with minimal difficulty via an endoscopic approach. Once the entire uterine body has been freed from its vascular pedicles, the remaining portion of the procedure can be performed by the vaginal route (or by complete laparoscopy) (Nezhat and Nezhat, 1990).

• Postoperative complications appear to be no different from the complete vaginal hysterectomy. However, since the procedure is relatively new, the long-term outcome of the patient and postoperative complications still need to be evaluated.

The techniques for laparoscopically assisted vaginal hysterectomy are based on several different approaches (see Table 8.1). The enhanced view that the surgeon can achieve using laparoscopy aids speed and safety and eliminates many of the unseen risks, for example, accidentally clamping other vital structures such as the bowel during the extraction of the uterus.

Table 8.1: Classification system (criteria compiled from several contributors: Stovall T, Reich H, Della Badia C, Grochmal S and Lyons T).

1	Laparoscopically-assisted vaginal hysterectomy: the infundibulopelvic ligaments and round ligaments are ligated laparoscopically.
2	Laparoscopic hysterectomy: the infundibulopelvic, round and broad ligaments and uterine arteries are ligated laparoscopically, the uterus is removed vaginally. Note: the vaginal cuff may be closed abdominally.
3	Total laparoscopic hysterectomy: same as 2 above except the uterus is morcellated and removed abdominally and the cuff closed abdominally.
4	Supracervical technique: (a) same as 2 above except only the uterine corpus is removed vaginally or abdominally. (b) CASH procedure. Same as 2 above with the exception of removing the majority of the cervix which allows greater support to the vaginal vault. All ligaments are suture-ligated laparoscopically and the uterus may be morcellated through the abdominal approach.

Footnote: No one classification has been accepted worldwide.

However, even though patients request and insist upon more minimal access procedures, laparoscopically assisted vaginal hysterectomy is still a major operation. Therefore, many patients will still request the more minimal access procedures of endometrial ablation and resection. Laparoscopically assisted vaginal hysterectomy will be most useful in those patients who have failed initial therapy with endometrial ablation or resection techniques, or when the surgeon wishes to convert a difficult abdominal hysterectomy to a vaginal hysterectomy. Some surgeons may prefer not to operate vaginally. For them, the total laparoscopic hysterectomy may be suitable. Other variations, particularly the supracervical hysterectomy and CASH procedure, offer the endoscopic surgeon alternatives to the traditional approach. Despite these variations, the standard vaginal hysterectomy is still the procedure of choice.

The use of the endoGIA (*see* Figure 8.17) has greatly helped the gynaecologist in attempting to extract the uterus and its appendages via the vaginal route (Reich *et al.*, 1992). Recently, there have been attempts to extract the uterus using a totally endoscopic procedure. The limiting factor, as with all new aggressive operative endoscopic procedures, is the lack of proper instrumentation. The ability to morcillate or grind up the uterus is now the major problem. Present morcillators are manually operated and it is extremely difficult to remove an entire uterus using a manual tissue extractor. However, many developments are underway to provide an automated, safe method of grinding up the tissue into small fragments and extracting them either through the electronic grinder or collecting them in a small specimen bag. The use of the Semm 'tissue extraction system' has been successful in morcellating uterine tissue up to 20 weeks gestation.

Current operating times for endoscopic removal of a uterus are 2–6 hours. There comes a point where endoscopic vanity outweighs the benefits provided to the patient and it becomes necessary to use one's judgement in determining whether or not the procedure should continue as an endoscopic one (Stovall *et al.*, 1992). Until proper instrumentation is developed, the totally endoscopic hysterectomy will be possible but difficult. Alternatively, upon development of the needed instrumentation, it will provide treatment for a large number of women who suffer from various problems presently necessitating removal of their uterus.

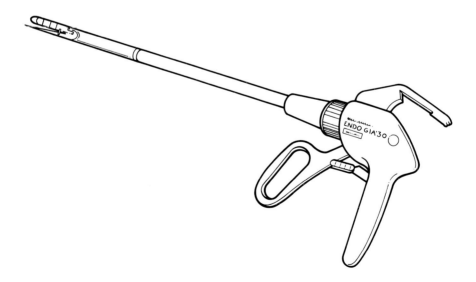

Figure 8.17: EndoGIA multifire endoscopic stapler. (Reproduced with the kind permission of US Surgical Corporation, USA.)

Microlaparoscopy

As described with intrauterine operative procedures, microendoscopy can play a useful adjunct to diagnosis and operative procedures as a truly minimal access endoscopic manipulation. This laparoscope originated from the more popular microendoscope or optical catheter (produced by Medical Dynamics, Englewood, Colorado). Using the Adair/Verres needle, creation of pneumoperitoneum and visualization of the peritoneal cavity can be achieved via a 1.6 mm semi-rigid endoscope. This microendoscope, or optical catheter, utilizes fibreoptic transmission of light and electronic imaging data which can be passed through the abdominal wall and visualization of the peritoneal cavity and its contents easily achieved. The recent introduction of 10 000 element fibres within the 1.6 mm telescope diameter provides an image almost equivalent to a large 10 mm diagnostic laparoscope. Although the visual image is small, digitized zooming of the image can be achieved with an acceptable clarity. This technique allows one to perform an entire laparoscopic procedure with a microendoscope.

The advantage of this system is that it allows the gynaecologist to perform easily more second-look laparoscopies for infertile patients and those with extensive endometriosis. Due to the small size of the introducing sheath and laparoscope itself, this procedure leaves minimal scarring in the abdomen, and is a more palatable approach for a quick second-look procedure than conventional laparoscopy (Grochmal and Lomano, 1992). It also leads to better patient compliance and as it is truly minimal access is more appealing to patients than conventional laparoscopy and the procedures may be accomplished using iv sedation.

As new technology is developed, the applications not only in gynaecology but also in other surgical specialities will be increased to take advantage of this miniaturized endoscopic system (Curlik and Grochmal, 1993).

Evaluation of the Fallopian tube is the one procedure which has always remained elusive for both the gynaecologist and the operative endoscopist. Falloposcopy, or evaluation via the fimbrial side of the Fallopian tube using flexible optical catheters as small as 0.3 mm in diameter, can take place using a secondary trocar site during conventional large laparoscopy. The ability to manipulate the optical catheter within the fimbrial ostium and beyond can be done by injecting saline solution (via an overlying cannula) into the Fallopian tube as the tube is passed over the cannula with atraumatic grasping forceps. The optical catheter is then advanced, while the liquid medium is injected into the Fallopian tube, and a falloposcopy performed directly visualizing the tubal lumen.

Alternatively, using the hysteroscopic approach, these optical catheters can be placed within the tubal ostium from the uterine cavity. Prior to insertion of the optical catheter a steerable guidewire can be inserted through the proximal end of the Fallopian tube and the entire tube examined in this fashion. This is preferably done under laparoscopic guidance, so as to prevent possible perforation of the tubal serosa. Once the cannula has been firmly situated within the tubal lumen, the optical catheter is passed through using saline as a distension fluid, the outside cannula sheath is removed and a retrograde tuboscopy is performed by pulling the optical catheter back towards the proximal end of the tube from its distal location (Lomano and Grochmal, 1992). As this is new technology and still under development, it will not become an active part of the gynaecologist's armamentarium within the near future. However, results of preliminary studies and evaluations of these video tuboscopies certainly leads one to believe that the minimal access evaluation of the reproductive tract may be a reality soon.

The optical catheter system can be used for both in-office (clinic) and theatre procedures, both diagnostically and surgically. Using the outer sheath of the microlaparoscope, it can be passed into the uterus without the need for cervical dilation or local anaesthesia of the cervix. Saline can be passed through the cannula as the distension medium and the area quickly becomes visible. More recently, the introduction of the micro-operation sheath has made possible the taking of biopsies, the performing of polypectomies and even myoma resections with the use of the laser (contact Nd:YAG) as in-office (clinic) procedures (*see* Figure 8.18). These developments mean that hysteroscopic surgical procedures can now be performed in the gynaecologist's office or clinic, which is more convenient for both patient and physician and is most cost effective (*see* Table 8.2).

Table 8.2: Applications of optical catheter technology.

Microhysteroscopy	Microlaparoscopy
• Cervical stenosis	• Pneumoperitoneum
• Endometrial biopsy	• Endometriosis
• Polyps, fibroids	• Adhesiolysis
• Septum, adhesions	• Tubal evaluation
• Tuboscopy	• GIFT procedures

As we approach the end of the 1990s it is obvious that the possibilities are limitless for operative endoscopy. As once stated by Kurt Semm; '*by the year 2000 the majority of procedures will be done endoscopically*'. We are truly entering a 'minimal access odyssey', and it is up to every operative endoscopist to make the most of current technology and techniques and provide the best of care for his or her patients. It is also important that we remember to continue to strive towards more progressive operative endoscopic procedures, that will

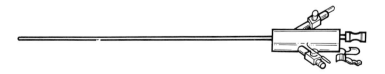

Figure 8.18: Multiple operation port micro catheter sheath with an outside diameter of approximately 3.9 mm. (Reproduced with the kind permission of Medical Dynamics Inc, USA.)

allow the patient the benefit of shorter hospital stay and recuperation time, as well as an improved outcome in their general well-being.

References

Baggish MS and Daniell JF (1989a) Death caused by air embolism associated with Nd:YAG laser surgery and artificial sapphire tips. *Am. J. Obstet. Gynecol.* **161**: 877–878.

Baggish MS and Daniell JF (1989b) Catastrophic injury secondary to the use of coaxial gas-cooled fibres and artificial sapphire tips for intrauterine surgery: a report of five cases. *Lasers Surg. Med.* 9: 581–584.

Corson SL and Brooks PG (1991) Resectoscopic myomectomy. *Fertility and Sterility.* 55: 1041–1044.

Curlik M and Grochmal S (1993) *Urologic applications for microendoscopy techniques.* In: Gomella G *et al.*, (Eds) Laparoscopic urologic surgery. Raven Press, New York.

Dubuisson JB *et al.*, (1991) Myomectomy: a preliminary report on 43 cases. *Fertil. Steril.* 56: 827–830.

Fedele L *et al.*, (1990) Treatment with GNRH agonists before myomectomy and the risk of short term myoma recurrence. *Br. J. Obstet. Gynae.* 97: 393–396.

Frydman R *et al.*, (1987) Uterine evaluation by microhysteroscopy in IVF candidates. *Human Reprod.* 2: 481–485.

Gary R, Erian J and Grochmal SA (1991) A multi-centre collaborative study into the treatment of menorrhagia by Nd:YAG laser ablation of the endometrium. *Br. Obstet. and Gynaec.* 98: 357–360.

Gary R *et al.*, (1992) A uterine distension system to prevent fluid absorbtion during Nd:YAG laser endometrial ablation. *Gyne. Endos.* 1: 23–27.

Goldrath MH, Fuller TA and Segal S (1981) Laser photovaporization of endometrium for the treatment of menorrhagia. *Am. J. Obstet. and Gynec.* 104: 14.

Grochmal S (1987) *Improved pregnancy notes after hysteroscopic septum resection.* Abstract from the AGGL clinical meeting, San Francisco.

Grochmal SA (1988) Endometrial ablation safely treats uterine bleeding. *Clinical Laser Monthly.* September: 15–4.

Grochmal S and Lomano J (1992) New microendoscopic technique reduces scars and recuperation time. *Clin. Laser.* 1: 125–126.

Istre O *et al.*, (1992) Changes in serum electrolytes transcervical resection of endometrium and submucous fibroids with use of glycine 1.5% for uterine irrigation. *Obstet. Gyne.* 80: 218–222.

Liu CY (1992) Laparoscopic hysterectomy: a review of 72 cases. *J. Repro. Med.* 37: 351–354.

Loffer FD (1990) Removal of large symptomatic intrauterine growths by the hysteroscope resectoscope. *Obstet. Gynecol.* 76: 836.

Lomano JM (1986) Ablation of the endometrium with the Nd:YAG laser: a multicenter study. *Colposc. Gynecol. Laser Surgery.* 2: 203–207.

Lomano J and Grochmal S (1992) *Microendoscopy: a new generation of in-office procedures.* Abstract of the 40th clinical meeting of ACOG, Las Vegas.

Magge G *et al.*, (1990) Laparoscopic management of cystic adenexal masses. *J. Gyne. Surg.* 6: 71–79.

Magos AL, Bauman R and Turnbull AC (1989) Transcervical resection of endometrium in women with menorrhagia. *BMJ.* 298: 1209–1212.

Magos A (1991) Laparoscopic assisted vaginal hysterectomy. *The Lancet.* 338: 1091–1092.

Neuwirth RX and Amin HV (1976) Excision of submucous fibroids with hysteroscopic control. *Am. J. Obstet. Gynecol.* 126: 95.

Nezhat C and Nezhat F (1990) Laparoscopic hysterectomy and bilateral salpingoo-pherectomy using the multi fire GAI surgical stapler. *J. Gynec. Surg.* 6: 287–288.

Reich H, Decaprio and McGynn F (1992) Laparoscopic hysterectomy. *J. Gynec. Surg.* 5: 213–215.

Ripps B and Martin DC (1991) Focal pelvic tenderness, pelvic pain and dysmenorrhea in endometrosis. *J. Repro. Med.* 36: 470–472.

Semm K (1978) Tissue puncher and loop ligation: new aide for surgical – therapeutic pelviscopy (laparoscopy) – endoscopic intra-abdominal surgery. *Endoscopy.* 10: 119.

Semm K and Mettler L (1983) Technical progress in pelvic surgery via operative laparoscopy. *Am. J. Obstet. Gynecol.* 138: 121.

Semm K (1987) *Operative manual for endoscopic abdominal surgery.* Year Book Medical Publishers, Chicago.

Stovall T, Edler RF and Ling F (1989) Predictors of pelvic adhesions. *J. Repro. Med.* 34: 345.

Stovall T, Summit R, Lipscomb G and Ling F (1992) *Randomized comparison of LAVH versus standard vaginal hysterectomy in an outpatient setting.* Abstract of the 40th clinical meeting of ACOG, Las Vegas.

Townsend DE *et al.*, (1990) 'Rollerball' coagulation of the endometrium. *Obstet. Gynecol.* 76: 310.

Vancaillie TG (1989) Electrocoagulation of the endometrium with ball end resectoscope (Rollerball). *Obstet. Gynecol.* 74: 425.

Vasilev S *et al.*, (1988) Serum CA125 levels in preoperative evaluation of pelvic masses. *Obstet. Gyne.* 71: 751–756.

9

Vascular Surgery

FRANK CROSS

Introduction

If it can be said that there are fashions in surgery, then this certainly applies to the introduction and subsequent abandoning of various devices designed to open blocked blood vessels by the percutaneous route. This chapter outlines the history of minimal access vascular surgery, and describes the use of some of the many devices now currently available for helping the surgeon and radiologist to avoid operating on the patient. All of these devices have been tested and used clinically in the peripheral circulation. However, some are now primarily used in the coronary vessels, and consequently a description of coronary work is occasionally included in this chapter, which otherwise principally addresses peripheral vascular disease. No particular directions are given in the practical use of these devices, as almost all of them are experimental and not widely used.

Percutaneous vascular access

The majority of percutaneous vascular procedures performed today, whether diagnostic or interventional, rely on the Seldinger technique (Seldinger, 1953) for access to the arterial or venous circulation. The underlying principle is the placement of a guidewire in the circulation via an easily accessible peripheral vessel such as the femoral artery. The wire is steered into the affected part of the circulation, and either a diagnostic catheter or a therapeutic device can then be placed at the target over the wire. The lumen of the artery chosen for access, is first entered with a hollow needle, through which a guidewire is threaded. The needle is then withdrawn and a series of graduated dilators are then passed, until the arteriotomy is large enough to admit a soft plastic sheath, which is closed with a punctured rubber bung through which devices can be placed. The great advantage of the technique is that it provides watertight access to the circulation, and devices can be exchanged without submitting the blood vessel wall to further trauma.

Investigative techniques

Advances in investigative techniques have paralleled the introduction of minimal access vascular techniques, and have actually made some of them possible. Investigations have become progressively less invasive as technological improvements have made more information available to the surgeon.

Advances in radiological techniques

Improved radiological imaging techniques such as biplanar screening are designed to enhance catheter localization, particularly during coronary procedures, and charge-coupled device (CCD) technology improves picture resolution and reduces the dose of ionizing radiation to the patient. In addition, the more recent provision of digital subtraction angiography (DSA) techniques allow the procurement of high quality arteriograms with much smaller doses of contrast medium, which may even be given intravenously where fine detail is not required, such as for graft surveillance (Harries *et al.*, 1991).

Angioscopy

The angioscope has been under development for 50 years, but it is only in the last three years that useful devices have been marketed. Improvements in fibre-optic technology have made this possible. The main uses for the device include the inspection of anastomoses and balloon dilatation sites (Mehigan and Olcott, 1986; White *et al.*, 1990), and the interior of *in-situ* vein grafts (Seeger and Abela, 1986; Fleisher *et al.*, 1986). Indeed, identification of patent venous tributaries and their subsequent closure with wire coils via the angioscope (Stierli and Aeberhard, 1991), can be said to be one of the few truly minimal access vascular procedures. Alternatively, the tributaries can be tied through small incisions made over the percutaneous transillumination from the 'scope at the site of the identified tributary.

Recently introduced disposable fibre-optic balloon catheters of 4.3 French diameter allow inspection of the coronary arteries after balloon or laser angioplasty to exclude intimal flaps, and this device has recently been used in 24 patients to determine the cause of recent coronary artery occlusion, together with post angioplasty inspection (Ramee *et al.*, 1991; White *et al.*, 1991). The main drawbacks of the technique are interruption of the blood flow by balloon inflation, and fluid overload associated with the flushing of saline to improve visualization. However, these problems have largely been overcome by video angioscopy, where a short flush of saline is followed by a video recording, which can then be studied at leisure. Angioscopy has not proved to be particularly useful as a guidance system for laser angioplasty, since the system only shows the operator where the catheter tip is, not where it is going.

Duplex ultrasound imaging

Real-time flow measurements combined with vessel imaging by pulsed colour-coded Doppler ultrasound, have made the selection of patients for angioplasty and the peroperative monitoring of angioplasty techniques possible. In a group of 134 patients with peripheral vascular disease, 110 were investigated by duplex alone, and 60 of these went on to arteriography. The outcome of balloon angioplasty was the same in both groups (Edwards et al., 1991). The diagnosis and treatment of arteria profunda femoris stenoses by balloon angioplasty has also been monitored by duplex in 103 patients (Strauss et al., 1991), and the peak flows in the stenoses, measured before and after the procedures, to confirm a satisfactory result.

Intravascular ultrasound

Imaging the blood vessel to be treated from within the lumen is a recent development, and there is much promise in the ability of ultrasound to identify plaque and its position in the vessel wall. There are two ways of doing it. The first consists of a conventional ultrasound probe mounted within a catheter. This produces readily identifiable images (Aretz et al., 1990), and computer generated three-dimensional imaging is possible. The device has been used to search for residual atheroma after coronary angioplasty in 27 patients (Tobis et al., 1991), and was shown to be capable of finding atheroma in areas where the arteriogram was normal. Werner et al., (1991a) have demonstrated the presence of plaque fissuring and flap formation in balloon dilated coronary arteries in 11 out of 14 cases. It can also be used intraoperatively to assess the quality of femoropopliteal vein grafts (The et al., 1991). The clinical benefits of this kind of imaging have not yet been demonstrated, but data is accruing in a number of centres. The current drawback is that the devices are quite bulky and produce a radial scan without much information distal to the catheter tip.

The second method relies on the acoustic shockwave from a laser pulse to produce an image in conjunction with a detector at the catheter tip (Bhatta et al., 1989). If the many problems associated with this method can be overcome, a small and manoeuvreable device will result. It has been used to produce acoustic signals which will differentiate between normal vessel wall and plaque, but no direct images have so far been obtained, and it is still at the experimental stage. Such a device would be a great advance, used in combination with some way of directing the laser fibre at the identified atheroma.

Therapeutic techniques

Intraluminal dilatation

The suggestion that arterial lesions could be dilated either percutaneously or intraoperatively, thus avoiding either direct surgery to the stenosing lesion or a bypass procedure, was first made by Charles Dotter (Dotter and Judkins, 1964). Dotter's balloon devices worked reasonably well for short lesions in the superficial femoral artery, but the catheter suffered from materials deficiencies and could not be made small enough or rugged enough to be effective percutaneously. It was nearly 10 years before the required modification was made to allow this technique to become more useful.

Balloon angioplasty

A percutaneously introduced double-lumen balloon catheter, which could be placed within an arterial stenosis over a wire, and then inflated to dilate the lesion, was first demonstrated by the Swiss physician Andreas Grüntzig (Grüntzig and Hopff, 1974). He presented his first five year follow-up (Grüntzig and Kumpe, 1979) at about the same time as his announcement of the first few coronary balloon angioplasty patients. Long-term follow-up on these patients was published in 1983 (Grüntzig and Meier, 1983).

Balloon angioplasty is supreme in the iliac vessels, where primary recanalization rates are good and long-term patency is high (Cumberland, 1983). Careful application of this technique can reduce the need for aortoiliac surgery (Davies et al., 1990; Walker et al., 1991). Whilst a great deal of effort has gone into laser and other recanalization methods, there have been steady advances in balloon catheter design. These have resulted in an improvement in the results from balloon angioplasty of total occlusions, both in the peripheral and coronary vessels. For example, in a recent series (Morgenstern et al., 1989) of 70 patients undergoing balloon angioplasty for total SFA occlusions varying from 1–10 cm in length, the primary success rate was 94%, compared with a previous figure of 74% from the same group (Martin et al., 1981). This compares very favourably with extant laser angioplasty series. These figures are reflected in other recent papers on coronary angioplasty for occlusion. There was little improvement in the primary success rate of around 50% between 1983 and 1987 (Meier, 1989), but figures are now beginning to improve, and this is attributed to improvements in balloon and guidewire design, such as the introduction of ultra low profile 'balloon-on-a-wire' probe devices. In small series of coronary lesions, these have been shown to bring the primary success rate in stenoses up to nearly 70% (Little et al., 1989), and in occlusions up to 53% (Hamm et al., 1990). There is no doubt that, whatever the improvements in balloon and guidewire technology, the long (more than 10 cm) femoral artery occlusion remains a problem, both in terms of primary success rates and reocclusion figures. The improvement in this area is not so good – only 25% patency at three years in occlusions, with one or no patent calf vessels (Jeans et al., 1990). Results in the crural vessels are even more dismal, but recent work with the low-profile probes suggests that a primary success rate of 96% can be achieved, although no follow-up figures are reported (Horvath *et al.*, 1990). Schwarten (1991) has shown that the results from tibial artery dilatation are as good as for femorodistal bypass, but that only 20–30% of such patients are suitable for balloon angioplasty.

Disease elsewhere in the body is becoming amenable to balloon angioplasty. Results have been reported in the treatment of renovascular disease (Schwarten, 1980; Englund and Brown, 1991), visceral disease (Levy *et al.*, 1987), subclavian stenosis or occlusion (Nicholson *et al.*, 1991) and other upper limb vessels (Insall *et al.*, 1990). Case reports are beginning to appear of carotid balloon angioplasty (Theron *et al.*, 1990), and the technique can be applied to venous disorders such as inferior vena cava obstruction (Sato *et al.*, 1990).

Other catheter-based interventions

Interventional radiological techniques also include embolization of blood vessels to control bleeding or to reduce tumour size preoperatively, and catheter placement for the administration of intra-arterial drug therapy. These techniques are dealt with elsewhere (Sutton, 1987).

Thrombolysis has been attempted for years, but has only recently become an established technique. Thrombolytic enzymes such as streptokinase, urokinase or tissue plasminogen activators can be used to clear a recently thrombosed vessel (Barr *et al.*, 1991; Dawson *et al.*, 1991). The drug is delivered as closely to the point of thrombosis as possible by catheter; it is important to remember that the vessel has nearly always thrombosed as a result of poor flow, so that the stenosing lesion must be dealt with at the same time or else the vessel will reocclude (Scott *et al.*, 1991).

Thrombolysis is important in the early therapy of acute myocardial infarction, and is often now given to such patients before their arrival in hospital by ambulance paramedics (Collins and Julian, 1991).

Laser angioplasty

This novel method for clearing arteries was first suggested in 1963 (McGuff *et al.*), but its immediate application was limited by shortcomings in fibre-optic and catheter technology, so it was not until 1984 (Ginsburg *et al.*) that case reports began to appear. A number of different lasers have been used. Continuous wave lasers are the most widespread, but suffer from the problem of causing distant tissue damage. Pulsed lasers produce less damage, because the tissue cools down between pulses and more of the laser energy is used to vaporize the tissue with each high powered pulse (Cross and Bowker, 1987). Thermal laser angioplasty can be carried out by mounting a metal tip on the end of the catheter, which heats up and melts its way through the tissue. A bare optical fibre causes perforation of the vessel wall and modified fibretips or multifibre over-the-wire ring catheters can overcome this problem.

Continuous wave systems

Argon ion

The light from an argon laser is blue-green and is well absorbed in the tissue. Its clinical use has been restricted to two modified systems. The first of these uses a multifibre shielded catheter (Strikwerda et al., 1986; Richards-Kortum et al., 1989). The laser light is shone down the fibres and a low power spectroscopic identification beam first identifies plaque by spectroscopic means. The argon ablation only fires when the probe tip is in contact with atheroma. The second system uses a single optical fibre which is centred inside the vessel within a balloon catheter, and which has a distal lens assembly which defocuses the beam to increase the area over which tissue ablation takes place (Nordstrom et al., 1988). Presented results (Nordstrom et al., 1989) show that in 33 SFA occlusions the initial success rate was 90%, but the restenosis rate was 29%, with a maximum follow-up of one year, and complications occurred in one third of cases. Some recent work has shown that, whilst fatty streaks absorb argon laser light better than normal vessel wall, fibrous white plaque is more resistant to ablation than normal tissue (Torres et al., 1990). Since most occlusions involve white fibrous plaque, this suggests that the argon ion laser may not be as safe or effective for laser angioplasty as was originally thought. Nevertheless, clinical work continues to be published.

Nd:YAG

Light from the Nd:YAG laser is in the near infrared and is very poorly absorbed in tissue. The first laser angioplasty to be reported from Europe was carried out using the continuous wave Nd:YAG and bare fibre delivery (Geschwind et al., 1984), but this is not a viable delivery system and only one group in Europe now seems to be using it (Neubauer et al., 1988). A 400 or 600 μm bare fibre is introduced into the vessels, using a double lumen rounded end catheter, containing both the optical fibre and a guidewire. The optical fibre is not allowed to protrude beyond the end. This system has been used in 132 SFA stenoses and occlusions with a 100% recanalization rate and 1.5% perforation rate. The mean stenosis was reduced from 87% to 54% without balloon angioplasty, and this is probably not enough to maintain adequate flow in the SFA. Late patency rates are not stated.

The majority of centres using continuous wave Nd:YAG laser light deliver it through artificial sapphire fibretips. Recent work has shown these actually to be made of quartz (Verdaasdonk et al., 1990a). They have a scattering surface which allows them to heat up in use, and this increases their efficiency, especially if they become contaminated with blood products (Verdaasdonk et al., 1990b). Although a number of groups have clinical experience with these devices (Fourrier et al., 1988; Wilms et al., 1990), the major experience comes from Austria. No series have been reported from the USA since the Food and Drug Administration (FDA) does not allow the use of a non-disposable device in the circulation. In a preliminary comparison of the sapphire with the hot tip in 88 patients (Lammer et al., 1988), the recanalization rate was 82%

with the sapphire and 78% with the hot tip. However, the perforation rate with the sapphire (8%) was significantly lower than that for the hot tip (14%), and the former was therefore selected for further work. Of 33 SFA occlusions or tight stenoses treated with the Nd:YAG laser and sapphire tips in a longitudinal series (Pilger *et al.*, 1988), 89% were open at 24 hours. Two vessels subsequently reoccluded at 48 hours and there was one late reocclusion at six months, the maximum extent of the follow-up at that time. A cumulative follow-up at three years shows an overall patency rate of 63% in the successful cases, but of 167 procedures attempted, 35 failed primarily (Pilger *et al.*, 1991).

Carbon dioxide (CO₂)

The CO_2 laser emits in the mid-infrared. It clearly ablates vascular tissue quite efficiently in pigs (Van Stiegmann *et al.*, 1984), but has not been a contender for laser angioplasty, because the light is not transmissible down quartz fibres. Silver halide fibres do exist, and they have been used clinically (Eldar *et al.*, 1986), but they are brittle and expensive, and tend to discolour in use. Their protagonists are optimistic (Gal and Katzir, 1987), but a commercially viable system is still awaited.

Pulsed systems

Pulsed Nd:YAG

Three groups have used the pulsed Nd:YAG clinically, two with sapphire fibretips and one with a ball-tipped device. Michaels *et al.*, (1989a) treated 40 superficial femoral artery occlusions in 34 limbs with an initial success rate of 67%, and a two-year follow-up patency of 53%. In Czechoslovakia (Kvasnicka *et al.*, 1991), a 100 µs pulsed Nd:YAG laser has been used with sapphire fibretips to recanalize 30 lesions in 22 patients. Lesions were in four sites in the leg. The procedure was successful in 67% cases, and was followed by balloon dilatation. The ankle/brachial pressure index rose significantly. There were no reocclusions at six months. Another group (White *et al.*, 1990) using the Lumonics pulsed Nd:YAG laser with a new ball-tipped device (Michaels *et al.*, 1989b) in 10 patients with SFA occlusions, produced satisfactory recanalization and objective improvement in symptoms in nine of them, with subsequent balloon angioplasty.

Pulsed infrared gas and solid state lasers

A whole range of lasers operating in the infrared region between 1.06 µm and 10.6 µm have been assessed for possible use in laser angioplasty. The best of these appear to be variants of the Nd:YAG laser using different elements, as the laser medium now compete with these systems. In particular, the Holmium:YAG laser at 2.01 µm and the Erbium:YAG laser at 2.94 µm are being looked at as possible lasers for angioplasty. The attraction is the target chromophore, which is tissue water. This absorbs the light from these lasers very strongly. There is very little published on the use of the Ho:YAG in laser angioplasty. The laser is pulsed with a low repetition rate and quite a high pulse energy. Some work (Oz et al., 1989) has shown that this laser is capable of making holes in calcified atheroma in vitro, and that each pulse ablated a consistent amount of tissue. Healing studies in the rabbit aorta showed marked similarities with the healing response to CO_2 laser light. The Ho:YAG has also been shown to be capable of vaporizing cardiac valve calcium (Lilge et al., 1989), without causing significant surrounding tissue damage. Clinical coronary trials with the Ho:YAG are in progress in some parts of Europe, and the early results of one of these (Geschwind et al., 1991), using a multifibre device in 23 patients with coronary stenosis or occlusion, shows an initial success rate in 20, with subsequent balloon dilatation being required in 17, one abrupt closure at 24 hours and no other complications.

Pulsed dye

There is preferential absorption of light in atheroma in the region 425–550 nm, due to the presence of carotenes (Prince et al., 1986), and this wavelength 'window' is easily matched by the pulsed dye at 504 nm in the blue. This effect is mitigated by the presence of blood (Gregory et al., 1990). The suggestion that carotenes given as a dietary supplement may enhance selective ablation still further has been demonstrated clinically (LaMuraglia et al., 1989), but does not seem to have been taken up therapeutically. The clinical use of the pulsed dye laser has largely been tied up with the use of spectral identification of plaque, and this is dealt with below. Murray et al., (1989) have used this laser to treat SFA occlusions without a 'smart' guidance system, but have markedly improved their initial success rate by introducing the ball-tipped fibres at an arterial cut-down, rather than percutaneously. This means that flush origin occlusions of the SFA can be dealt with, and the results show an improved primary recanalization rate over percutaneous techniques. Latest results (Mitchell et al., 1992) in 78 superficial femoral artery occlusions, causing rest pain or severe claudication in 71 patients, suggest a primary technical success rate of 74%, with clinical improvement in 59%. One year cumulative patency in the technical success group was 45%. Another series presented by a surgeon (Veith et al., 1991) showed that out of 415 lower limb arteriograms, 94 patients responded to conventional balloon angioplasty treatment, 218 patients were not suitable for either balloon or laser angioplasty and underwent a bypass procedure, and only 11 patients were both suitable for and underwent a laser angioplasty; three of these vessels were closed within six months, and all had long occlusions of the femoral artery. This kind of comprehensive audit perhaps puts laser angioplasty in a more realistic perspective, and the figures are confirmed elsewhere in relation to balloon angioplasty (Holm et al., 1991).

Excimer

The Excimer laser emits in the ultraviolet. It produces extraordinarily sharp craters in tissue (Grundfest et al., 1985; Isner et al., 1985; Bowker et al., 1986), and this is probably due to the short pulse length and high tissue absorption. Fibre-optic transmission is a problem, and clinical use of the Excimer laser therefore depends on the combination of a long pulse length and a relatively long wavelength, focused down a multifibre catheter which contains a guidewire.

The first clinical trials of the Excimer were in peripheral arteries. One of these (Litvack *et al.*, 1989) showed a recanalization rate of 77% in 31 patients with SFA occlusion and stenoses, using the long pulse Excimer and multifibre over-the-wire catheter. Subsequent balloon angioplasty was carried out in 28 patients. The restenosis rate at nine months was 29%. The system quickly moved to the coronary arteries, where the same authors conducted a large multicentre clinical series on coronary artery stenoses (Goldenburg *et al.*, 1990). This is an over-the-wire system and so it will not address anything other than stenoses or very short occlusions. The trial as presented in January 1990 outlined results in 210 cases, with treatment of 228 stenoses and 27 occlusions. A successful result was defined as an increase of 25% in the lesion diameter. The initial success rate was 85% and balloon angioplasty was subsequently used in 66% of the successful cases. Complications were few. Similar results have been presented from groups in Germany (Werner *et al.*, 1991b) and the USA (Sanborn *et al.*, 1991) using similar devices. No controlled trials have been performed, and the long-term results are no better than balloon angioplasty with a similar restenosis rate. There has been a suggestion that the device may not always reach the energy threshold required for tissue ablation, and may be working as a simple dilatation catheter (Ischinger *et al.*, 1990a).

Laser thermal angioplasty

The so-called 'hot tip' device was the first to gain widespread use, following the disappointing clinical results seen with the argon laser/bare fibre combination in two centres (Ginsburg *et al.*, 1985; Cumberland *et al.*, 1986). A small metal probe made of nickel steel is crimped on to the end of the optical fibre and all the laser light is absorbed by the tip and turned into heat. No laser light therefore reaches the tissue.

The choice of laser, although confined to continuous wave devices, is less critical in this application. The early use of the argon laser soon gave way to the much more reliable solid state continuous wave Nd:YAG. Experimental work has shown beyond reasonable doubt that the hot tip reaches unacceptably high temperatures in blood (Verdaasdonk, 1987), that a considerable amount of particulate debris enters the circulation during their use (Keogh *et al.*, 1989), and that their clinical use in the coronary arteries seems to lead to ECG and enzyme changes (Cumberland *et al.*, 1986). There is an isolated case report of distal embolus due to thermal damage (Delcour *et al.*, 1990).

Nevertheless, the device is installed in a number of centres, many of which have reported results (Fletcher *et al.*, 1989; Enge *et al.*, 1988; White *et al.*, 1989a; Fleisher *et al.*, 1987) not dissimilar to those of Cumberland, always allowing for differences in analysis of results. Only one controlled trial of the device has been performed (Jeans *et al.*, 1989), comparing laser with balloon.

Recanalization rates in the laser group were the same as in the balloon only group. Current opinion leads away from this device (Greenfield, 1991).

Alternative research lies with the Spectraprobe, which is a hybrid probe incorporating a small sapphire window, which lets about 20% of the laser light through to interact directly with the tissue. Like the original 'hot tip', this device may be used with either the argon or Nd:YAG laser. Use is fairly widespread, but work from two centres in particular is interesting. In the first, the device is used in critically ischaemic limbs in patients who would otherwise not be suitable for surgery (Seeger et al., 1990). Seventeen patients were treated; 13 had angina or were unsuitable for surgery because of various other reasons, and four had severe infrapopliteal disease. The laser probe was introduced percutaneously in seven patients, and via a cut-down in the remainder. Laser recanalization was successful in nine patients. None of the patients who underwent infrapopliteal laser recanalization improved. Surgery was attempted in five of the eight laser failures but was only successful in two of these. Four of the nine successful cases had angiographic evidence of restenosis at one year, but had not developed symptoms. Seeger's conclusion is that even in severe disease the laser can help to salvage limbs, but if the disease is infrapopliteal, the prospects are grim. In Sheffield (Belli et al., 1990), the device was first demonstrated to be safe and effective in the recanalization of 37 iliac or SFA occlusions, with a primary success rate of 81%, and a randomized trial is now in progress between balloon angioplasty alone and spectraprobe laser angioplasty for SFA occlusions. Coronary laser angioplasty has been attempted with this device (Rosenthal et al., 1988), but current coronary therapy also now lies elsewhere.

Other laser applications

Spectroscopic guidance for laser angioplasty

A number of attempts to improve the results from laser angioplasty by localizing atheromatous disease by spectroscopic techniques have been made. Human tissue can be made to fluoresce under irradiation from ultraviolet or short wavelength visible light, and this fluorescence can be detected by light sensitive diodes and analysed using multichannel devices. Different kinds of tissue produce a different fluorescence signal, and the difference in the signals obtained from normal vessel wall and atheroma can form the basis of a fluorescence guided system, or 'smart' laser. One such system (now unavailable for commercial reasons) uses a He:Cd laser (325 nm) as a probe and a pulsed dye laser for ablation. A probing pulse is initially sent down the laser fibre when the distal end is in contact with the occlusion. The return fluorescence is analysed and, if the spectrum suggests atheroma, an ablation pulse is transmitted. If normal tissue is identified, the laser is prevented from firing. An automatic computer-controlled system based on this principle has been in use for some time, but the results have not been as good as was hoped. Initial work was promising (Leon et al., 1990), achieving recanalization in 85% of SFA occlusions, the failures being in calcified lesions. Similar work carried out in France by Geschwind (1991) in 66 patients with femoropopliteal occlusions not amenable to conventional treatment, reveal an 83% initial success rate but there were seven immediate occlusions and eight perforations. This last figure is of major concern, as the laser is supposed to switch itself off if normal arterial wall is encountered. These results show that the complication rate with this 'smart' system is surprisingly high, and that there is clearly much more work to do before a safe laser angioplasty system, based on spectroscopic identification of plaque, becomes widely available.

Similar systems based on Excimer lasers, where the probe pulse is a low energy pulse from the same laser which then ablates at a much higher energy, are being investigated. Early *in vitro* work is promising (Laufer *et al.*, 1988), and clinical results are awaited.

Hot balloon

The concept of laser balloon angioplasty was first suggested by Spears (Hiehle *et al.*, 1985; Spears *et al.*, 1988). It is a completely different therapeutic modality from laser angioplasty, aimed at preventing restenosis after conventional balloon angioplasty. Instead of using laser light to vaporize tissue, it is used diffusely, shone through the expanded dilating balloon in the coronary artery, to weld the intima in place, preventing flap formation and, it is hoped, reducing restenosis, which is currently running at 30% at six months after conventional angioplasty. One such device is the subject of a multicentre trial which is reported from time to time, and a randomized clinical trial in the coronary arteries, with 200 patients entered at present, is in progress. The device appears to be useful where conventional PTCA has failed because of restenosis or flap formation (Jenkins *et al.*, 1990). It may also be used for the treatment of coronary spasm (Bowker *et al.*, 1990). The desired end-point is a reduction in coronary restenosis and this result is awaited. A similar system, with thermal feedback control, is in use in Germany (Ischinger *et al.*, 1990b). All the evidence points to no improvement in restenosis rates at all over conventional balloon angioplasty (Reis *et al.*, 1991). Radiofrequency heated balloons as an alternative to laser devices are under development.

Laser welding

The use of a laser beam to assist in microvascular anastomosis by tissue welding has been extensively investigated. The process seems to work by the welding of collagen in the vessel wall (Schober *et al.*, 1986), and healing at the join is relatively uncomplicated. It is important not to let tissue temperatures rise to the point where vaporization occurs. Early work in rat femoral arteries (Neblett *et al.*, 1986) using a milliwatt CO_2 laser to carry out end-to-end anastomoses, with sutured anastomoses as a control, showed the procedure to be feasible with a patency rate of 95% and good weld strength at 21 days. Aneurysm formation was observed in 7% of the laser group against 11% in the controls. The use of tissue staining, with indocyanine green stained fibrinogen, seems to increase the weld strength immediately after the procedure when a semiconductor laser is used. The use of chromophores also seems to enhance the weld strength for the Nd:YAG laser (Brooks *et al.*, 1990). Finally, the argon laser has been used clinically to fashion Cimino fistulae in 10 renal failure patients (White *et al.*, 1989b). The radial artery and vein were opened and brought together with four stay sutures, and the edges then welded together with 0.5 W. The procedure is limited by the length of weld which is possible – currently about 5 mm. All anastomoses were satisfactory and no aneurysms were reported at up to 20 months.

Endocardial ablation

The use of a catheter to ablate abnormal cardiac conduction pathways, instead of dysrhythmia surgery, is attractive. Endocardial mapping at open surgery departs from the physiological situation, and closed methods may well be more accurate. This can be achieved either electrically or with a laser. There are a number of experimental techniques in both fields and the procedures, at least experimentally, are not without hazard (Bogen *et al.*, 1987). As far as the laser is concerned, heat is used to destroy conducting pathways and this can either be applied by direct laser irradiation using the Nd:YAG (Weber *et al.*, 1990) or argon laser, with the hot tip (Rosenthal *et al.*, 1989), or indirectly by a hot balloon (Schuger *et al.*, 1990) in the coronary sinus. Early clinical results are now becoming available (Geschwind *et al.*, 1990).

Mechanical recanalization devices

Atherectomy

The Simpson atherectomy catheter (Simpson *et al.*, 1985) is similar to a Crosby capsule. The catheter has at its distal end a metal tube with a window down the full length of one side. A rotating cutter (2000 rpm) can be moved down the window. When the device is in place within a stenosis, a balloon on the opposite side of the window is inflated, and atheroma is pressed into the tube. The rotating knife is then advanced, and the atheroma is sliced off and held within the tube. The catheter is withdrawn after three or four passes and the tube emptied. The procedure is often referred to as directional atherectomy. There is fairly extensive experience with this device. Belli and Cumberland (1989) used it in 14 SFA stenoses or occlusions of less than 1 cm in length. All lesions were successfully negotiated and cleared, with a mean reduction in stenosis from 88% to 15%. It will deal with hard or calcified lesions. Follow-up was limited to a mean of nine months with one recurrence. Simpson himself reported a series of 41 lesions treated in 21 patients (Höfling *et al.*, 1988). Five of these were iliac, 35 in the SFA and one in the popliteal artery. Only four lesions were totally occluded. All but three of the lesions were successfully treated, with a significant reduction in stenosis and consequent improvement in walking distance. Follow-up is short at six months with one recurrence successfully retreated. In a much larger series (Dorros *et al.*, 1989) of 195 lesions treated in 131 patients, the device worked in 98% of the 139 stenoses and all of the 56 occlusions, which had a mean length of 10.5 cm. 99 of the lesions underwent subsequent balloon angioplasty. Complications included local thrombosis and distal embolus, but no patient was made worse. Again, follow-up was short but recurrence rates low.

Atherectomy is also used in the coronary arteries where preliminary results are good (Kaufmann *et al.*, 1989), but restenosis rates approach 50% at one year (Garratt *et al.*, 1990). The device is somewhat limited in that it is very rigid, and is best applied to stenoses rather than occlusions (Hinohara *et al.*, 1991; Maynar *et al.*, 1990). It is very useful from a morphological point of view, in that it provides histological specimens of atheroma.

Drills

These devices are properly known as rotational angioplasty devices. They drill their way through atheromatous plaque leaving a channel which can then be balloon dilated. The best known of these is the Kensey catheter (Kensey *et al.*, 1987) which rotates at a high speed, breaking down the plaque into an emulsion which can be dispersed in the distal circulation without danger of distal embolization. A catheter is introduced into the occluded vessel. The bevelled metal tip is made to rotate at 80 000 rpm with a saline flush to prevent frictional heating, and the debris is reduced to particles of 10–20 μm in diameter. The device is supposed to remove hard material and leave soft vessel wall untouched, much like a plaster saw. Early clinical results were promising, with peripheral recanalization rates of up to 85% (Desbrosses *et al.*, 1990), but restenosis rates are fairly high. In addition, there is a case report (Wholey *et al.*, 1989) of intractable distal thrombosis after the use of the device in the SFA, which led to a below knee amputation. Results in the coronary vessels are becoming available (Bertrand *et al.*, 1990), and the incidence of acute occlusion with myocardial infarction is about 6% of lesions treated. A similar rotational device has been used in Germany (Steckmeier *et al.*, 1989) to recanalize seven out of 10 SFA occlusions successfully. The use of an embolectomy catheter to remove particulate debris, immediately before patency is finally achieved, is recommended. Angioscopic examination of recanalized vessels shows a very high intimal flap formation rate (Gehani *et al.*, 1990).

There are at least two similar devices which rotate at much lower speeds to produce the same result; one of these (Vallbracht *et al.*, 1989), which rotates at 1–200 rpm, has been used in 83 patients with arterial occlusions. The aim is for the device to remove soft material selectively, making a channel through which a balloon can be passed to deal with the hard material. 56 patients had SFA occlusions, 21 had popliteal disease and six had occluded iliac vessels. The device is used with heparin and urokinase infusion. In the SFA, 20 out of 21 lesions of less than 10 cm length were opened, and 29 out of 39 longer than 10 cm. This represents an overall recanalization rate of 80%. There were six dissections and one embolization.

Transluminal extraction devices are designed to break up the plaque and remove it by suction. A double-bladed cutter at the tip of a 7 or 9 French catheter rotates at 700 rpm, drilling its way through the atheromatous occlusion. Debris is removed by applying suction down the catheter to the tip. Wholey *et al.*, (1989), in a series of 126 lesions in 95 patients, report a 95% success rate in the SFA, with a 90% clinical improvement rate. The concomitant use of urokinase with this device, in patients with a previous failed angioplasty, is also reported (Starck and Wagner, 1991), with a primary success rate of 96%. These devices are not by any means in widespread use and there is little long-term follow-up.

Non-laser thermal devices

If a heated metal device will recanalize arteries, it may not need to be heated up by a laser to be effective, and a number of devices were quickly announced which were variously heated by catalyst-stimulated chemical reaction (Lu *et al.*, 1987), electrical heating (Lu *et al.*, 1986) or radio-frequency heating. These suffer from the same problems as the laser hot tip, in that to be effective they need to reach high temperatures which is difficult to achieve in a non-bulky device. There is also the problem of particulate embolization. Some work on the radio-frequency heated tip (Verdaasdonk *et al.*, 1990c) suggests that it does not reach a high enough temperature to produce tissue ablation. None of these devices are in widespread clinical use.

Ultrasonic ablation

Ultrasonic disruption of atheroma is possible using a high-powered ultrasonic transmitter at the tip of a catheter. The device generates ultrasound at 20 KHz at a power output of up to 25 W cm^{-2}, and has been shown to be effective in recanalizing atheromatous, totally occluded femoral vessels *in vitro* (Rosenschien *et al.*, 1991), and stenosed vessels *in vivo* (Siegel *et al.*, 1990), but it is too early to say whether this is a viable treatment option.

Intraluminal stents

Stents are designed as a metal latticework which is introduced into a stenosis on the end of a catheter. Once open, they are intended to hold a ballooned stenosis or occlusion open, thus reducing the restenosis rate (Sigwart, 1990). They are of two types – self-expandable and balloon-expandable. The first type springs open under its own tension when released, and the second requires the inflation of a balloon for proper deployment. There has been quite extensive clinical use of both types. Animal experiments have suggested that immediate thrombosis is a likely complication unless anticoagulation is used (van der Giessen *et al.*, 1990). Preliminary results of a multicentre study using the Palmaz-Schatz balloon-expandable stent in the coronary arteries in 226 patients show that anticoagulation does prevent early closure, and that the restenosis rate at six months in this group is acceptable (Schatz *et al.*, 1991). Results from the placement of 117 intracoronary metal self-expanding stents (Serruys *et al.*, 1991) were less encouraging, with an early reocclusion rate of 25%. The coating of stents with anticoagulant drugs, or even endothelial cells, to prevent the rather high restenosis rate, has been suggested (Pompa and Ellis, 1990). Stents have also been used in the iliac vessels (Sikrit *et al.*, 1991), the portal vein (Lopez *et al.*, 1991) and even the urethra (Sarramon *et al.*, 1990).

The advent of the stent may make the treatment of simple small infrarenal aortic aneurysms which have not yet leaked, a percutaneous possibility. Early work has shown that it is quite possible to stent the abdominal aorta following balloon angioplasty (el Ashmaoui *et al.*, 1991), and the stenting of aortic dissections and aneurysms is already being undertaken in some centres (Yoshida *et al.*, 1991). The limiting factor for these stents appears, at the moment, to be the inability to make a stent which is strong enough to contain an aneurysm when expanded to the large diameter required, whilst still making it small enough when closed to be safely introduced percutaneously. This is unlikely to remain a problem for very long.

Conclusions

There are many new devices in experimental use for angioplasty as an alternative to open surgery in both peripheral and coronary vascular surgery. It is probably true to say that none of these has been shown to be safe, effective and reliable, with the possible exception of balloon angioplasty. In particular, a major dearth of controlled clinical trials has prevented the clear delineation of their place in therapeutic angiology. None of these devices can be recommended for widespread routine use until the results of such trials have become available. The future of minimal access vascular surgery probably lies in a combination of a recanalization device and a drug to prevent restenosis. A number of these are now under early evaluation (Lungergan *et al.*, 1991; Lindner and Reidy, 1991; Sahni, 1991). Endoluminal treatment of aneurysms is an exciting possibility, and the endoluminal preparation of the long saphenous vein for *in-situ* grafting is an important advance. Already the introduction of non-sutured grafts for abdominal aortic aneurysm repair is reducing the difficulty of this type of surgery (Harris, 1992). To date, no-one has yet suggested the laparoscopic approach for the management of the dilated or occluded abdominal aorta, but even this unlikely prospect merits serious attention when the range of organs already removed through the laparoscope is considered.

Physician accountability

There is a tendency in general surgery for minimal access techniques to pass into the province of the physician rather than the surgeon, and this can lead to obvious problems both in relation to patient selection and in the event of postoperative complications requiring surgery. This is particularly the case with vascular surgery. The patient should always be seen by the vascular surgeon who takes the decision to treat. The surgeon can then liaise with the radiologist, who can perform the percutaneous surgery at a time when the surgeon is available to co-operate and deal with any complication.

References

Aretz HT (1990) Intraluminal ultrasound guidance of transverse laser coronary atherectomy. *SPIE Vol 1201–Optical Fibers in Medicine*. 68–78.

Barr H *et al.*, (1991) Intra-arterial thrombolytic therapy in the management of acute and chronic limb ischaemia. *Br. J. Surg.* 78: 284–287.

Belli AM and Cumberland DC (1989) Percutaneous atherectomy–early experience in Sheffield. *Clin. Radiol.* 40: 122–126.

Belli AM *et al.*, (1990) Peripheral arterial occlusions: initial results from percutaneous angioplasty with a hybrid laser probe. *Radiology*. 174: 447–449.

Bertrand ME *et al.*, (1990) Percutaneous coronary rotary ablation. *Herz*. 15: 285–291.

Bhatta KM, Rosen DI and Dretler SP (1989) Acoustic and plasma-guided laser angioplasty. *Lasers Surg. Med.* 9: 117–123.

Bogen DK *et al.*, (1987) Is catheter ablation on target? *Am. J. Cardiol.* 60: 1387–1392.

Bowker TJ *et al.*, (1986) Excimer laser angioplasty. Quantitative comparison in vitro of three ultraviolet wavelengths on tissue ablation and haemolysis. *Lasers in Medical Science*. 1: 91–99.

Bowker TJ *et al.*, (1990) Clinical coronary laser balloon angioplasty: effect on ergonovine responsiveness. *SPIE Vol 1201–Optical Fibers in Medicine*. 87–94.

Brooks SG *et al.*, (1990) Laser welding for coronary artery anastomosis: techniques, temperature profiles and the role of chromophores. *SPIE Vol 1201–Optical Fibers in Medicine*. 99–105.

Cikrit DF *et al.*, (1991) Early experience with the Palmaz expandable intraluminal stent in iliac artery stenosis. *Ann. Vasc. Surg.* 5: 150–155.

Collins R and Julian DG (1991) British Heart Foundation surveys (1987 and 1989) of United Kingdom treatment policies for acute myocardial infarction. *Br. Heart J.* 66: 250–255.

Cross FW and Bowker TJ (1987) The physical properties of tissue ablation with Excimer lasers. *Medical Instrumentation*. 21: 226–230.

Cumberland DC (1983) Percutaneous transluminal angioplasty–a review. *Clin. Radiol.* 34: 25–38.

Cumberland DC, Tayler DI and Procter AE (1986) Laser-assisted percutaneous angioplasty: initial clinical experience in peripheral arteries. *Clin. Radiol.* 37: 423–428.

Davies AH *et al.*, (1990) Recent changes in the treatment of aortoiliac disease by the Oxford Regional Vascular Service. *Br. J. Surg.* **77**: 1129–1131.

Dawson KJ *et al.*, (1991) Results of a recently instituted programme of thrombolytic therapy in acute lower limb ischaemia. *Br. J. Surg.* **78**: 409–411.

Delcour C *et al.*, (1990) Embolization hazard of laser hot-tip catheters and coated guidewires. *Br. J. Radiol.* **63**: 76.

Debrosses D *et al.*, (1990) Percutaneous atherectomy with the Kensey catheter: early and midterm results in femoropopliteal occlusions unsuitable for conventional angioplasty. *Ann. Vasc. Surg.* **4**: 550–552.

Diethrich EB, Timbadia E and Bahadir I (1989) Applications and limitations of laser-assisted angioplasty. *Eur. J. Vasc. Surg.* **3**: 61–70.

Dorros G, Lewin RF, Sachdev N and Mathiak L (1989) Percutaneous atherectomy of occlusive peripheral vascular disease. *Cath. Cardiovasc. Diagn.* **18**: 1–6.

Dotter CT and Judkins MP (1964) Transluminal treatment of arteriosclerosis obstruction. Description of a new technic and a preliminary report of its application. *Circulation.* **30**: 654–670.

Edwards JM, Coldwell DM, Goldman ML and Strandness DE Jr (1991) The role of duplex scanning in the selection of patients for transluminal angioplasty. *J. Vasc. Surg.* **13**: 69–74.

el Ashmaoui A *et al.*, (1991) Angioplasty of the terminal aorta: follow-up of 20 patients treated by PTA or PTA with stents. *Eur. J. Radiol.* **13**: 113–117.

Eldar M *et al.*, (1986) The effects of varying lengths and powers of CO_2 laser pulses transmitted through an optical fiber on atherosclerotic plaques. *Clin. Cardiol.* **9**: 89–91.

Enge IP and Schilvold A (1988) Recanalization of occluded peripheral vessels by laser assisted PTA. *Ann. Radiol.* **31**: 74–76.

Englund R and Brown MA (1991) Renal angioplasty for renovascular disease: a reappraisal. *J. Cardiovasc. Surg. Torino.* **32**: 76–80.

Fleisher HL III *et al.*, (1986) Angioscopically monitored saphenous vein valvulotomy. *J. Vasc. Surg.* **4**: 315–320.

Fleisher HL *et al.*, (1987) Human percutaneous laser angioplasty. *Am. J. Surg.* **154**: 666–670.

Fletcher JP and Wonk KP (1989) Early experience with laser-assisted thermal angioplasty for peripheral vascular disease. *Med. J. Aust.* **151**: 372–379.

Fourrier JL *et al.*, (1988) Novelle méthode d'angioplastie laser par saphir de contactdes artères périphériques: résultats préliminaires. *Arch. Mal Ceour.* **81**: 253–258.

Gal D and Katzir A (1987) Silver halide optical fibers for medical applications. *IEEE J. Quantum Electron.* QE-23: 1827–1835.

Garratt KN *et al.*, (1990) Restenosis after directional coronary atherectomy: differences between primary atheromatous and restenosis lesions and influence of subintimal tissue resection. *J. Am. Coll. Cardiol.* 16: 1665–1671.

Gehani AA *et al.*, (1990) Experimental and clinical percutaneous angioscopy experience with dynamic angioplasty. *Angiology.* 41: 809–816.

Geschwind HJ *et al.*, (1984) Percutaneous transluminal laser angioplasty in man. *The Lancet.* 1: 844.

Geschwind H and Dubois-Rande JL (1990) Laser and arterial recanalization. *Rev. Prat.* 40 (26): 2448–2454.

Geschwind HJ *et al.*, (1991) Results and follow-up after percutaneous pulsed laser-assisted balloon angioplasty guided by spectroscopy. *Circulation.* 83: 787–796.

Geschwind HJ *et al.*, (1991) Percutaneous coronary mid-infrared laser angioplasty. *Am. Heart J.* 122: 552–558.

Ginsburg R *et al.*, (1984) Salvage of an ischemic limb by laser angioplasty: description of a new technique. *Clin. Cardiol.* 7: 54–58.

Ginsburg R *et al.*, (1985) Percutaneous transluminal laser angioplasty for treatment of peripheral vascular disease. *Radiology.* 156: 619–624.

Goldenburg T *et al.*, (1990) Percutaneous Excimer laser coronary angioplasty *SPIE Vol 1201–Optical Fibers in Medicine.* 190–194.

Greenfield AJ (1991) Hot tip laser. Results and complications. *Circulation.* 82 (2 Suppl): 194–196.

Gregory KW *et al.*, (1990) Effect of blood on the selective ablation of atherosclerotic plaque with a pulsed dye laser. *Lasers Surg. Med.* 10: 533–543.

Grundfest WS *et al.*, (1985) Pulsed ultraviolet lasers and the potential for safe laser angioplasty. *Am. J. Surg.* 150: 220–226.

Grüntzig AR and Hopff H (1974) Perkutane Rekanalisation chronischer arterieller Verschlusse mit einem neuen Dilationskatheter. Modifikation der Dotter-Technik. *Deutsche. Med. Wochenschr.* 99: 2505–2505.

Grüntzig A and Kumpe DA (1979) Technique of percutaneous transluminal angioplasty with the Grüntzig balloon catheter. *Am. J. Roentgenol.* 132: 547–552.

Grüntzig AR and Meier B (1983) Percutaneous transluminal coronary angioplasty. The first five years and the future. *Int. J. Cardiol.* 2: 319–323.

Hamm CW *et al.*, (1990) Recanalization of chronic, totally occluded coronary arteries by new angioplasty systems. *Am. J. Cardiol.* 66: 1459–1463.

Harries S et al., (1991) An evaluation of intravenous digital subtraction angiography in assessing lower limb ischaemia. Eur. J. Vasc. Surg. 5: 205–207.

Harris PL (1992) An intraluminal non-sutured graft for aortic aneurysm repairs. In: The cause and management of aneurysms, ed, Harris PL.

Hiehle JF Jr et al., (1985) Nd-YAG laser fusion of human atheromatous plaque – arterial wall separation in vitrol. Am. J. Cardiol. 56: 953–957.

Hinohara T et al., (1991) Effect of lesion characteristics on outcome of directional coronary atherectomy. J. Am. Coll. Cardiol. 17: 1112–1120.

Höfling B et al., (1988) Percutaneous removal of atheromatous plaques in peripheral arteries. The Lancet. 20: 384–386.

Holm J et al., (1991) Chronic lower limb ischaemia. A prospective randomized controlled study comprising the 1-year results of vascular surgery and percutaneous transluminal angioplasty (PTA). Eur. J. Vasc. Surg. 5: 517–522.

Horvath W, Oertl M and Haidinger D (1990) Percutaneous transluminal angioplasty of crural arteries. Radiology. 177: 565–569.

Insall RL et al., (1990) Percutaneous transluminal angioplasty of the innominate, subclavian and axillary arteries. Eur. J. Vasc. Surg. 4: 591–595.

Ischinger T et al., (1990a) Angioscopic findings after Excimer laser angioplasty: laser or 'Dotter' effects. Circulation. 82 (Suppl 3): 671.

Ischinger T et al., (1990b) Laser balloon angioplasty: technical realization and vascular tissue effects of a modified concept. Lasers Surg. Med. 10: 112–123.

Isner JM et al., (1985) The Excimer laser: gross, light microscope and ultrastructural analysis of potential advantages for use in laser therapy of cardiovascular disease. J. Am. Coll. Cardiol. 6: 1102–1109.

Jeans WD et al., (1990) Randomized trial of laser-assisted passage through occluded femoro-popliteal arteries. Br. J. Radiol. 63: 19–21.

Jeans WD et al., (1990) Fate of patients undergoing transluminal angioplasty for lower limb ischaemia. Radiology. 177: 559–564.

Jenkins RD and Spears JR (1990) Management of failed angioplasty with laser balloon angioplasty. SPIE Vol 1201–Optical Fibers in Medicine. 80–86.

Kaufmann UP et al., (1989) Safety and results of coronary atherectomy during the inital experience at Mayo clinic. Cathet. Cardiovasc. Diagn. 17: 66.

Kensey KR et al., (1987) Recanalization of obstructed arteries with a flexible, rotating tip catheter. Radiology. 165: 387–389.

Keogh Be et al., (1989) Intravascular delivery of laser energy with metal-capped optical fibres: the potential hazard of distal embolism. Am. Heart J. 118: 47–53.

Kvasnicka J et al., (1991) Percutaneous laser angioplasty with a pulsed Nd:YAG laser. Initial clinical experience and early follow-up. *Int. Angiol.* 10: 29–33.

Lammer J and Karnel F (1988) Percutaneous transluminal laser angioplasty with contact probes. *Radiology.* 168: 733–737.

LaMuraglia GM et al., (1989) Enhancing the carotenoid content of atherosclerotic plaque: implications for laser therapy. *J. Vasc. Surg.* 9: 563–567.

Laufer G et al., (1988) Excimer laser-induced simultaneous ablation and spectral identification of normal and atherosclerotic arterial tissue layers. *Circulation.* 78: 1031–1039.

Leon MB et al., (1990) Fluorescence-guided laser-assisted balloon angioplasty in patients with femoropopliteal occlusions. *Circulation.* 81: 143–155.

Levy PJ, Haskell L and Gordon RL (1987) Percutaneous transluminal angioplasty of splanchnic arteries: an alternative method to elective revascularisation in chronic visceral ischaemia. *Eur. J. Radiol.* 7: 239–242.

Lilge L, Radtke W and Nishioka N (1989) Pulsed holmium laser ablation of cardiac valves. *Lasers Surg. Med.* 9: 458–464.

Lindner V. and Reidy MA (1991) Proliferation of smooth muscle cells after vascular injury is inhibited by an antibody against basic fibroblast growth factor. *Proc. Natl. Acad. Sci.* 88: 3739–3743.

Little T, Pichard AD and Lindsay J (1989) Probe angioplasty of total coronary occlusion using an intracoronary probing catheter. *Cathet. Cardiovasc. Diagn.* 17: 218–223.

Litvack F et al., (1989) Percutaneous Excimer laser assisted angioplasty of the lower extremities: results of initial clinical trials. *Radiology.* 172: 331–335.

Lopez RR et al., (1991) Expandable venous stents for treatment of the Budd-Chiari syndrome. *Gastroenterology.* 100 (5 pt 1): 1435–1441.

Lu DY, Leon MB and Bowman RL (1986) Electrical thermal angioplasty in an atherosclerotic rabbit model. *Circulation.* 74 (Suppl 2): II–8.

Lu DY, Leon MB and Bowman RL (1987) A prototype catalytic thermal tip catheter: design parameters and in vitro tissue results. *J. Am. Coll. Cardiol.* 9: 187A.

Lundergan CF, Foegh ML and Ramwell PW (1991) Peptide inhibition of myointimal proliferation by angiopeptin, a somatostatin analogue. *J. Am. Coll. Cardiol.* 17: (6 Suppl B) 132B–136B.

Martin EC, Fankuchen EI and Karlson KB (1981) Angioplasty for femoral artery occlusion: comparison with surgery. *Am. J. Radiol.* 137: 915–919.

Maynar M et al., (1990) The Simpson atherectomy catheter in the management of complete obstructions. *ROFO.* 153: 547–550.

McGuff PE *et al.*, (1963) Studies of the surgical applications of laser (Light Amplification by Stimulated Emission of Radiation). *Surg. Forum.* 14: 143–145.

Mehigan JT and Olcott C (1986) Video angioplasty as an alternative to intraoperative arteriography. *Am. J. Surg.* 152: 139–145.

Meier B (1989) Chronic total coronary occlusion angioplasty. *Cathet. Cardiovasc. Diagn.* 17: 212–217.

Michaels JA *et al.*, (1989a) Laser angioplasty with a pulsed Nd:YAG laser: early clinical experience. *Br. J. Surg.* 76: 921–924.

Michaels JA *et al.*, (1989b) Assessment of a new device for laser angioplasty. *Eur. J. Vasc. Surg.* 3: 71–77.

Mitchell DC *et al.*, (1992) Laser-assisted angioplasty for arterial occlusion of the lower limb: initial results and follow-up. *Br. J. Surg.* 79: 81–85.

Morgenstern BR *et al.*, (1989) Total occlusions of the femoropopliteal artery: high technical success rate of conventional balloon angioplasty. *Radiology.* 172: 937–940.

Murray A and Wood RFM (1989) Peripheral laser angioplasty with pulsed dye laser and ball-tipped optical fibres. *The Lancet.* Dec 23/30: 1471–1474.

Neblett CR, Morris JR and Thomsen S (1986) Laser-assisted microsurgical anastomosis. *Neurosurgery.* 19: 914–934.

Neubaur T, Klepzig M and Strauer BE (1988) Perkutane transluminale Laser-angioplastie bei peripherer arterieller Verschlußkrankheit–Entwicklung eines neuen Laserkathetersystems. *Z. Kardiol.* 77: 245–250.

Nicholson AA *et al.*, (1991) Percutaneous transluminal angioplasty of the subclavian artery. *Ann. Roy. Coll. Surg. Eng.* 73: 46–52.

Nordstrom LA *et al.*, (1988) Direct argon laser exposure for recanalization of peripheral arteries: early clinical results. *Radiology.* 168: 359–364.

Nordstrom J, Haugland M and Strauss GS (1989) Direct laser angioplasty: clinical results of 53 consecutive human peripheral and five coronary cases. *Lasers Surg. Med.* S1: 7 (A).

Oz MC *et al.*, (1989) A fibreoptic compatible midinfrared laser with CO_2 laser-like effect: application to atherosclerosis. *J. Surg. Res.* 47: 493–501.

Pilger E *et al.*, (1988) Laser angioplasty with a contact probe for the treatment of peripheral vascular disease. *Cardiovasc Res.* 22: 149–153.

Pilger E *et al.*, (1991) Nd:YAG laser with sapphire tip combined with balloon angioplasty in peripheral arterial occlusions. Long-term results. *Circulation.* 83: 141–147.

Pompa JJ and Ellis SG (1990) Intracoronary stents: clinical and angiographic results. *Herz.* **15**: 307–318.

Prince MR *et al.*, (1986) Preferential light absorbtion in atheromas in vitro. Implications for laser angioplasty. *J. Clin. Invest.* **78**: 295–302.

Ramee SR *et al.*, (1991) Percutaneous angioscopy during coronary angioplasty using a steerable microangioscope. *J. Am. Coll. Cardiol.* **17**: 100–105.

Reis GJ *et al.*, (1991) Laser balloon angioplasty: clinical angiographic and histologic results. *J. Am. Coll. Cardiol.* **18**: 193–202.

Richards-Kortum R *et al.*, (1989) Spectral diagnosis of atherosclerosis using an optical fiber laser catheter. *Amer. Heart J.* **118**: 381–391.

Rosenschein U *et al.*, (1991) Ultrasonic angioplasty in totally occluded peripheral arteries. Initial clinical, histological and angiographic results. *Circulation.* **83**: 1976–1986.

Rosenthal E *et al.*, (1988) Percutaneous laser thermal angioplasty: early experience in peripheral and coronary arteries. *Heart and Vessels.* **4**: 59 (A).

Rosenthal E *et al.*, (1989) His bundle ablation with the laser thermal probe ('hot tip'): a feasibility study. *PACE.* **12**: 812–822.

Sahni R *et al.*, (1991) Prevention of restenosis by lovastatin after successful coronary angioplasty. *Am. Heart J.* **121** (6 Pt 1): 1600–1608.

Sanborn TA *et al.*, (1991) Percutaneous coronary Excimer laser-assisted angioplasty: initial multicenter experience in 141 patients. *J. Am. Coll. Cardiol.* **17**: 169B–173B.

Sarramon JP *et al.*, (1990) Use of the Wallstent endourethral prosthesis in the treatment of recurrent urethral strictures. *Eur. Urol.* **18**: 281–285.

Sato M *et al.*, (1990) Percutaneous transluminal angioplasty in segmental obstruction of the hepatic inferior vena cava: long-term results. *Cardiovasc. Intervent. Radiol.* **13**: 189–192.

Schatz RA *et al.*, (1991) Clinical experience with the Palmaz-Schatz coronary stent. Initial results of a multicenter study. *Circulation.* **83**: 148–161.

Schober R, Ulrich F and Sander T (1986) Laser-induced alteration of collagen substructure allows microsurgical tissue welding. *Science.* **232**: 1421–1422.

Schuger CD *et al.*, (1990) Percutaneous transcatheter laser balloon ablation from the coronary sinus: implications for the Wolff-Parkinson-White syndrome. *Lasers Surg. Med.* **10**: 140–148.

Schwarten DE *et al.*, (1980) Transluminal angioplasty of renal artery stenosis: 70 experiences. *Am. J. Roentenol.* **135**: 969–974.

Schwarten DE (1991) Clinical and anatomical considerations for nonoperative therapy in tibial disease and the results of angioplasty. *Circulation.* **83 (2 Suppl):** 186–190.

Scott DJ *et al.,* (1991) Intra-arterial streptokinase infusion in acute lower limb ischaemia. *Br. J. Surg.* **78:** 732–734.

Seeger JM and Abela GS (1986) Angioplasty as an adjunct to arterial reconstructive surgery: a preliminary report. *J. Vasc. Surg.* **4:** 315–320.

Seeger JM *et al.,* (1990) Laser recanalization in high risk patients. *Lasers Surg. Med.* **10:** 105–111.

Seldinger S (1953) Catheter replacement of the needle in percutaneous arteriography. *Acta Radiologica.* **39:** 368–376.

Serruys PW *et al.,* (1991) Angiographic follow-up after placement of a self-expanding coronary artery stent. *New Eng. J. Med.* **324:** 13–17.

Siegel RJ *et al.,* (1990) Percutaneous peripheral ultrasonic angioplasty. *Herz.* **15:** 329–334.

Sigwart U (1990) Coronary endoprostheses (stents). *Herz.* **15:** 319–328.

Simpson JB *et al.,* (1985) Transluminal atherectomy: a new approach to the treatment of atherosclerotic vascular disease. *Circulation.* **72 (Suppl. 3):** 146.

Spears JR *et al.,* (1988) Plaque-media rewelding with reversible tissue optical property changes during receptive CW Nd-YAG laser exposure. *Lasers Surg. Med.* **8:** 477–485.

Starck EE and Wagner HJ (1991) Rotation aspiration thromboembolectomy. *Deutsche. Med. Wochenschr.* **116:** 1–6.

Steckmeier B *et al.,* (1989) Erfahrungen mit der Rotationsatherotomie und der Atherektomie. *Herz.* **14:** 43–51.

Stierli P and Aebelhard P (1992) In situ femorodistal bypass: novel technique for angioscope-assisted intraluminal side-branch occlusion and valvulotomy. A preliminary report. *Br. J. Surg.* **78:** 1376–1378.

Strauss AL, Schaberle W, Rieger H and Roth FJ (1991) Use of duplex in the diagnosis of arteria profunda femoris stenosis. *J. Vasc. Surg.* **13:** 698–704.

Strikwerda S *et al.,* (1986) Ablation of obstructive atherosclerosis by argon-ion laser radiation delivered through an optical shield laser catheter. *Lasers Med. Sci.* **1:** 310.

Sutton D (1987) *A textbook of radiology and imaging,* 4th Edition. Churchill Livingstone, Edinburgh.

The SHK *et al.,* (1991) Femoropopliteal vein bypass grafts studied by intravascular ultrasound. *Eur. J. Vasc. Surg.* **5:** 523–526.

Theron J et al., (1990) New triple coaxial catheter system for carotid angioplasty with cerebral protection. *Am. J. Neuroradiol.* **11**: 869–874.

Tobis JM et al., (1991) Intravascular ultrasound imaging of human coronary arteries in vivo. Analysis of tissue characterizations with comparison to in vitro histological specimens. *Circulation.* **83**: 913–926.

Torres JH, Motamedi M and Welch AJ (1990) Disparate absorption of argon laser radiation by fibrous versus fatty plaque: implications for laser angioplasty. *Lasers Surg. Med.* **10**: 149–157.

Vallbracht C et al., (1989) Rotationsangioplastik–Klinische Erfahrungen bei 83 Patienten mit chronischen arteriellen Gefäßverschlüssen. *Herz.* **14**: 39–42.

Van der Giessen WJ et al., (1990) Arterial stenting with self-expandable and balloon-expandable endoprostheses. *Int. J. Card. Imaging.* **5**: 163–171.

Van Stiegmann G et al., (1984) Endoscopic laser endarterectomy. *Surg. Gynecol. Obstet.* **158**: 529–534.

Veith FJ et al., (1991) Early experience with the smart laser in the treatment of atherosclerotic occlusions. *Am. Heart J.* **121**: 1531–1538.

Verdaasdonk RM et al., (1987) Laser angioplasty with a metal laser probe ('hot tip'): probe temperature in blood. *Lasers Med. Sci.* **2**: 153–158.

Verdaasdonk RM and Borst C (1990a) Beam profile analysis of optically modified fiber tips. In: *Laser angioplasty with modified fiber tips.* Verdaasdonk RM, PhD Thesis, University of Utrecht, p 111–112.

Verdaasdonk RM, Jansen ED, Holstege FC and Borst C (1990b) Optically modified fiber tips penetrate tissue only when 'dirty'. *SPIE Vol 1201–Optical Fibers in Medicine.* 129–136.

Verdaasdonk RM, Holstege FCP, Jansen ED and Borst C (1990c) In vitro comparison of a radio frequency heated and a laser heated metal probe for angioplasty. In: *Laser angioplasty with modified fiber tips.* Verdaasdonk RM, PhD Thesis. University of Utrecht, p 67–79. *Investigative Radiology*, in press.

Walker PJ, Harris JP and May J (1991) Combined percutaneous transluminal angioplasty and extra-anatomic bypass for symptomatic unilateral iliac artery occlusion with contralateral iliac artery stenosis. *Ann. Vasc. Surg.* **5**: 209–216.

Weber H et al., (1990) Effects of Nd:YAG laser coagulation of myocardium on coronary vessels. *Lasers Surg. Med.* **10**: 133–139.

Werner GS et al., (1991a) Intravascular ultrasound imaging of human coronary arteries after percutaneous transluminal angioplasty: morphologic and quantitative assessment. *Am. Heart J.* **122** (1 Pt 1): 212–220.

Werner GS et al., (1991b) Excimer laser angioplasty in coronary artery disease. *Eur. Heart J.* **12**: 24–29.

White CJ *et al.*, (1990) Laser angioplasty using a lensed-fiber delivery system and a pulsed Nd:YAG laser: early clinical results. *SPIE Vol 1201–Optical Fibers in Medicine.* 206–210.

White CJ *et al.*, (1991) Percutaneous coronary angioscopy in patients with restenosis after coronary angioplasty . *J. Am. Coll. Cardiol.* **17 (6 Suppl B)**: 46B – 49B.

White GH *et al.*, (1990) Endoscopic intravascular surgery removes intraluminal flaps, dissections and thrombus. *J. Vasc. Surg.* **11**: 280–286.

White RA and White GH (1989a) Laser thermal probe recanalization of occluded arteries. *J. Vasc. Surg.* **9**: 598–608.

White RA *et al.*, (1989b) Initial human evaluation of argon laser-assisted vascular anastomoses. *J. Vasc. Surg.* **9**: 542–547.

Wholey M and Jarmolowski CR (1989a) New reperfusion devices: the Kensey catheter, the atherolytic reperfusion wire device and the transluminal extraction catheter. *Radiology.* **172**: 947–952.

Wilms G *et al.*, (1990) La recanalisation artérielle au laser Nd:YAG avec sonde à pointe saphir. *J. Radiol.* **71**: 103–107.

Yoshida H *et al.*, (1991) Transcatheter placement of an intraluminal prosthesis for the thoracic aorta. A new approach to aortic dissections. *ASAIP Trans.* **37**: 272–273.

10

The Urinary Tract

JUSTIN VALE, TIMOTHY CHRISTMAS, ROGER KIRBY and HUGH WHITFIELD

Introduction

Development of minimal access surgery in the lower urinary tract began in the 19th century, when it was first realized that there were enormous advantages to be gained from dealing with intravesical pathology via the urethra as opposed to an open suprapubic incision. In the early years of this century, the first attempts were made to deal with prostatic obstruction endoscopically; now 98% of the 400 000 prostatectomies performed annually in the USA are accomplished transurethrally. Renal stone surgery has undergone an even more dramatic transformation, from open surgery to percutaneous surgery and now extracorporeal shockwave lithotripsy (ESWL). In this chapter we will briefly review the enormous impact of minimal access philosophy, instrumentation and technique on the management of the many diseases of the urinary tract.

The kidney

There can be few fields of surgery in which the move towards minimal access surgery has been as rapid as in renal surgery. In 1941 the first percutaneous nephrolithotomy was performed (Rupel and Brown, 1941), using a cystoscope inserted through a nephrostomy track established at open operation. Subsequently, a number of similar procedures were reported, but in all cases the nephrostomy track was created at open operation. The first description of a technique for the entirely percutaneous removal of renal stones was in 1976 (Fernström and Johnson). Since then progress has been rapid with the development of the first commercially-available nephroscopy instrumentation systems (Günther *et al.*, 1979; Barbaric, 1979), and the development both of ultrasonic (Kurth *et al.*, 1977) and electrohydraulic lithotripsy probes (Raney, 1975a,b).

Anatomical considerations

Percutaneous renal surgery is facilitated by the position of the kidneys, with their posterior and lateral margins being immediately subjacent to the lateral abdominal wall. Thus there are no intervening organs liable to injury, and the only structure that is really at risk is the pleura. The lower line of this usually crosses the twelfth rib at the lateral border of the erector spinae muscle, and therefore posterior to this the pleura is actually below the twelfth rib. There is little risk of pleural injury with punctures below the twelfth rib and two finger-breadths lateral to the lateral border of erector spinae, but with supracostal approaches puncture of the pleura is highly likely.

The renal artery, the renal vein, and the majority of their main branches and tributaries are anterior to the renal pelvis, and are safe provided the needle is not advanced beyond the collecting system (Figure 10.1). The most notable exception to this general rule is the posterior segmental artery. This usually crosses posterior to the pelvis at the level of the upper pole infundibulum, and then runs downwards parallel to the hilar rim. It is only at risk if the kidney

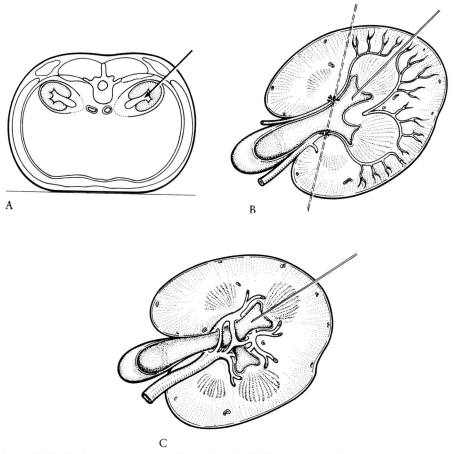

Figure 10.1: Ideal access to a posterior calyx (A). This is a relatively avascular approach (B), and by entering the calyx at its cusp the large veins around the calyceal infundibulum (C) are avoided. (Reproduced with the kind permission of Churchill Livingstone.)

is punctured too medially.

The correct siting of a nephrostomy track is essential to successful percutaneous renal surgery (Figure 10.2). A lower pole calyx permits good access to the renal pelvis and upper pole calyces, but not necessarily to the pelvi-ureteric junction (PUJ) and neighbouring lower pole calyces. A middle pole calyx may afford better access to the PUJ. With solitary calyceal stones it is essential to create a track into the relevant calyx, and this is often best achieved by relying on the feel of the percutaneous needle when it strikes stone. Otherwise, it is possible to create a tract into a calyx which has a parallel lie to the stone-containing calyx, and the stone is inaccessible. Understanding the spatial orientation of the calyceal system is essential to percutaneous renal surgery. In the normal kidney, the anterior and posterior calyces are arranged at angles of 70° and 20° to the coronal plane (Kaye, 1983). Thus on a standard intravenous urogram, the anterior calyces appear as the lateral extensions of the collecting system, and the posterior calyces will be in an orthotopic projection due to the overlying pelvis.

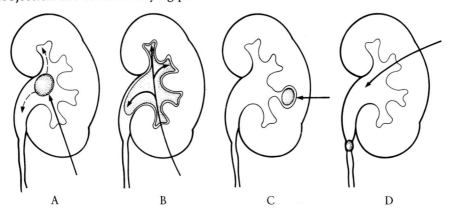

| A | B | C | D |

Figure 10.2: Percutaneous access. A track through a lower pole calyx will provide good access to a stone in the pelvis (A) and to most upper pole calyceal extensions of a staghorn calculus (B). For a solitary stone in a middle pole calyx (C), direct puncture into that calyx is necessary. An upper pole calyx or middle pole calyx gives best access to the ureter (D). (Reproduced with the kind permission of Churchill Livingstone.)

Tracks into the kidney must be straight and follow a transparenchymal course. If the pelvis is punctured directly, extravasation is common. Likewise, the calyx entered should be one which has a satisfactory infundibulum, so permitting passage of a guidewire and subsequent dilatation. Some experts in the field have described transparenchymal access from one calyx to another (Wickham and Miller, 1983), but this carries a significant risk of haemorrhage.

The potential risks of percutaneous renal surgery relate mainly to vascular complications, and this is reflected in the only real contraindications, which include renovascular malformations (for example renal artery aneurysms) and uncorrected clotting disorders.

Percutaneous nephrolithotomy (PCNL)

Preoperative preparation

In view of the ability of many renal stones to harbour infection, all patients undergoing percutaneous renal stone surgery should have a preoperative mid-stream urine analysis. Following this, antibiotic prophylaxis can be directed to any organisms cultured. In the absence of a positive urine culture, the patient should receive prophylaxis using an effective urinary anti-microbial agent such as gentamicin.

Procedure

General anaesthesia and endotracheal intubation are essential. With the patient in the supine position, a ureteric catheter (7 French) is passed up the ureter. This can be used subsequently for injection of contrast prior to fluoroscopy, and in addition, reduces the likelihood of any stone fragments passing into the ureter. The patient is then turned carefully into the prone-oblique position (Kellet, 1983). A number of alternative positions have been recommended, including the prone (Marberger, 1983) and supine-oblique positions (Günther et al., 1979). The advantage of the prone-oblique position, with the patient rotated 30–45°, is that it shifts the skin puncture site to lie directly over the best point of entry into the pelvicalyceal system in the normal kidney. Thus with vertical beam fluoroscopy the two points are superimposed, and puncture can be performed in a vertical direction parallel to the beam of the fluoroscope. The disadvantage of this is that depth of puncture is difficult to assess, but this can be overcome by rotation of the C-arm of the fluoroscope – if this type of fluoroscope is used – or gentle rotation of the patient during screening.

Renal puncture is performed initially using a skinny needle (20 gauge). This is useful for determining the direction of puncture for best access, and is very safe because of the small calibre of the needle. The ideal site for skin puncture for lower pole calyceal entry is on the dorsolateral aspect of the flank below the twelfth rib, with the needle angled at 45° to the sagittal plane. It is helpful at this stage to opacify the collecting system by injecting contrast through the ureteric catheter. Once the pelvicalyceal system has been entered and the direction of puncture established, a standard sheathed needle is inserted in the same direction. Entry of the needle into the renal parenchyma can be confirmed by observing paradoxical movement of the projecting needle on respiration. Entry into the collecting system is confirmed by removing the needle from the sheath, and aspirating urine.

If the position of the needle is satisfactory on fluoroscopy, a 0.035 inch semirigid Lunderquist guidewire with a 10 cm flexible J tip is inserted and advanced through the calyceal infundibulum into the renal pelvis. Once this stage is reached, the tract can be established by dilatation. A number of dilator types are available including semirigid Teflon dilators, coaxial polyethylene dilators, metal telescopic dilators, and balloons. We use semirigid Teflon dilators (Amplatz, Cook), starting with size 8 French and increasing in increments of 2 French or 4 French to 30 French. Each dilator is passed over the guidewire, and inserted using a twisting motion in the line of the guidewire. It is important to check the dilator position using fluoroscopy, as it is possible to force the dilator through the collecting system and out the other side. The final stage in establishing the tract is to pass a 30 French Amplatz sheath over the 30 French dilator. The sheath is not only invaluable for maintaining the track, but also reduces bleeding by a tamponade action.

With the track now established, the nephroscope can be inserted and the operation commenced. There is a considerable range of rigid nephroscopes available, the essential features of which are that they have a 0–5° offset telescope, and a good sized instrument channel. We use a Wolf nephroscope; this has a 0° obliquely offset telescope, an overall size of 21 French and an instrument channel of 4 mm in diameter. The latter is very important, because if the nephroscope is used without its sheath, the same channel will be used for both irrigation and insertion of graspers/lithotripsy probes. Thus if the channel is inadequate, insertion of instruments may preclude good visibility. By virtue of using an Amplatz sheath to maintain our track, we allow the saline irrigant to spill out into a bag attached to the side of the operating table and drapes. In some centres, a continuous irrigation system is used, with the nephroscope sheath being employed instead of an Amplatz sheath. Flexible nephroscopes are also available, but are of limited value currently. They have an instrument channel of only 2–2.6 mm, and because this channel is also the only means of irrigation, the view becomes very poor if there is any bleeding. In addition, there is only a relatively limited range of flexible graspers available, and rigid ultrasonic lithotripsy probes cannot be used. At the current time, the only potential value of a flexible scope is to reach stones in inaccessible calyces, and even this consideration is becoming increasingly obsolete with the advent of ESWL.

Once the nephroscope is inserted, the first requirement is one of orientation. Fluoroscopy can be helpful at this stage, and the injection of methylene blue-containing saline through the ureteric catheter can help in localizing the PUJ.

Stone retrieval

It may be possible to remove stones from the pelvicalcyeal system intact. There are a number of graspers available (Figure 10.3), the most useful of which are the alligator and tri-radiate graspers. Removal of stones intact is clearly ideal, because it leaves no residual fragments to block the ureter. However, it is only possible with small stones; the sheath versus stone size is the limiting factor. In practice, the largest stone that can be removed through a 30 French sheath is about 0.9 cm diameter.

Stone disintegration

Mechanical

Stone crushing forceps and 'punch' lithotrites are of little value in the upper tract. The mechanical strength required from them makes them

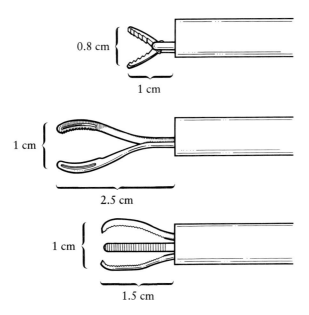

Figure 10.3: Stone manipulation forceps for use with the rigid nephroscope. The figures quoted demonstrate that quite a large amount of space is required to operate them. (Reproduced with the kind permission of Churchill Livingstone.)

bulky and cumbersome to use, and there is insufficient space for them in the non-dilated pelvicalyceal system. They have been largely superseded by ultrasonic, electrohydraulic and laser lithotripsy.

Ultrasonic lithotripsy

This technique of stone disintegration was first used in the kidney in 1977 (Kurth *et al.*, 1977), using sonotrodes designed for vesical calculi. These instruments were not suitable for use through the working channel of a nephroscope, and the first purpose-built ultrasonic probes for use in the kidney were introduced in 1982 (Marberger *et al.*).

The mechanism of stone disruption is not actually due to the ultrasound itself, but rather the effect of ultrasound at a frequency range of 20–27 kHz on a steel probe which is an integral part of the sonotrode. The ultrasound sets up a high frequency sinus vibration of the steel probe which, when in contact with the stone, acts like a drill. There is a hollow channel within the centre of the sonotrode through which the stone debris is aspirated. The resulting flow of stone-containing irrigant through the sonotrode is essential for cooling, and if this irrigant flow is interrupted, the sonotrode will heat up to temperatures over 40°C within seconds. Theoretically this may cause a thermal injury to the patient, and in addition, it may cause the sonotrode to fracture.

Ultrasonic lithotripsy is the disintegration mechanism of choice in the upper tract (Figure 10.4). It has minimal adverse effects; the maximal sound intensity at the tip is less than 0.35 W/cm², and this decays rapidly within millimetres of the tip. Its drawbacks are that it is rigid, and therefore can only be used on stones with straight access, and it may not break very smooth hard calculi – usually uric acid or some calcium oxalate stones.

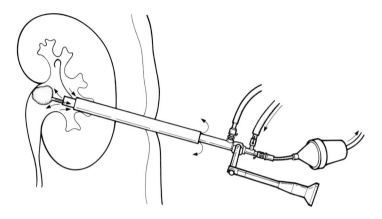

Figure 10.4: Stone disintegration using the ultrasonic lithotripsy probe. The probe is inserted through the instrument channel of the nephroscope. A simple irrigation system is being used, with irrigant spilling out from the Amplatz sheath. (Reproduced with the kind permission of Churchill Livingstone.)

Electrohydraulic lithotripsy (EHL)

This was first developed for use on bladder stones (Goldberg, 1969), and was first used on renal calculi in 1975 (Raney and Handler). The electrohydraulic (EH) probe consists of a coaxial cable with an axial inner and tubular outer electrode. When a high voltage discharge is applied underwater, a short but steep pressure impulse is generated of amplitude up to 500 Bar. This spreads spherically in water at a velocity of 1500 m/s. There is a rapid decay in the pressure curve from the point of discharge, and therefore, as with ultrasonic lithotripsy, contact of the probe on the stone is essential. As well as causing stress forces within the stone, there is some reflection of the pressure impulse from the stone resulting in rebound phenomena. The latter generate high strain forces and cavitation within the stone, which also contributes to stone disintegration.

The advantages of EHL over the ultrasonic technique are that it is more efficient and will break harder stones. In addition, the probes are flexible and can be used with the flexible nephroscope to treat stones in remote calyces. However, it has the major disadvantage that any tissue within 5 mm of the tip will receive high energy shock waves, and these have the potential to cause injury similar to the 'blast' effect of an explosion (Terhorst et al., 1975; Pelander and Kaufman, 1980). In addition, stone fragments are blasted like shrapnel into the mucosa (Webb and Fitzpatrick,

1985a), with further potential to cause injury. To help reduce these hazards, modern EHL probes have multiple power levels and a high degree of control over impulse frequency and pulse duration. Full optical control is essential, and at discharge the tip must be within 1 mm of the calculus, and at least 5 mm from all soft tissues and the endoscope – which it may otherwise shatter!

Lasertripsy

Two types of laser have been used to disintegrate renal calculi: the Q-switched Nd:YAG laser and the pulsed-dye laser. With lasertripsy, the shock waves are generated by the rapid rise and collapse of the plasma bubble at the site of action. However, lasers have a very small focal area and treatment is therefore time-consuming. They have the advantage of being thin and flexible enough for use with the flexible nephroscope, but as discussed earlier these are themselves of limited value in the kidney.

Postoperative care

All percutaneous renal procedures should be drained postoperatively. The drain serves two purposes: firstly it reduces any bleeding from the track by a tamponade effect, and secondly it drains the renal collecting system in the event of a stone fragment causing ureteric obstruction. We use a 28 French nephrostomy tube secured with a suture and tape. It is easily inserted through the Amplatz sheath, its position being checked by fluoroscopy.

The nephrostomy tube is routinely left for 24 hours, at which time it is clamped unless postoperative ESWL is planned. If the patient remains pain-free when the tube is clamped, it is removed. If clamping precipitates pain, a nephrostogram is performed.

Patients remain on antibiotics until the nephrostomy tube has been removed. Early ambulation is encouraged, and most patients leave hospital within 2–3 days.

Complications

Mortality

Percutaneous nephrolithotomy is safe, provided it is avoided in patients with known renovascular abnormalities and uncorrected clotting disorders. In a series of 1500 procedures, Marberger (1991) reported only one death, and this followed a vascular complication in an elderly patient with a solitary kidney.

Pleural puncture

This occurs almost exclusively with supra-twelfth rib punctures, and patients undergoing these high procedures should have a chest X-ray before leaving theatres. If there is evidence of a pneumo- or hydro-thorax, a chest drain can be inserted.

Haemorrhage

Haemorrhage requiring intervention should occur in less than 1% of procedures. If bleeding sufficient to obscure vision develops during a procedure, there is no point in proceeding and a large-bore nephrostomy should be inserted to tamponade the track (Alken et al., 1983). If bleeding continues through the tube, the tube can be clamped.

If haemorrhage continues necessitating transfusion of more than four units, an arteriogram should be performed. Any arterial lesions demonstrated are best treated by super-selective embolization. Unless essential to stabilize the patient's condition, open surgery should be avoided as it will almost inevitably result in nephrectomy.

A rare complication of percutaneous renal surgery is late haemorrhage due to an iatrogenic pseudoaneurysm or arteriovenous malformation (Patterson et al., 1984). Once again, arteriography and super-selective embolization are indicated.

Perforation of the collecting system

Small isolated perforations of the collecting system occur frequently, and are of no significance provided there is adequate drainage postoperatively. If a larger perforation is created and recognized at the time of surgery, it is best to establish drainage and abandon the procedure. There has been a reported fatality from a transurethral resection (TUR) type syndrome following percutaneous nephrolithotomy (Shultz et al., 1983). This can only arise if electrolyte-free irrigants are used, and these are unnecessary. Normal saline is the safest irrigant.

Septicaemia

This is not a problem if antibiotic prophylaxis is used and obstruction is avoided by adequate drainage.

Residual stones

With large complex staghorn calculi, some residual stones are almost inevitable. With the availability of ESWL, these can often be treated without recourse to further surgery.

Results of percutaneous nephrolithotomy (PCNL)

The stone-free rate following PCNL will depend largely on the size of stones treated and the experience of the operator. However, with multiple interventions and the selective use of ESWL for residual calculi, stone-free rates of 95% have been achieved in many centres (Alken *et al.*, 1983; Segura, 1985).

Percutaneous pyelolysis

This is the endoscopic division of the PUJ to treat PUJ obstruction. The technique requires general anaesthesia and passage of a retrograde ureteric catheter as for PCNL; the latter is invaluable for marking the site of the PUJ. A track is then created as for PCNL, but it is advisable to use a middle or upper pole calyx as this will give better access to the PUJ. It may be necessary to use a supra-twelfth rib approach.

An incision is then made posterolaterally at the PUJ using the Sachse urethrotome. It should extend over a length of 2.5 cm and penetrate through the full thickness of the ureteric wall so that peri-ureteric fat is seen. Two J-J stents are then inserted antegradely into the ureter, and their positions checked using fluoroscopy. A nephrostomy drain is left *in-situ* for 48 hours. The J-J stents are removed after six weeks.

Debate is rife as to whether or not this endoscopic procedure is a satisfactory alternative to dismembered pyeloplasty for primary PUJ obstruction. However, overall success rates of about 60% have been reported (Ramsay *et al.*, 1984). In the series mentioned, success was defined as the absence of symptoms and no evidence of obstruction on a radio isotope renogram a mean of 18 months postoperatively. The technique is certainly of value for secondary PUJ obstructions.

Percutaneous surgery for transitional cell carcinoma of the renal pelvis

Transitional cell carcinoma (TCC) affecting the upper tract is uncommon, but when present poses a therapeutic dilemma. TCC is a panurothelial disease (Gowing, 1960), and therefore may develop in the other kidney at any time. Therefore, eradicating the disease without recourse to nephroureterectomy would be highly desirable. Furthermore, there are some patients who have already undergone nephrectomy on the contralateral side. With this in mind, percutaneous renal surgery for renal pelvis TCC has been performed in a limited series of patients (Woodhouse *et al.*, 1986).

A track is created in exactly the same way as for PCNL, using a calyceal approach suitable for accessing the site of the tumour. If feasible, the tumour is then resected using a standard 24 French resectoscope, and a nephrostomy tube is left *in-situ*. The latter can be used to introduce an iridium wire postoperatively, and so deliver interstitial irradiation to the urothelium of the collecting system, and also destroy any tumour cells which may have seeded the track.

In the small series of patients treated in this way, there were no major complications and all of the tracks healed following removal of the nephrostomy tube and wire.

Laparoscopic nephrectomy

This is a new technique which has only recently become possible. There were three major problems which had to be overcome before laparoscopic nephrectomy could be attempted.

1 Reliable vascular control.
2 Some method of organ isolation to enable the operator to morcellate the kidney without disseminating bacteria or cancer cells around the abdominal cavity.
3 A fast safe morcellator to mince up the tissue into fragments small enough to remove through an 11 mm laparoscopic port.

These problems have all been overcome. The vessels may be first localized preoperatively by arteriography, and the renal artery embolized. At laparoscopy, the kidney is approached transabdominally, the peritoneal fold of the colon is incised, and the colon reflected medially. A ureteric catheter inserted retrogradely is used to tent up the ureter. The vessels are secured with Liga clips. The kidney is then fully mobilized, and the ureter clipped and divided following removal of the catheter. The kidney is placed in a tough flexible impermeable sac, introduced through another portal. The mouth of the sac is manoeuvred to one of the 11 mm portals, the morcellator introduced, and the kidney morcellated and aspirated until the sac can be withdrawn from the abdominal cavity.

In a recent series (Clayman et al., 1991), a total of eight nephrectomies have been performed in this way. The main drawbacks of the technique were that it was very time-consuming, and if used for tumour-bearing kidneys, histopathology was limited to a diagnosis of type of tumour with no information on stage.

Renal haemorrhage

Persistent haemorrhage from the kidney leading to haematuria may occur in cases of adenocarcinoma of the kidney, transitional cell carcinoma of the renal pelvis, arteriovenous malformations, haemangiomata (Holmes, et al., 1991) and angiomyolipoma of the kidney (Noble et al., 1989). Renal malignancy, even in the least fit patients, is best treated by nephrectomy. Renal tumours have been treated by selective arteriographic embolization using gelfoam or metallic coils. However, such techniques are often unsuccessful in stemming the haemorrhage, and may be complicated by infarction of normal renal tissue and migration of the material used for embolization to other arteries, which has resulted in occlusion of iliac vessels leading to intermittent claudication, and even gangrene necessitating foot amputation. Furthermore, even successful selective embolization is almost always accompanied by a postinfarction syndrome consisting of loin pain, fever and hypertension (Swanson, 1983). For these reasons, preoperative renal embolization for renal carcinoma has largely been abandoned, and is now also rarely used as a palliative treatment.

The ureter

Most endoscopic surgery on the ureter is performed for calculus disease. Since the 1940s, it has been possible to remove over 80% of ureteric stones requiring treatment by retrograde manipulation of baskets and loops under fluoroscopic control (Dourmashkin, 1945; Dormia, 1982). However, a number of other approaches to ureteric stones are now available, including endoscopic ureterolithotomy, antegrade ureterolithotomy, push-percs, push-bangs and even *in-situ* ESWL.

Anatomical considerations

The normal ureter is up to 34 cm long, and follows a tortuous course. Early attempts at ureteroscopy utilized rudimentary flexible instruments which had no steering mechanism and no system of irrigation (Marshall, 1964; Takayasu *et al.*, 1970). A major breakthrough in ureteroscopy was the realization that due to its mobility and distensibility, the ureter can be negotiated with a rigid endoscope. The first purpose-built rigid ureteroscope was produced as recently as 1980 (Perez-Castro *et al.*, 1980).

The amount of surgical distension that the ureter can withstand was another key issue in the development of ureteroscopes. In rabbits (Ford, *et al.*, 1984), minipigs (Boddy *et al.*, 1988), and dogs (Hasun *et al.*, 1990) it has been shown that the ureter can be dilated to twice its baseline luminal diameter before rupture. Most human ureters admit an 8 French catheter with ease, and therefore theoretically, can be safely dilated to 16 French. The speed of dilatation also has a significant effect on distensibility. Clayman *et al.*, (1987) demonstrated that the porcine ureter could be dilated slowly with a balloon to 24 French, but if this was performed rapidly over 10 seconds, extravasation occurred.

During ureteroscopy, the sites where the endoscope is most likely to stick are the narrowest points of the ureter – the ureterovesical junction (UVJ), the pelvic brim, and the PUJ. In practice, the UVJ/intramural ureter is the most difficult area to negotiate, but should normally accept an 8–9 French catheter. Catheters/guidewires with an angulated tip are the easiest to insert, as gentle twisting will encourage the catheter to follow the course of the ureter. Force should be avoided; the medial wall of the intramural ureter has only a thin muscle layer and is easily perforated.

Retrograde ureterolithotomy

This technique can be used for ureteric stones at any level, but in practice is largely reserved for stones in the lower third of the ureter. The procedure can be performed under fluoroscopic control only, or with a combination of ureteroscopy and fluoroscopy.

Fluoroscopic retrograde ureterolithotomy

As with PCNL, preoperative urine cultures and antibiotic prophylaxis are mandatory. The patient is given a general anaesthetic and placed in either the lithotomy or Lloyd-Davies position. A cystoscope is inserted into the bladder, and a stone extraction basket passed through the instrument channel. There are many types of basket available, the Dormia 4-wire helical basket being the most common. The basket is passed through the ureteric orifice and up the ureter to beyond the stone. The basket is then opened, and gently withdrawn under fluoroscopic control until it engages the stone. Subsequently, the basket can be closed to entrap the stone (Figure 10.5), or it can be withdrawn in its open state in the hope that it will 'trawl' the stone down the ureter. The advantage of the latter technique is that it minimizes the risk of catching and damaging the ureteric wall. If the basket sticks, it should be advanced up the ureter again and the process of withdrawal repeated. Very occasionally, the basket becomes immovable. If this is at the level of the ureteric orifice, it can be freed by making a 3–4 mm incision in the roof of the orifice. If the basket becomes trapped higher up the ureter, open surgery is necessary to remove it. Any attempt to force a trapped basket may result in ureteric avulsion.

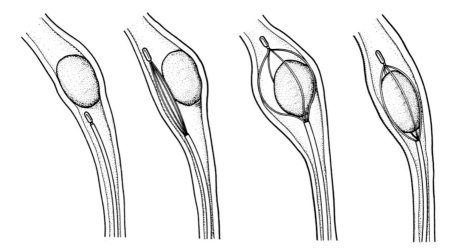

Figure 10.5: Use of a wire basket for removing a calculus from the ureter. The basket can either be closed around the stone or used to 'trawl' the stone down the ureter. (Reproduced with the kind permission of Churchill Livingstone.)

Using this technique, success rates of over 80% have been reported for stones of diameter less than 8 mm, impacted in the lower third of the ureter (Drach, 1983). However, failure and complication rates increase dramatically when higher stones are manipulated (Furlow and Bucchiere, 1976).

Endoscopic ureterolithotomy

The principles of this are very similar to those of fluoroscopic ureterolithotomy, but it has a number of advantages. Firstly, the operator can visualize the stone and any attempts to extract it, and secondly, lithotripsy probes can be used to disintegrate a large stubborn stone.

There is a vast range of ureteroscopes available. For ureterolithotomy, essential features include a 0–5° offset telescope and an instrument channel of sufficient size to accept a sonotrode (1.9 mm diameter). Short ureteroscopes (28 cm) are sufficient for stones in the lower half of the ureter, with a sheath of 10.5 or 11.5 French. Such instruments will enter 75% of ureters without formal dilatation of the ureteric orifice (Webb and Fitzpatrick, 1985b; Stackl and Marberger, 1986). However, if the ureteric orifice is too small to accept the instrument, a standard 24 French cystoscope is used to pass a guidewire into the ureter and a series of Teflon dilators are passed over the guidewire, starting at 8 French and increasing to 12 French. This is the largest dilator which will fit through the instrument channel of the cystoscope, but is sufficient to permit subsequent insertion of an 11.5 French ureteroscope. If a ureteric stenosis is encountered higher up the ureter, this is best treated using an angioplasty balloon dilatation catheter. This is slowly inflated within the narrow segment under fluoroscopic control, and left inflated for 2–3 minutes. If this fails to achieve adequate dilatation, the procedure is best abandoned and a J-J stent inserted. Sufficient ureteric dilatation will occur around the stent to permit a further attempt at ureteroscopy a few days later.

There are a number of devices available for ureteroscopic stone retrieval, including alligator forceps and baskets. Although these are often successful for stones up to 6 mm in diameter, larger stones are best fragmented *in situ*. The ultrasonic probe can be passed through the instrument channel of the ureteroscope, and is the ideal implement for disintegrating ureteric stones, as long as good stone contact can be achieved. The EHL probe has been used in the ureter (Green and Lytton, 1985), but is of very limited value. There is insufficient space to maintain a distance of 5 mm between the tip of the probe and the ureteric wall.

A particularly exciting development is the use of lasertripsy in the ureter. The thin quartz fibres can be used with flexible instrumentation, and because laser energy acts only where it is absorbed, it should not damage surrounding soft tissue (Watson *et al.*, 1988). Two systems are under evaluation; the Q-switched Nd:YAG laser and the flash-lamp excited dye laser (Candela). The importance of lasertripsy is likely to increase with the current trend back towards flexible ureteroscopes. The latter are clearly preferable in a tortuous tube such as the ureter, but in the past they have suffered on the grounds of expense, lack of durability, and small instrument channels. Perhaps with advances in peripheral equipment they may gain in popularity.

Postoperative care

Unless ureteric surgery has been traumatic, routine insertion of J-J stents is unnecessary. Most patients can be discharged home on the day of surgery or the following day.

Complications

Perforation

This occurs in about 10% of ureterolithotomies, and is more likely in ureters which have been subject to previous surgery or pelvic irradiation. Provided the perforation is detected at the time of surgery, and a J-J stent inserted, it usually seals within 1–3 days and is rarely the cause of long-term morbidity. It has been suggested that secondary extravasation can lead to periureteric fibrosis and ureteric strictures in up to a third of patients (Kramolowsky, 1987). However, this has not been confirmed by other operators (Stackl and Marberger, 1986; Lytton *et al.*, 1987), and the true stricture rate is probably below 5% (Amar *et al.*, 1981).

It is often possible to complete stone extraction in the presence of a small perforation. However, if the hole is larger, or at a point which makes further stone manipulation difficult, the procedure should be abandoned and a stent inserted with a view to reoperation some weeks later.

Ureteric avulsion

This is the most serious ureteric injury, and is usually caused by careless use of a basket. The mechanism is either one of trapping of the ureteric wall within the basket, or else an overzealous attempt to remove a stone which is too large to pass through narrower stretches of the ureter. Ureteric avulsion should be wholly avoidable if basket closure is always performed under direct vision, and if extraction is stopped whenever the basket or stone becomes trapped.

If ureteric avulsion does occur and is recognized, primary surgical repair – usually ureteric reimplantation – is the best treatment.

Ureteric strictures

Theoretically, these may develop as a result of direct trauma to the mucosa of the ureter, thermal damage due to prolonged activation of the ultrasonic lithotriptor, or periureteric fibrosis following perforation and extravasation. The incidence of such strictures has been variably reported, from 0% (Lyon *et al.*, 1984; Stackl and Marberger, 1988) to 5% (Kramolowsky, 1987), and almost all develop within the first six weeks.

The best treatment of these iatrogenic strictures depends upon their site. Scarring of the ureteric meatus and intramural ureter can often be divided with endoscopic scissors or an endoscopic knife, whilst strictures of the PUJ are best treated by pyelolysis. Strictures of the intervening segments of the ureter can either be dilated using an angioplasty balloon, or incised using special ureteroscopic blades. However, a prerequisite for all these techniques is the passage of a guidewire and, if this is not feasible, open surgery is necessary.

Antegrade ureterolithotomy

The development of this technique was an entirely logical progression from PCNL, and it provides excellent access for stones in the upper ureter. The first stage of the procedure is to create a track similar to that used for PCNL, but utilizing a middle or even upper pole calyx. These relatively high punctures are necessary to establish a track through which a rigid instrument can be passed down the ureter. If this is not possible, flexible instrumentation is used.

Once an adequate track has been established and the PUJ negotiated ureteroscopically, stone retrieval using a basket, or disintegration using ultrasonic lithotripsy, can be performed. Before commencing the latter, a balloon catheter should be passed retrogradely to prevent stone fragments disappearing down the ureter in front of the advancing probe.

Results of ureteroscopic stone manipulation

With careful consideration as to the most appropriate approach (antegrade versus retrograde), it is possible to achieve 95% stone-free success rates regardless of position within the ureter.

The bladder

Introduction

The urinary bladder is one of the best examples of an organ in which minimal access surgery has made a huge impact on surgical practice. In the early days of surgery, open operations on the bladder, either via a transabdominal or transperineal approach, were frequently complicated by sepsis and urinary fistulae. At the time of Samuel Pepys, bladder calculi were common and were often treated by transperineal lithotomy, a procedure that was performed rapidly over approximately two minutes with considerable morbidity and almost 30% mortality. The greatest single advance in minimal access surgery of the bladder was the development of the cystoscope. Adequate illumination was the main problem with early cystoscopes. In 1806, Bozzini attempted to deflect candle-light down a cystoscope, using a mirror attached to the forehead. However, it was not until 1887, that intravesical illumination developed, when a heated platinum wire bulb was fitted to the tip of a cystoscope by Nitze (Murphy, 1972). The next great advance was the development in 1954 of the flexible glass-fibre along which light could be transmitted (Hopkins and Karany, 1954). This was later adapted, by Professor Harold Hopkins, to produce a rod-lens telescope (Figure 10.6) – an ideal arrangement for a cystoscope, permitting both illumination of the bladder and attachment of a flexible teaching aid. Contemporary rigid cystoscopes incorporate a rod-lens, an irrigating channel to permit adequate vision by flushing blood and other material away from the field of vision, and electrocautery apparatus to enable the operator to resect or cauterize intravesical tissue (*see* TURP, page 230). Further technological advance has

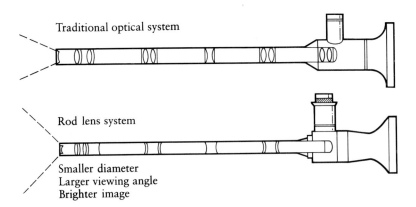

Traditional optical system

Rod lens system

Smaller diameter
Larger viewing angle
Brighter image

Figure 10.6: The rod lens system introduced by Professor Harold Hopkins in 1956. The upper telescope is a conventional rigid cystoscope with air spaces between the relay and field lenses. The lower instrument has a rod-lens system.

produced small-calibre flexible cystoscopes which are now in routine use throughout the world (Fowler, 1984).

Cystoscopy

Endoscopic examination of the urethra and bladder is an important diagnostic procedure in routine urological practice. In patients presenting with macroscopic or microscopic haematuria, it is our practice to perform intravenous urography (IVU) and send urine for cytological examination. If IVU and urine cytology are normal, we proceed to flexible cystoscopy under local anaesthesia. If the IVU suggests an intravesical abnormality, or cytological examination suggests the presence of a transitional cell carcinoma, we proceed to cystoscopy under general anaesthesia using a rigid cystoscope. Other indications for endoscopic examination of the bladder include follow-up of patients with a previous history of transitional cell carcinoma of the bladder or kidney, unexplained frequency of micturition or difficulty passing urine, pain thought to originate from the bladder, and investigation of an intravesical abnormality apparent on IVU or bladder ultrasound. It is our practice to perform the majority of such endoscopic examinations using the flexible cystoscope.

Rigid cystoscopy is usually performed under general anaesthesia, although recently such procedures have been performed under sedoanalgesia as day cases (Miller *et al.*, 1990). The patient is placed in the lithotomy position and, under direct endoscopic vision, the urethra and bladder are carefully examined. It is usual practice to endoscope using a 30° telescope. In order to visualize the anterior wall of the bladder adequately, especially at the bladder neck, it is often necessary to switch to 70° or 120° telescopes.

Flexible cystoscopy is usually performed as a day case procedure using local anaesthesia. In males, the procedure is performed in the supine position, whilst in females, the legs are flexed and abducted. Lignocaine gel is inserted through the urethral meatus, and in male patients, a penile clamp is applied for two minutes to allow the anaesthetic to take effect. As with rigid cystoscopy, the whole urethra and bladder are examined. One of the advantages of the flexible cystoscope, apart from the ease with which the procedure may be performed under local anaesthesia, is that excellent retrograde views of the bladder neck may be obtained by coiling the cystoscope up within the bladder. Similarly, bladder diverticula may be examined by feeding the cystoscope through the neck of the diverticulum, and manipulating the tip of the cystoscope to enable complete examination of the urothelium.

If for any reason the urethral approach to the bladder is impassable, cystoscopy can be performed via the suprapubic approach. A suprapubic puncture is made, and when the operator gains entry to the bladder by aspiration of urine, the tract is dilated, and either a rigid or flexible cystoscope can be passed antegradely and the bladder inspected.

Cystoscopic biopsy

At rigid or flexible cystoscopy, lesions of the urothelium may be apparent. It is usual practice to biopsy such areas using cold-cup biopsy forceps. The biopsy site may need to be electrocauterized to prevent haemorrhage. Small papillary carcinomas, carcinoma-*in-situ* and areas of interstitial cystitis or more unusual lesions of the bladder may be biopsied, and a diagnosis made using this technique.

Bladder tumour resection

Small transitional cell carcinomas of the bladder may be destroyed on an out-patient basis using a flexible cystoscope and a Nd:YAG laser (Fowler and Boorman, 1986). However, laser equipment is expensive and not widely available. In the majority of cases, bladder tumours are treated by transurethral resection, which may be performed under sedoanalgesia (Miller *et al.*, 1990) or general anaesthesia. Using the same resectoscope electrocautery loop as used for transurethral prostatectomy, and irrigating with isotonic glycine solution, the bladder tumour may be removed piece-meal (Figure 10.7), siphoned from the bladder using the Ellick's evacuator and sent for histological examination. Superficial tumours are readily resected using this technique. In order to stage the tumour, the base of the tumour, including detrusor muscle, should be resected and submitted separately for histological examination. This should permit determination of the stage and grade of the tumour, both of which are important determinants for treatment and prognosis. Following resection of the bladder tumour, and when haemostasis has been achieved, a three-way irrigating urethral catheter should be passed. Irrigation may be discontinued when the drained fluid becomes clear of blood and the urethral catheter can be removed soon after.

The stages of transitional carcinoma of the bladder and the contemporary modes of treatment are shown in Table 10.1. In the early stages, (Tis/Ta/T1) bladder carcinoma may be managed by minimal access techniques. However, more advanced tumours are now often treated by cystectomy and total

Stage	Definition	Treatment
Tis	flat, carcinoma-*in-situ*	local treatment, intravesical BCG therapy
Ta	non-invasive, papillary	transurethral resection
T1	invades lamina propria	transurethral resection
T2	invades superficial detrusor	cystectomy ± chemotherapy (or external beam radiotherapy)
T3a	invades deep detrusor	cystectomy ± chemotherapy (or external beam radiotherapy)
T3b	invades perivesical fat	cystectomy ± chemotherapy (or external beam radiotherapy)
T4	invades adjacent structures	external beam radiotherapy ± chemotherapy

Table 10.1: Transitional cell carcinoma – staging and treatment.

bladder reconstruction, using small or large bowel or a combination of the two, with or without radiotherapy.

All cases of transitional cell carcinoma of the urinary tract should be followed up indefinitely, since there is a high incidence of metachronous urothelial tumours within the bladder, and also the upper urinary tract.

Cystodistension

Cystodistension was first advocated as a treatment for superficial transitional cell bladder carcinoma. In patients with florid growth of superficial papillary transitional cell carcinoma of the bladder, a special catheter with a large inflatable balloon at the tip may be inserted into the bladder, and inflated at a pressure equal to the patient's systolic blood pressure for 1–3 hours, under spinal or epidural anaesthesia – resulting in pressure necrosis of the bladder tumour. Subsequent transurethral resection of residual tumour is usually necessary (Helmstein, 1972). Balloon cystodistension has also been advocated as a treatment for low functional bladder capacity due to detrusor instability (Dunn *et al.*, 1974), and for interstitial cystitis (Dunn *et al.*, 1977), but the long-term efficacy of this treatment is very limited.

Bladder haemorrhage

Protracted and gross haematuria from the bladder may occur with carcinoma of the bladder, especially after a course of radiotherapy. Also, treatment with the cytotoxic agent cyclophosphamide may lead to haemorrhagic

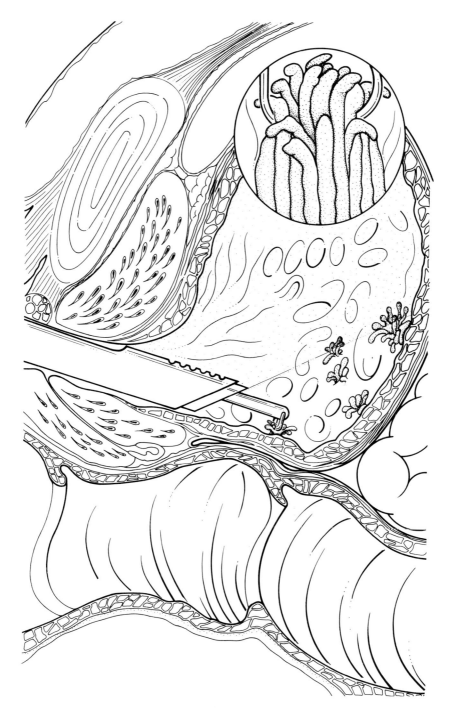

Figure 10.7: Transurethral resection of a bladder tumour.

cystitis. Such haemorrhage may be difficult to control by endoscopic surgery. Attempts are sometimes made to stem such haemorrhage by local cauterization which may be successful. Intravesical instillation of formaldehyde or alum solution may be used to stop the haemorrhage. If this fails, an alternative technique is selectively to embolize the superior and inferior vesical arteries, although in the authors' experience, this manoeuvre is rarely successful. In some instances, ligation of the internal iliac arteries, or even emergency cystectomy, may be required to stem the haemorrhage.

Subureteric injection of Teflon for ureteric reflux

Many cases of ureteric reflux resolve spontaneously by the time puberty is reached. Those which suffer breakthrough infections in spite of antibiotics, or persist beyond puberty, are considered candidates for surgery. Open ureteroneocystostomy is now being challenged by the minimal access option of trigonal subureteric injection of Teflon through specially developed applicators. This technique changes the angle of the ureteric orifice, and has produced good results in a considerable number of cases. More recently, a number of alternative injectable substances have been developed.

The prostate

The prostate is the organ of the body most commonly afflicted by disease in the ageing male. Benign prostatic hyperplasia (BPH) is present histologically in the prostate in 70% of 70-year-old men, and produces symptoms of outflow obstruction in more than half of them (Garraway *et al.*, 1991). Adenocarcinoma of the prostate is now the most common cause of cancer death in men over 60 years in the USA. Minimal access surgery has had a considerable impact in both these diseases.

Benign prostatic hyperplasia (BPH)

BPH was only recognized as a specific disease entity in the 18th century, and for many years after this, the effects of outflow obstruction were thought to be the result of 'bladder atony' and treated by intermittent catheterization. The first prostatectomy operations were performed around 1886 by, among others, Magill of Leeds and Belfield in the USA, but the technique was popularized and improved in 1901 by Sir Peter Freyer. Not long afterwards Hugh Hampton Young (1905), working at Johns Hopkins University in Baltimore, described the punch resectoscope for transurethral resection of both benign and malignant obstructing prostatic tissue. A further advance in instrumentation came with the development of the Stern-McCarthy resectoscope, which permitted removal of larger portions of prostatic tissue and improved haemostasis. With subsequent refinements, transurethral prostatectomy (TURP) has become the method of choice for dealing with all except the largest of benign obstructing glands.

Worldwide, transurethral prostatectomy is performed in more than half a million individuals each year, at an estimated cost of 4.5 billion dollars in the USA alone.

While there is no question that prostatectomy is the gold standard method of relieving bladder outflow obstruction due to BPH, there is also an effect on ejaculatory function which many patients regard as undesirable. There is, in addition, a small but significant mortality and reoperation rate, which inevitably complicates TURP. It must be remembered that it is often performed in elderly men with a considerable number of comorbid conditions (Roos *et al.*, 1989). These factors have provided the impetus for the development of a number of minimal access alternatives to prostatectomy.

Balloon dilatation of the prostate

The concept that it is not always necessary to remove the prostate physically to relieve outflow obstruction is largely due to Deisting (1956), who used a specially developed metal dilator to distend the prostatic urethra. The technique, however, was soon surpassed by improvement in resectoscopes and gradually fell into abeyance. With the development of high pressure balloon technology for intraluminal angioplasty in the 1980s, interest was rekindled in the concept. Studies in dogs (Burhenne *et al.*, 1984) and humans (Casteneda *et al.*, 1987), showed that over dilatation of the prostatic urethra could be achieved without serious side-effects, and with some improvement in symptoms and uroflow. Currently, two basic types of high pressure prostatic

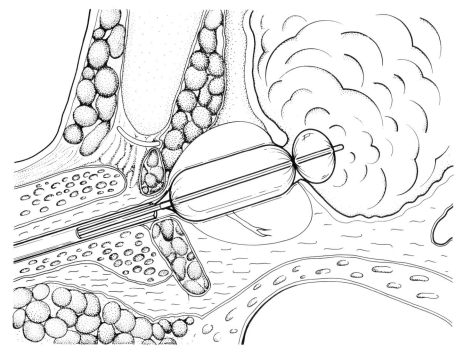

Figure 10.8: Balloon dilatation of the prostate. The balloon is left inflated for 10 minutes at 3 atmospheres – the balloon diameter is 25 mm at this pressure.

balloons are available: the ASI system which employs a disposable endoscopic placement system to ensure the distal sphincter is not dilated, and the AMS (Optilume) and Microvasive systems. Both of these latter systems use a nodule below the sphincter which is palpable per rectum for correct balloon localization. Once correctly sited, the balloon is inflated to 3 atmospheres, which effectively expands the prostatic urethra to 75 French (25 mm) (Figure 10.8). This dilatation ruptures the anterior prostatic commissure in the majority of cases. A urethral catheter is then inserted and retained for 24–48 hours. A number of authors have reported reasonably encouraging results with this technique – especially in patients with small prostates and reasonable bladder function (McLoughlin et al., 1991; Klein and Lemming, 1989). However, not all patients respond to this therapy. Most authors report about a 70% response rate, and longer term follow-up in many patients shows a tendency to return to pre-dilatation values. Symptomatic improvement, however, is reasonably well maintained.

Insertion of intraprostatic stents

Fabian (1980) was the first to advocate the use of an intraprostatic metal stent – the urospiral – to relieve prostate obstruction in patients unfit for, or unwilling to undergo, surgery. Since then, a number of removable stents have been developed and modified, to prevent the dual problems of encrustation and displacement, but these have not found a widespread usage because of these twin problems. In an attempt to get round these difficulties, two permanently implantable metallic stents have been developed, which are localized in the prostatic urethra and then expanded to fix them in position (Figure 10.9). After 3–6 months, the majority of these stents become epithelized (Figure 10.10), which should reduce their tendency to encrust – at least in the longer term. We have currently inserted 27 of the ASI titanium stents and followed the patients up for up to 20 months (Figure 10.11). Reasonable results have been obtained (Kirby et al., 1992), mirroring those achieved with the AMS optilume stainless steel device (Chapple et al., 1990). However, the long-term consequences of leaving a metallic foreign body within the prostatic urethra, even if epithelized, have not yet been defined.

Microwave hyperthermia

Hyperthermia has been used as an adjunctive therapy for conditions such as head and neck tumours for some time. The technique relies on the differential susceptibility of malignant tissues, compared with normal tissue, to heating. BPH tissue is probably no more sensitive to heating than normal prostate, but hyperthermia does seem to produce symptomatic improvement in patients with this disease, although the mechanism for this effect is still unclear.

Hyperthermia may be administered as a multiple dosage regimen by the transrectal route, or in single or thrice repeated dosages via transurethral applicators. There are theoretical disadvantages in the transrectal route, in that the rectal wall, Denonvilliers' fascia and posterior prostate absorb much of the energy, when the obstructing tissue in BPH is mainly periurethral in location. Using sophisticated catheters, combining a microwave applicator

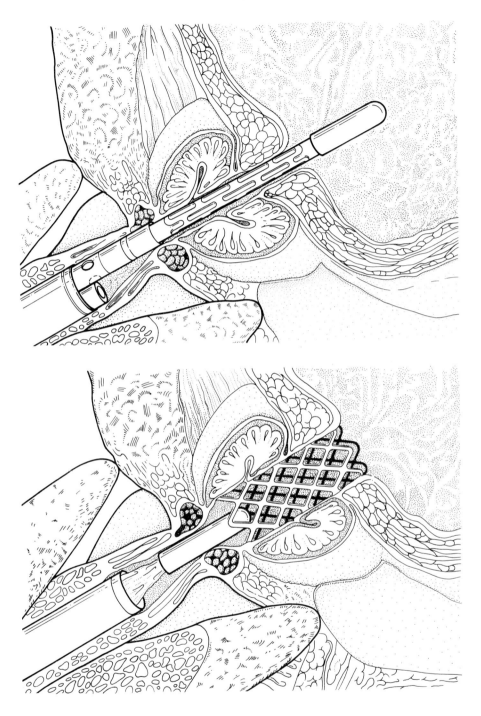

Figure 10.9: Insertion of a titanium wire mesh stent. The upper figure shows cystoscopic stent localization. A balloon is then inflated to expand and release the stent from its introducer. The lower diagram shows an expanded stent in perfect position.

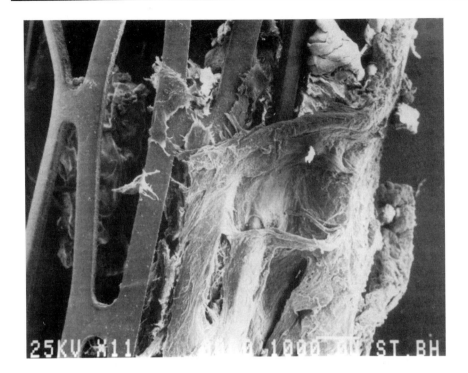

Figure 10.10: Scanning electron micrograph to show early stent epithelization.

and a cooling system, which preserves the urethra as well as rectal temperature probes to ensure the rectal wall is not damaged, the Technomed 'Prostatron' apparatus is capable of achieving temperatures within the obstructing transition zone of the prostate of above 46°C. This temperature is cytotoxic to smooth muscle cells, and may also damage sensory nerve endings within the prostate. Symptomatic relief is achieved in more than 70% of patients treated with this device, and flow rates improve by a mean of 30% with some reduction of residual urine. Whether or not these improvements are maintained in the longer term, and whether further treatment courses can be administered, is yet to be determined.

Other energy sources as therapy for BPH

A number of other energy sources have been assessed as a means of destroying obstructing prostatic tissue. Laser prostatectomy is now feasible, although still undergoing clinical trials. Focused ultrasound can be delivered extracorporeally and produce accurate high tissue destruction, and it may be possible in the future to use this or other modalities to relieve symptoms and obstruction in this most prevalent of diseases of elderly men.

Carcinoma of the prostate

Carcinoma of the prostate is an increasing health issue in the ageing societies of both the developing and developed world. Considerable controversy exists

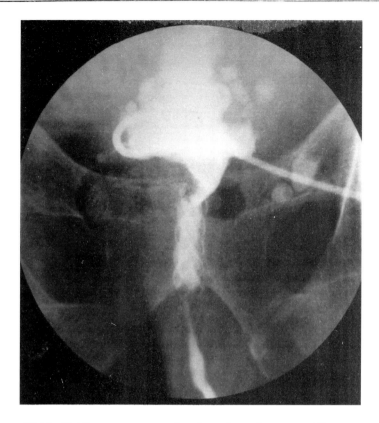

Figure 10.11: Voiding cystogram after insertion of a stent. The contrast has been introduced through a suprapubic catheter, which we insert routinely to cover the immediate postoperative period.

over the optimum treatment for localized disease, which is now increasingly detected before metastatic spread has occurred. External beam radiotherapy is not reliably curative, and radical prostatectomy involves major surgery in a population who are not always fit. Laser ablation of small posteriorly placed adenocarcinomata has been described, and the focused ultrasound tissue destruction described above may also have an application in this disease.

In addition, laparoscopic dissection of the internal iliac lymph nodes is now a practical proposition, and allows detection of those patients with lymph node involvement without the need for laparotomy. These cases are then referred for radiotherapy rather than radical prostatectomy. Although minimal access techniques have not made a major impact on prostatic cancer surgery, there seems little doubt that rapidly improving technology will lead to developments in this area before too long.

The urethra

Urethroscopy

In all cases, the urethra should be carefully endoscoped at the time of cystoscopy. The most likely abnormality that might be detected is a urethral stricture, particularly in the male. Unusually, calculi can become impacted within the urethra, and even less commonly, malignant tumours may be seen.

Urethral strictures

In the male, urethral stricture may be congenital or occur following external trauma, infective urethritis (particularly with gonococcus) or transurethral instrumentation with a catheter or endoscope. The bulbar urethra is commonly involved. Patients usually complain of a gradual diminution of the urinary stream, but in severe cases, can present with acute retention of urine. It is our practice to assess all cases with urethral strictures by ascending and descending urethrography prior to surgery. The alternative modes of treatment are blind urethral dilatation using sounds or bougies, optical urethrotomy, urethroplasty or insertion of a metallic intraurethral stent. Urethral dilatation is less likely to cure the problem, since the trauma of the procedure, by circumferentially tearing the scar tissue, almost inevitably leads to recurrent stricturing, and may exacerbate the process leading to a longer and tighter stricture in the long term. Optical urethrotomy is performed through a standard panendoscope, fitted with a sharp scalpel blade, mounted on two carrying rods. Through a side arm in the endoscope, a fine-bore ureteric catheter is passed through the stricture, and then the stricture is divided by upward cutting movements, with the blade following the course of the catheter. Most strictures may be divided in this way, and it is usual practice to leave a urethral catheter *in-situ* for 24 hours after this procedure. Although the clean cut made at optical urethrotomy is less likely to lead to recurrent stricture than blind dilatation, it is common for urethral strictures to recur after this procedure. It is our practice to undertake urethroplasty in the more complex urethral strictures, since in our hands the recurrence rate is minimal, although the duration of in-patient care is usually seven days as opposed to two days. It could, however, be argued that an anastomotic urethroplasty with 90% cure rate (Kirby and Christmas, in press) is worth a prolonged single hospital stay compared to the option of multiple urethrotomies, which are more likely to lead to recurrent stricture and may ultimately necessitate more complex procedures, such as pedicled-island penile skin inlay urethroplasty (Turner-Warwick, 1972). A new exciting minimal access alternative treatment for urethral strictures is stainless steel stents, which may be inserted after optical urethrotomy, and become incorporated into the urethra since they cover with urothelium within 3–6 months (Milroy *et al.*, 1988). The long-term consequences of stainless steel urethral stent insertion is not known, although in the short-term they appear to prevent recurrence of urethral strictures effectively. Although they are valuable for the management of short bulbar strictures, they are less useful for strictures of the pendulous urethra or pelvic fracture strictures. Currently, work is being done on the development of stents which eventually become absorbed. These may have a particular place in urethral as well as ureteric strictures in the future.

The testis

Minimal access surgery has a limited role in the management of diseases of the testis and scrotal contents. Vasectomy is performed in most centres through a small scrotal incision and the ends of the vas ligated and folded over to prevent recanalization. Hydrocele of the testis and epididymal cysts do not often require surgical intervention, but the best current treatment is open surgery. The management of cryptorchidism is, however, now potentially less invasive, since maldescended or ectopic testes can usually be located by computerized tomography or magnetic resonance imaging (MRI) scanning. Intra-abdominal testes may be located at laparoscopy, and since their ectopic location predisposes them to malignant transformation, they are best removed, and this can now be performed through the laparoscope (Castilho *et al.*, 1991).

Varicoceles are a common finding in males, and treatment of these lesions may be indicated when associated with oligozoospermia, pain or discomfort. We favour the Palomo operation – the left spermatic vein is approached through a high incision between the anterior superior iliac spine and the umbilicus. Through an extraperitoneal approach, the spermatic vein is identified and ligated. An alternative laparoscopic technique in which the spermatic veins are ligated at the internal inguinal ring, has recently been described (Mehan *et al.*, 1991), and this minimal access procedure is likely ultimately to replace other more invasive operations in the future.

Conclusions

Urological surgeons have always been quick to adopt new technologies for the benefit of their patients. There is no question that further advances will be made in the laudable aim of reducing the morbidity associated with the large 'entry and exit' wounds of conventional surgical approaches. The prospects for further developments are exciting as we move towards the new millenium.

References

Alken P *et al.*, (1983) Percutaneous nephrolithotomy–a routine procedure? *Br. J. Urol.* **Suppl 1.**

Amar AP *et al.*, (1981) Ureteral stricture following ureterolithotomy. *J. Urol.* 105: 416.

Barbaric ZL (1979) Interventional uroradiology *Radiol. Clin. N. Amer.* 17: 413.

Boddy SM *et al.*, (1988) Acute ureteric dilatation for ureteroscopy. An experimental study. *Br. J. Urol.* **61**: 27.

Burhenne HJ, Chisholm RJ and Quenville F (1984) Prostatic hyperplasia: radiological intervention. *Radiology.* **152**: 655–657.

Castenada F *et al.*, (1987) Benign prostatic hypertrophy: retrograde transurethral dilatation of the prostatic urethra in humans. Work in progress. *Radiology.* **163**: 649–653.

Castilho LN *et al.*, (1991) Laparoscopic orchiectomy. *J. Urol.* **145**: 206A.

Chapple CR, Milroy EJG and Rickards D (1990) Permanently implanted urethral stent for prostatic obstruction in the unfit patient. *Br. J. Urol.* **66**: 58 – 65.

Clayman RV *et al.*, (1987) Experimental extensive balloon dilatation of the distal ureter: immediate and long-term effects. *J. Endour.* **1**: 19.

Clayman RV *et al.*, (1991) Laparoscopic nephrectomy: initial case report. *J. Urol.* **146**: 278–282.

Deisting W (1956) Transurtheral dilatation of the prostate: a new method of treatment of benign prostatic hypertrophy. *Urol. Int.* **2**: 158–171.

Dormia E (1982) Dormia basket: standard technique observations and general concepts. *Urology.* **20**: 437.

Dourmashkin RL (1945) Cystoscopic treatment of stones in the ureter with special reference to large calculi based on a study of 1550 cases. *J. Urol.* **54**: 245.

Drach GW (1983) Transurethral ureteral stone manipulation. *Urol. Clin. N. Amer.* **10**: 709.

Dunn M *et al.*, (1974) Prolonged bladder distention as a treatment of urgency and urge incontinence. *Br. J. Urol.* **46**: 645–652.

Dunn M *et al.*, (1977) Interstitial cystitis, treated by prolonged bladder distension. *Br. J. Urol.* **49**: 641–645.

Fabian KM (1980) Der Intraprostatische 'partie ile Katheter'. *Urologe.* **(A) 19**: 236–238.

Fernström I *et al.*, (1977) Percutaneous puncture nephrostomy. In: *Encyclopedia of urology, V/1.* Eds: Andersson L *et al.*, Springer, Berlin.

Ford TF *et al.*, (1984) Clinical and experimental evaluation of ureteric dilatation. *Br. J. Urol.* **56**: 460.

Fowler CG (1984) Fibrescopes in urology. *Br. J. Hosp. Med.* **32**: 202–205.

Fowler CG and Boorman LS (1986) Out-patient treatment of superficial bladder cancer. *The Lancet.* **i**: 38.

Furlow WL and Bucchiere JJ (1976) The surgical fate of ureteral calculi: review of the Mayo clinic experience. *J. Urol.* **116:** 559.

Garraway WN, Collins CN, and Lee RJ (1991) High prevalence of benign prostatic hypertrophy in the community. *The Lancet.* 338: 469–471.

Goldberg BB (1969) Electrohydraulic lithotripsy. In: *Proceedings of Kiev. Conference of Russian Urologists*, Moscow.

Gowing NFC (1960) Urethral carcinoma associated with cancer of the bladder. *Br. J. Urol.* 32: 428–438.

Green DF and Lytton B (1985) Early experience with direct vision electrohydraulic lithotripsy of ureteral calculi. *J. Urol.* 133: 767.

Günther R *et al.*, (1979) Percutaneous nephropyelostomy using a fine-needle puncture set. *Radiology.* 132: 228.

Hasun R *et al.*, (1990) The effects of acute dilation in the canine ureter. *Urol. Res.* (In press.)

Helmstein K (1972) Treatment of bladder carcinoma by a hydrostatic pressure technique. *Br. J. Urol.* 44: 434–450.

Holmes SAV *et al.*, (1991) The management of intrarenal vascular abnormalities. *Br. J. Radiol.* 64: 16.

Hopkins HH and Karany NS (1954) A flexible fibrescope, using static scanning. *Nature.* 173: 39–41.

Kaye K (1983) Renal anatomy for endourological stone removal. *J. Urol.* 130: 647.

Kellet MJ (1983) Percutaneous access to the kidney. In: *Percutaneous renal surgery*. Eds. Wickham JEA and Mill RA. Churchill Livingstone, Edinburgh.

Kirby RS and Christmas TJ (1991) The results of anastomotic bulbar urethroplasty in 100 cases. (In press)

Kirby RS, Heard S, Christmas T, Vale J, and Bryan J (1992) Use of the ASI titanium stent in the management of bladder outflow obstruction due to BPH. *J. Urol.* (In press)

Klein LA and Lemming B (1989) Balloon dilatation for prostatic obstruction. *Urol.* 32: 198–201.

Kramolowsky EV (1987) Ureteral performation during ureterorenoscopy: treatment and management. *J. Urol.* 138: 36.

Kurth KH *et al.*, (1977) Ultrasound litholopaxy of a staghorn calculus. *J. Urol.* 117: 242.

Lyon ES *et al.*, (1984) Ureteroscopy and pyeloscopy. *Urology.* **Suppl 23:** 29.

Lytton B *et al.*, (1987) Complications of ureteral endoscopy. *J. Urol.* **137**: 649.

Marberger M *et al.*, (1982) Percutaneous litholopaxy of renal calculi with ultrasound. *Euro. Urol.* **8**: 236.

Marberger M (1983) Disintegration of renal and ureteral calculi with ultrasound. *Urol. Clin. N. Amer.* **10**: 729.

Marberger M (1991) Percutaneous stone manipulation. In: *Stone Surgery*. Marberger M, Fitzpatrick JM, Jenkins AD and Pak CYC (eds). Churchill Livingstone, Edinburgh.

Marshall VF (1964) Fibreoptics in urology. *J. Urol.* **91**: 11.

McLoughlin J *et al.*, (1991) Balloon dilatation of the prostatic urethra with 35 mm balloon. *Br. J. Urol.* **67**: 177.

Mehan DJ *et al.*, (1991) Laparoscopic varicocelectomy: preliminary report of a new technique. *J. Urol.* **145**: 242A.

Miller RA *et al.*, (1990) The impact of minimally invasive surgery and sedoanalgesia on urological practice. *Postgrad. Med. J.* **66**: 72–76 (suppl.).

Milroy EJG *et al.*, (1988) A new treatment for urethral strictures. *The Lancet.* i: 1424–1427.

Mundy AR (1983) Long-term results of bladder transection for urge incontinence. *Br. J. Urol.* **55**: 642–644.

Murphy LJT (1972) *The history of urology*, pp 180–193, 358–359. Thomas, Springfield, Illinois.

Noble JG *et al.*, (1989) Renal angiomyolipoma: a comparison of five cases diagnosed by CT scan. *J. Roy. Soc. Med.* **82**: 25–27.

Patterson DE *et al.*, (1985) The etiology and treatment of delayed bleeding following percutaneous lithotripsy. *J. Urol.* **133**: 447.

Pelander WM and Kaufman JM (1980) Experience with electrohydraulic disintegrator. *J. Urol.* **117**: 159.

Perez-Castro E *et al.*, (1980) Transurethral ureteroscopy – a current urological procedure. *Arch. Esp. Urol.* **33**: 445.

Ramsay JWA *et al.*, (1984) Percutaneous pyelolysis: indications, complications and results. *Br. J. Urol.* **56**: 586–588.

Raney AM (1975a) Electrohydraulic lithotripsy: experimental study and case reports with the stone disintegrator. *J. Urol.* **113**: 345.

Raney AM and Handler J (1975b) Electrohydraulic nephrolithotripsy. *Urology.* **6**: 439.

Roos MP, Wenberg JE and Malenk DJ et al., (1989) Mortality and reoperation and transurethral resection of the prostate for benign hypertrophy. *New Eng. J. Med.* 320: 1120–1124.

Rupel DE and Brown R (1941) Nephroscopy with removal of stone following nephrostomy for obstructive-calculus anuria. *J. Urol.* 46: 177.

Schultz RE et al., (1983) Percutaneous ultrasonic lithotripsy: choice of irrigant. *J. Urol.* 130: 858.

Segura JW (1985) Rigid nephroscopy and ultrasound lithotripsy. In: *Endourology.* Carson CC and Dunnick NR (eds). Churchill Livingstone, Edinburgh.

Stackl W and Marberger M (1986) Late complications of the management of ureteral calculi with the ureteroscope. *J. Urol.* 136: 386.

Swanson DA (1983) Management of renal cancer. In: *Principles and management of urologic cancer,* pp 522–537. Williams and Wilkins, Baltimore/London.

Takayasu H et al., (1970) Fibreoptic pyeloureteroscopy. In: *Proceedings of the 15th Congress of the International Society of Urology, vol II.* University of Tokyo Press.

Terhorst B et al., (1975) Der Einfluss von elektrohydraulischer Schallwelle und Ultraschall auf das Uroepithel. *Urologe.* 14: 41.

Turner-Warwick RT (1972) The use of pedicle grafts in the repair of urinary tract fistulae. *Br. J. Urol.* 44: 644–656.

Watson GM et al., (1988) An assessment of the pulsed dye laser for fragmenting calculi in the pig ureter. *J. Urol.* 138: 199.

Webb DR and Fitzpatrick JM (1985a) Experimental ureterolithotripsy. *World J. Urol.* 3: 33.

Webb DR and Fitzpatrick JM (1985b) Simple aid to ureteroscopy. *Euro. Urol.* 11: 57.

Wickham JEA and Miller RA (1983) *Percutaneous renal surgery.* Churchill Livingstone, Edinburgh.

Woodhouse CRJ et al., (1986) Percutaneous renal surgery and local radiotherapy in management of renal pelvic transitional cell carcinoma. *Br. J. Urol.* 58: 245–249.

11

Thoracic Surgery

DAVID ROSIN

Introduction

The rapid expansion in cardiac surgery over the last 20 years has led to something of an eclipse of the status of non-cardiac thoracic surgery. Thoracic surgical techniques can be more difficult to learn than cardiac surgery, most of which is limited in range.

Minimal access surgery is a natural consequence of the developments which took place in endoscopy during the late 1970s; at this time fibre-optic bronchoscopy was being used merely as a diagnostic tool. Rigid bronchoscopy has been used for many years, but the ability to remove foreign objects and take biopsies increased its role from being merely diagnostic to therapeutic as well. In 1959, mediastinoscopy was introduced, which by removing lymph nodes, was useful for staging lung cancer as well as being a diagnostic procedure. Jacobaeus, who performed the first laparoscopy (coelieoscopy), is also reported to have performed the first thoracoscopy in the first decade of this century. However, thoracoscopy proved an unpopular procedure for many years and was only used by very few surgeons.

The rapid development of thoracoscopy from an investigative to a therapeutic tool has been even more rapid than that of laparoscopic surgery. In both, the development is due to the ability to perform procedures using a video camera and screen.

Bronchoscopy

Bronchoscopy is fundamental to the management of patients with diseases involving the lungs and major airways. Two basic instruments are available: the fibre-optic scope and the rigid one. The rigid instrument is more suitable for the removal of foreign bodies and the aspiration of secretions. It allows safer biopsy of vascular tumours because it is easy to control bleeding. Also, the rigid nature of the instrument allows the endoscopist to assess the fixity of a tumour by proprioception.

The flexible endoscope can penetrate much further into the bronchial tree, and allows brushings and biopsies of very peripheral lesions. It has a wide angle of vision, particularly in the upper lobe. It is the instrument of choice for patients with cervical spine problems with a fixed small bite because of its flexibility. In addition, it can be easily passed through an endobronchial or tracheostomy tube.

The techniques involved in the use of each instrument are very different. A thoracic surgeon in training should endeavour to become expert in the handling of both of them.

The instruments

Rigid bronchoscope (Figure 11.1)

The Negus bronchoscope is that most frequently used in clinical practice, a variety of sizes being available for various age groups. Fibre-optic light cables are the best source of illumination; an attachment to both the bronchoscope and telescope should be available. The three principal telescopes used are 0°, 60° and 90°. Combined use of these allows inspection of all lobar bronchi and their segmental divisions. Additional necessary instruments include straight and angled forceps, Chevalier-Jackson forceps for foreign bodies and a straight metal sucker.

To ventilate the patient, the inspired gas is administered by a Venturi system. Oxygen is injected under pressure through a nozzle on the side of the bronchoscope. Air enters through the open proximal end of the bronchoscope, creating an oxygen-air mix.

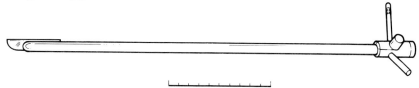

Figure 11.1: Rigid bronchoscope.

Fibre-optic bronchoscope (Figure 11.2)

Several models are available. They are all delicate and expensive instruments, and careful handling by trained staff is essential. The operating head of the endoscope has an adjustable eyepiece, and a finger and thumb control lever to direct the distal end of the instrument. A channel for the introduction of biopsy forceps, brush or Dormier basket is present with most models. There is a further port for suction on the side.

Bronchoscopy, either rigid or flexible, can be performed under general or local anaesthesia. The method of performing bronchoscopy is beyond the limit of this chapter and can be found in any standard thoracic surgery textbook.

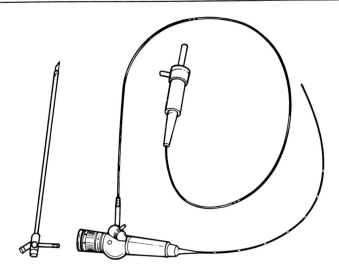

Figure 11.2: Fibre-optic bronchoscope.

Thoracoscopy

Thoracoscopy takes a mid position between needle biopsy and open surgery. It used to be a prerequisite that a pleural effusion or a free pleural space allowing for the creation of a pneumothorax was present. However, with modern techniques, this is not necessary if the anaesthetist has used a double lumen tube so that the lung can be deflated; artificial pneumothorax then can be obtained by insertion of a Verres needle using CO_2 to avoid embolism.

Indications and contraindications are listed in Table 11.1.

Procedure

Under general anaesthesia, with a double lumen endotracheal tube in place, the patient is positioned on the appropriate side. A small pneumothorax is induced using a Verres needle. If a pleural effusion is present, the needle can be inserted directly, and the effusion drained prior to introduction of CO_2. The choice of introduction site of the thoracoscope will depend on which part of the intrathoracic anatomy needs to be visualized.

In the lateral position it is usually inserted in either the third, fourth or fifth intercostal space, between the anterior and mid-axillary line. In the supine position, it is inserted in the second or third intercostal space in the mid-clavicular line.

In order to introduce the thoracoscope, a trochar and cannula are first inserted following introduction of the pneumothorax. This will usually be a 10 mm cannula. There are commercially available disposable cannulae or ports, with a safety shield which comes down over the trochar once it has passed through the thoracic wall. It is wise to use such a disposable port to ensure that no damage occurs to the underlying lung should it not have deflated. An incision just over 1 cm is necessary, and the trochar and cannula

---

Indications

1. The evaluation of a pleural effusion, to establish or exclude a malignant cause.

2. Evaluation and management of empyema cavities.

3. Assessment of mediastinal tumours.

4. Assessment of chest wall tumours.

Contraindications

1. Coagulopathies.

2. Recent myocardial infarction (within six weeks).

3. Severe impairment of pulmonary function (although this is not an absolute contraindication, great care must be taken).

4. Absence of a pleural space.

Table 11.1: Indications and contraindications to thoracoscopy.

are passed through this incision into the pleural cavity. Once the trochar is removed, the pneumothorax is maintained as the cannula is valved. Either a 0° or 30° telescope is then introduced. Intrapleural inspection can be made and biopsies taken.

At completion of thoracoscopy, the anaesthetist is asked to reinflate the lung, and if this occurs fully then there is usually no need for a drain. If the lung does not inflate completely, then a pleural drain should be inserted. As always for a chest drain, this should be attached to an underwater seal.

Mediastinoscopy

In 1959, in an attempt to identify patients preoperatively with mediastinal involvement from carcinoma of the lung who would not benefit from surgical resection, Carlins proposed the use of cervical mediastinal exploration (Cooper, 1986). Since then, this has been used for this purpose as well as for assessing other intrathoracic problems such as sarcoidosis. Thymic tumours and other anterior mediastinal tumours cannot be safely approached in this manner, because the tumour lies in front of the great vessels. Superior vena cava obstruction is not a contraindication as such.

There has been a resurgence of interest in this procedure since more widespread and enthusiastic application of the principles of staging of primary tumours prior to attempting resection. The presence of mediastinal lymph node involvement (N2 disease), has in turn altered the long-term prognosis for survival to such an extent that many surgeons will not consider proceeding to major pulmonary resection if N2 disease is present. More recent evidence suggests that prior evaluation with computerized tomography (CT) scanning is very helpful in deciding which patients require mediastinoscopy as a staging procedure. If no nodes are visible with contrast enhanced mediastinal CT scans, or all nodes are less than 1 cm, mediastinal biopsy is unnecessary.

Procedure

Mediastinoscopy is carried out under general anaesthesia. A sandbag is placed between the scapulae, and the head lowered to drop the shoulders and project the trachea forward. A 2.5 cm transverse incision is then made 1 cm above the upper border of the manubrium. The platysma muscle is divided and a retractor inserted. The midline between the sternothyroid muscles is then defined and this layer is incised. With blunt dissection beneath it, the anterior wall of the trachea is identified. If a common inferior thyroid vein is present, it should be divided (Figure 11.3).

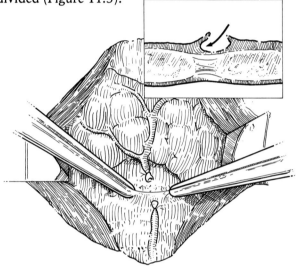

Figure 11.3: Division of the common inferior thyroid vein.

The pretracheal fascia is now elevated and incised. Blunt dissection extends downwards along the trachea and behind the innominate artery (Figure 11.4). Dissection is gradually extended along both sides of the trachea, although more so on the right. In this way, a bloodless paratracheal tunnel is developed, into which the mediastinoscope can be inserted. Dissection is continued with the tip of a metal sucker or with a blunt dissector.

Individual lymph nodes which have been identified by CT scan can be dissected out in this way, as far down as the right tracheobronchial angle and the carina. The lymph nodes in the right paratracheal group are contained within a firm fibrous envelope, and this must be disrupted prior to the individual nodes being identified.

If a large mass is present, a biopsy may be obtained from it. It is wise to precede this by aspiration with a large needle to exclude a vascular structure, particularly the superior vena cava right of the trachea, which could be adherent to the tumour. Indeed, if there is any doubt about the nature of the structure to be biopsied, it is wise to exclude a vascular structure by prior aspiration.

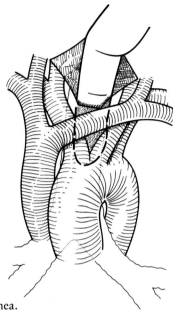

Figure 11.4: Blunt finger dissection along the trachea.

As many as possible of the abnormal lymph nodes should be biopsied or removed.

On completion of the procedure, haemostasis is secured by diathermy. The pretracheal muscles and the platysma are approximated, the mediastinoscope is removed and the skin incision closed.

Complications

Haemorrhage from the superior vena cava azygos vein, brachocephalic artery, arch of the aorta or even the right pulmonary artery is possible. Pneumothorax may also result, and therefore a routine chest X-ray should be taken after the procedure. Damage to the recurrent laryngeal nerves is possible, from excessive dissection around the sides of the trachea.

If major haemorrhage occurs, the wound should be packed. If bleeding cannot be controlled by this method, a mediastinotomy or thoracotomy will be necessary.

Oesophagoscopy

This procedure lies more in the domain of a gastrointestinal surgeon, although rigid oesophagoscopy is still performed by some thoracic surgeons – especially for removal of a large foreign body. Flexible fibre-optic oesophagoscopy is far safer and has been described in a previous chapter.

Minitracheostomy

In the early postoperative period, sputum retention can be life-threatening. A minitracheostomy can be very effective for aspirating sputum and obviating the need for intubation and ventilation. The complications following insertion of such a tube are very few, provided it is inserted carefully and accurately.

Early intervention while the patient still has adequate spontaneous ventilation will usually result in rapid improvement of the patient's condition, and obviate the need for bronchoscopy or ventilation. Therefore, insertion at the earliest sign of sputum retention, or even pre-emptively in a patient at high risk, is desirable.

Procedure

The patient is positioned supine with the head fully extended and a sandbag placed under the shoulders. It is possible to carry out the procedure with the patient sitting at 45° with the head extended over a pillow. To prevent undue reflex and movement of the lungs during the procedure, an assistant holds the chin firmly. The site of the cricothyroid membrane is identified and marked. The skin and tissue over this area are then infiltrated with local anaesthetic. This infiltration should extend through the cricothyroid membrane and a small amount of anaesthetic should be dribbled into the trachea. This will cause the patient to cough which will diffuse anaesthetic agent over the local tracheal epithelial area. A small transverse stab incision is made through the skin and underlying structures until the cricothyroid membrane has been punctured. A scalpel with a guarded blade is useful for this part of the procedure. The introducer is then passed through the wound and into the trachea (Figure 11.5.). The cannula is passed over the introducer and into the trachea, following which the introducer is withdrawn. There is a flange attached to the edge of the cannula to allow secure attachment of the surrounding skin with sutures (Figure 11.6). Suction can then easily be performed through the cannula.

Removal

The tube is simply pulled out and a light dressing placed over the wound. Within 2–3 days, the wound has closed securely without any sutures being necessary.

Therapeutic thoracoscopic procedures

Assisted thoracoscopic procedure – excision of first rib

Impression of the nervous or vascular structures, or both, in the gap between the first rib and the clavicle causes one of the thoracic outlet compression syndromes. The thoracic outlet contains a subclavian artery, subclavian vein and brachial plexus. Various skeletal abnormalities may lead to compression

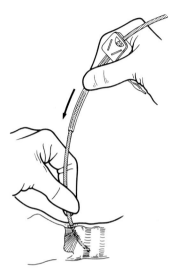

Figure 11.5: The minitracheostomy introducer.

of the contents of this thoracic outlet (Table 11.2). Removal of the first rib decompresses the floor of the outlet and ensures detachment of the muscles and fibrous bands, thus relieving any compression that may have occurred (Figure 11.7 and 11.8).

Procedure

The patient is placed in the lateral position and the arm raised to 90° flexed

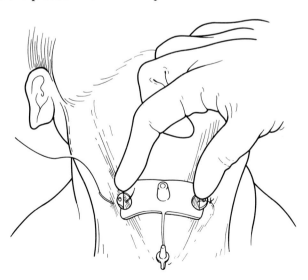

Figure 11.6: Attachment of the minitracheostomy.

1. Cervical rib.
2. Elongated transverse process from C7 vertebra.
3. Fibrous band from C7 transverse process to the first rib.
4. Excrescences and anomalies of the first rib.
5. Developmental abnormalities of the clavicle may reduce the costoclavicular space.
6. Compression by the scalene muscles.

Table 11.2: Causes of compression at the thoracic outlet.

at the elbow. General anaesthesia is used, and a double lumen endotracheal tube inserted by the anaesthetist. The lung on the affected side is deflated and an artificial pneumothorax induced, if necessary, as previously described.

A trochar and cannula is placed in the fourth intercostal space in the anterior axillary line, and a further one in the fifth or sixth intercostal space in the posterior axillary line. The first will be used for the telescope, with the video camera attached, and the second one for insertion of instruments.

The subclavian artery is seen clearly and an incision in the pleura made just below it. The brachial plexus can then be clearly seen.

A transverse incision is made at the inferior margin of the hairline parallel with the skin crease, through which the upper part of the chest wall is exposed and the first rib identified. An assistant raises the arm, and in so doing opens up the costoclavicular recess. The anterior and medial scalene muscles and subclavius muscles are separated from the first rib and at the same time are observed with the thoracoscope. The periosteum of the rib is then incised with a diathermy point, and a periosteal elevator is used to strip it first from the anterior and then from the superior surface of the rib. As the vessels and post-thoracic nerve are clearly seen by the thoracoscope, damage to these structures should not occur. The costoclavicular ligament anteriorly is then divided, and the anterior end of the rib divided with appropriately angled rib shears or bone nibblers. Dissection is then carried posteriorly beyond the tubercle of the rib, where it is divided with rib shears or nibblers. The rib is then removed and bony spicules trimmed with bone nibblers.

If a cervical rib is present, it is detached from the first rib, and resected at this stage. Similarly any cervical fibrous band is divided (Figure 11.7). The lung is inflated and, if no pneumothorax remains, no drain is necessary. Absorbable sutures are used to cover the subcutaneous layers over a Redivac drain. The skin is usually closed with a subcuticular absorbable suture.

Thoracoscopic cervicothoracic sympathectomy

This operation is indicated for hyperhidrosis of the hands and axillae and advanced cases of Raynaud's phenomenon. The procedure is effective, simple, cheap, and requires only an overnight stay. It can now be recommended as the treatment of choice for upper limb hyperhidrosis (Edmundson, Bannerjee and Rennie).

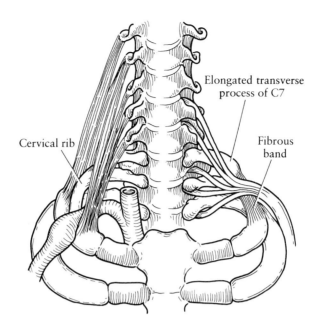

Figure 11.7: Anatomy of fibrous band and cervical rib.

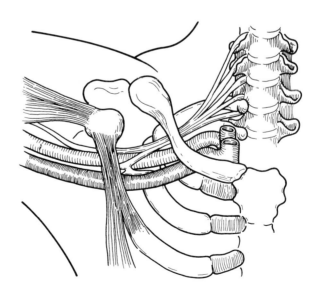

Figure 11.8: Thoracic outlet obstruction caused by the first rib.

Procedure

A double lumen endotracheal tube is used so that the lung on the affected side can be deflated prior to thoracoscopy. Ports are placed, following induction of a pneumothorax, in the second and fourth mid-axillary line thoracic spaces. The telescope, with the video camera attached, is usually used through the lower port whilst the upper port (5 mm) is used to transmit scissors and the hook diathermy.

The view obtained is better than with any conventional approach for this operation. The sympathetic chain is seen lying on the heads of the ribs beneath the parietal pleura. Incision is made just lateral to the chain over the uppermost rib seen, which would be the second rib and also over the third and fourth ribs. The sympathetic chain is picked up with the diathermy hook (Figure 11.9) and freed. The chain is divided by the head of the fourth rib and the ganglia there destroyed. The dissection is carried upwards and two rami communicantes, each going to the corresponding intercostal nerves, are seen and destroyed with the diathermy. The intercostal arteries and veins lie deep to the chain, but a few branches lie in front of it. These should be secured with diathermy, or the chain carefully dissected off them.

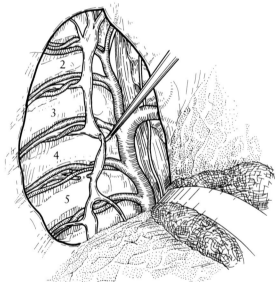

Figure 11.9: Anatomy of the thoracic sympathetic chain.

As the dissection proceeds upwards, the first rib is not seen and therefore there is no danger of causing a Horner's syndrome, but the overuse of the diathermy on the second rib, may cause arcing and give a transient Horner's syndrome.

Once haemostasis has been ensured, the lung is reinflated and, if no pneumothorax is present, the thoracoscope is removed and there is no need for a drain. The procedure takes 20–30 minutes and both sides can be done under the same anaesthetic.

Thoracoscopic pulmonary operations

All thoracoscopic procedures are performed under general anaesthesia and with a double lumen endotracheal tube in place.

Lung biopsy

This is indicated when transbronchial or needle biopsies are inadequate or unhelpful, due to insufficient tissue for a pathological diagnosis.

Obviously the thoracoscopy is performed on the side where the pathology is. A 10 mm port is inserted into the fifth intercostal space, through which the telescope and camera will be passed. In the seventh or eighth intercostal space, a 12 mm port is inserted, through which the endoGIA stapling device can be passed. These ports are placed in the mid-axillary line, and it is sometimes useful to use a 5 mm port posteriorly through the fourth or sixth intercostal space, through which a grasping forceps can be used. The area of lung which needs to be biopsied is grasped with the grasping forceps and an endoGIA sizer then passed across it. The correct size staple is then used on the endoGIA, and this is passed across the lung tissue leaving it closed with three rows of staples (Figure 11.10 and 11.11). The biopsy is removed via the 12 mm cannula. The lung is forcibly reinflated by the anaesthetist and, provided it obliterates the pleural cavity, there is no need for a drain. If an endoGIA is not available, the lung can be excised with scissors and oversewn with a continuous vicryl suture.

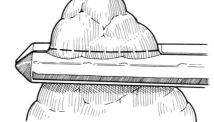

Figure 11.10: The endoGIA stapler placed across the lung.

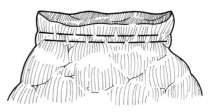

Figure 11.11: The staple line once the stapler has been fired.

Operation for spontaneous pneumothorax

This may be required for the management of chronic or recurrent pneumo-
thoraces. Pleurodesis or pleurectomy can be performed; pleurodesis by
abrasion can be performed thoracoscopically, and at the same time any
pulmonary bullae can be treated.

The same configuration of ports is used as for a lung biopsy, and the parietal
pleura is abraided using a small swab on the end of the forceps or by using the
forceps themselves. The abrasion is carried out vigorously until the pleural
surface is inflamed and bleeding. Following this procedure, the whole of the
lung must be inspected. If bullae are present, they can be closed easily, using
an endoGIA stapling device.

Lobectomies

Middle and lower lobectomies can be performed thoracoscopically, whilst
upper ones are more difficult anatomically. As the procedures, apart from
anatomical differences, are much the same, one lobectomy will be described.

Thoracoscopy is performed in the usual way through the fifth intercostal
space in the mid-axillary line. If the greater fissure is more or less complete,
the dissection should begin by exposing the pulmonary artery. This is usually
marked by a lymph node in the depth of the fissure. The artery is dissected
out completely, and the dissection is extended both proximally and distally to
display the arterial branches. In order to leave an adequate cuff of the pulmonary artery, it is usually necessary to ligate the common basal, apical lower and
middle lobe arteries separately for a middle and right lower lobectomy. If the
fissure is obliterated, the dissection begins with the inferior pulmonary vein,
accessible from the anterior or posterior aspect of the lung. To identify the
inferior pulmonary vein, the pulmonary ligament is divided and its vessels
secured with diathermy. This incision is continued up to the lower margin
of the inferior pulmonary vein. The lung is then retracted forwards and the
inferior pulmonary vein dissected out, together with its apical lower and
common basal branches. The vein is divided using an endoGIA.

The middle lobe vein is then identified and divided at its origin. Once
again, an endoGIA is used. The inferior segment of the lower lobe is then
separated from the posterior segment of the upper lobe, using blunt and
sharp dissections. If a small portion of lung resists separation, it can be
divided using the endoGIA stapler. The lower lobe is displaced forwards,
and the vagal nerve branches and bronchial arteries supplying the lobe are
identified and divided as they pass over the back of the bronchus. The
intermediate bronchus is now visible and the lymph node between it and
the lower margin of the upper lobe bronchus can be seen. The lobe is dissected
away from both the bronchi. The plane in which the instrument can be passed
around the intermediate bronchus is found, and the bronchus divided, using
the endoGIA at least 1 cm below the lower margin of the upper lobe bronchus.
The middle and lower lobes are now free and can be inserted into a bag in
which to morcellate them. The carinal lymph node and right paratracheal
nodes are dissected out for staging purposes. The bronchial suture line should

be tested by inflation with the bronchus under warm saline poured into the pleural cavity. Two drains are usually used, one for fluid at the base and one placed apically for any air.

If it proves difficult performing the lung dissection with three ports, a fourth or even a fifth can be introduced. Instruments with memory are very useful in passing around the arteries, veins and bronchi.

Although pneumonectomy has not been performed, it would be feasible through a thoracoscope, although time-consuming.

Thoracic oesophagus operations

Heller's operation for achalasia of the cardia

This operation is usually indicated whenever achalasia is diagnosed, to prevent complications associated with aspiration of the oesophageal contents into the lungs. If the condition is found to be associated with a hiatus hernia, repair of the hernia should be carried out at the same time.

The operation is carried out under general anaesthesia and a double lumen endotracheal tube is inserted to permit deflation of the lungs. A left thoracoscopic approach will be used, so the patient should be on their right side. Three ports are usually used, a 10 mm port being inserted to transmit the telescope and video camera, which is usually placed in the sixth intercostal space in the mid-axillary line. Two 5 mm ports are placed in the fourth and eighth intercostal spaces in the posterior axillary line. Obviously the lung is deflated prior to insertion of the ports, and once deflated, the lung is retracted upwards exposing the inferior pulmonary ligament (Figure 11.12) which is divided with scissors/diathermy close to the lung. This incision stops at the lower margin of the inferior pulmonary vein, which can be identified by the lymph nodes situated immediately below it. The enlarged, thick-walled oesophagus is clearly seen, and mobilized using the forceps. It is usual to place tapes around the lower end of the oesophagus, and these should be 12 mm moistened linen tapes which are passed close to the muscle of the oesophagus. These tapes are threaded through the 5 mm ports and do not preclude the continued use of the ports with the tape coming through them. If there is any problem, the port can be removed and the tape brought out through the small hole. The port can then be reinserted. By pulling on the tapes, the oesophagogastric junction is drawn up into the thorax and a narrow segment of oesophageal wall is clearly seen. It is our preference to use the Nd:YAG laser to divide the muscle wall, but scissors could be used or, preferably, the harmonic scalpel blade. A 5 cm incision is made in the long axis of the oesophagus, extending down to the oesophagogastric junction. As this incision deepens into the longitudinal muscle fibres, the deeper circular muscle comes into view (Figure 11.13). Diathermy should be avoided because of the risk of causing necrosis of the mucosa and subsequent perforation.

As the circular muscle fibres are divided, the blade of the knife or laser is rotated so that it cuts almost parallel to the surface. The mucosa bulges through once the deep muscle fibres have been divided. Any remaining constricting bands show up clearly and are divided. The muscle is then swept back on either side using the grasping forceps, sometimes with a bronchus swab. In this way, the mucosa is freed for half of the circumference. A nasogastric tube is not used, as this may erode through the very thin mucosa.

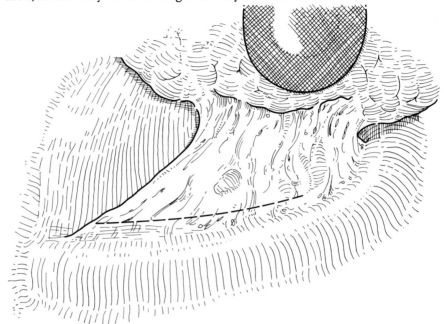

Figure 11.12: Exposure of the inferior pulmonary ligament.

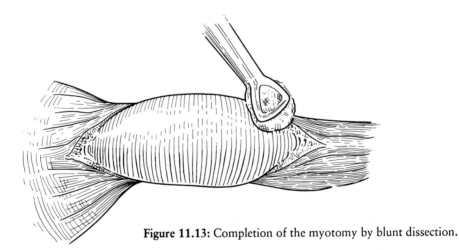

Figure 11.13: Completion of the myotomy by blunt dissection.

The instruments and tapes are removed and the lung reinflated. If it is fully inflated, there is no need for a drain. Everything is removed, and the skin closed with interrupted sutures.

Operations for hiatus hernia

These are usually performed laparoscopically, although fundoplication or a

Belsey mark IV operation could be performed thoracoscopically. They are described in detail elsewhere.

Thoracoscopic closure for perforations or spontaneous rupture of the oesophagus

Most perforations of the oesophagus occur after instrumentation. Small penetrating wounds may be treated non-operatively, but large wounds obviously need thoracoscopic drainage and repair.

Spontaneous rupture occurs more frequently in men than women and usually in late middle age. There is commonly a history of vomiting against a closed glottis.

The procedure can vary, but essential features are to drain the pleural space, expand the lung and prevent further contamination of pleural space. The site to be operated upon is determined by thin barium or gastrograffin swallow. Once this has been done, the patient is placed on the operating table with the site of the leak uppermost. Once again, general anaesthesia and a double lumen endotracheal tube are used.

Thoracoscopy is performed and the perforation is easily diagnosed. If it is a recent perforation, it can be closed using a continuous vicryl suture. If the perforation is not recent, then the pleural cavity is cleaned out and a large drain inserted.

Thoracoscopic management of leiomyoma of the oesophagus

These benign tumours are most commonly found in the wall of the oesophagus. They usually occur in the lower part of the oesophagus where the wall consists of smooth muscle. Frequently they are incidental findings at the time of surgery for other conditions. Occasionally they may cause dysphagia. Contrast radiographic studies usually reveal a smooth filling defect. At endoscopy, no mucosal lesion is visible and no biopsy should be taken, as a breach of the mucosal wall may lead to an oesophageal leak after surgical removal.

The patient is placed on his side, general anaesthesia having been induced and a double lumen endotracheal tube inserted. As stated, the tumours usually lie in the lower part of the oesophagus where the smooth muscle is to be found, and therefore a thoracoscopic approach is made through the posterior axillary line in the eighth intercostal space. Two further 5 mm ports are inserted, to aid excision of the tumour. Whilst the oesophagus is mobilized, moistened linen tapes can be placed around it to stabilize it, and the outer thin adventitial layer and muscular layer are then incised. The leiomyoma can almost always be enucleated with blunt dissection, although the initial incision can be carried out precisely using an Nd:YAG laser. If the mucosa is breached, it should be repaired with an absorbable suture. The muscle wall can be approximated using loose interrupted sutures, once the tumour has been excised.

The tumour, if small enough, can be delivered through the 10 mm port, but if large, it is best placed in a bag and then morcellated prior to removal. A small chest drain may be inserted, following which the ports are removed and the skin closed with sutures.

Carcinoma of the oesophagus

Over the last 10 years it has been my practice to perform transhiatal oesophagectomies (Orringer), taking the stomach up to the neck for anastomosis to the cervical oesophagus. As there is no anastomosis in the thorax, postoperative radiotherapy can be given safely.

The advent of thoracoscopic mobilization of the oesophagus was a great advantage. Transhiatal oesophagectomy meant blind dissection, and the presence of the operative hand mobilizing the oesophagus behind the heart, always disturbed both patient and anaesthetist. There is no doubt that thoracoscopic mobilization of the oesophagus is not only safer, because it is carried out under direct vision, but probably also gives a better clearance than blind dissection.

In 1989, Buess introduced the technique of transcervical endoscopic dissection using a modified rigid endoscope (Figure 11.14), introduced into the mediastinum by a left cervical approach. The entire length of the oesophagus is dissected out close to the oesophageal wall. Whilst avoiding the trauma of thoracotomy, and the dangers of blind transhiatal dissection, mobilization is very close to the oesophagus, and therefore the paraoesophageal lymphatic system is not removed.

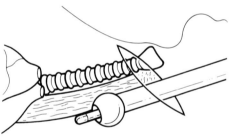

Figure 11.14: Buess' modified rigid endoscope.

Thoracoscopy is performed through the right chest, and the patient is positioned under general anaesthetic with a double lumen endotracheal tube, as for a right thoracotomy. The right lung is deflated and a 10 mm port inserted into the right sixth intercostal space in the mid-axillary line. A telescope with camera attached is inserted through this port, and initial evaluation of the lung and pleural cavity is carried out.

Four more thoracic ports are inserted under direct vision – usually two in the axillary line and two in the posterior axillary line. It is usual to use a 5 and 10 mm port anteriorly and a 5 and 12 mm port posteriorly.

The 10 mm cannula is used for the insertion of the endoclip and the 12 mm for the endoGIA. The surgeon stands on the right of the patient, together with the camera assistant, and a second assistant is placed opposite so that he can retract the lung. Incision of the triangular ligament, down to the inferior pulmonary vein, allows retraction of the right lung to be effected.

Resectability of the oesophagus is once again assessed, especially with respect to local extension into the mediastinum. The mediastinal pleura is then opened posteriorly along the azygos vein, and along the right uppermost aspect of the spine. Anteriorly, it is divided along the pericardium with inferior pulmonary vein, the right main bronchus and the trachea. Pleural incisions meet at the apex of the pleural cavity and lower margin at the hiatus.

It is usual to commence the dissection of the oesophagus at the hiatus. If one intends to mobilize the stomach laparoscopically, then the hiatus must not be opened. If the thoracic duct is clearly seen, it can be clipped and divided. The dissection is then continued following the aorta. The arch of the azygos vein is dissected out, and then divided using the endoGIA (Figure 11.15) which is introduced through the 12 mm port. Similar dissection continues by clipping and coagulating small oesophagobronchial branches. Anteriorly, dissection follows the pericardium as far as the left pleura. It then continues upwards posteriorly to the anterior pulmonary vein and the right main bronchus. At this level, the right bronchial artery, originating from the right intercostal artery and crossing the oesophagus, usually has to be clipped and divided. The posterior bronchial plane is followed as far as the left main bronchus. All intertracheobronchial nodes are removed, and the dissection then proceeds along the posterior aspect of the trachea. Dissection extends upwards along the plane of the pleura to the inferior aspect of the aortic arch.

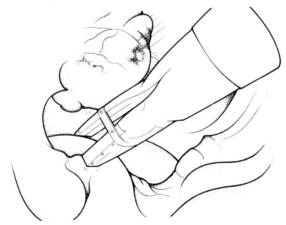

Figure 11.15: Division of the azygos vein.

Both vagi are divided. On the left side, the recurrent laryngeal nerve has to be identified prior to dividing the vagus below it. The oesophagus above the aortic arch is mobilized right up to the level of the clavicles.

Once the mobilization is complete, lavage is carried out with saline, and haemostasis is secured. A chest drain is inserted through the 12 mm trochar. The position is confirmed using the thoracoscope, and the right lung is then fully re-expanded. The small skin wounds are closed with interrupted sutures.

Obviously, this thoracoscopic mobilization of the oesophagus must be followed by mobilization of the stomach and mobilization of the cervical oesophagus. The mobilized stomach can then be pulled up to the neck, the oesophagus having been fully mobilized as described.

It has been my practice to perform a laparoscopy prior to the thoracoscopic mobilization of the oesophagus, to ensure that there is no widespread disease or other reason for not continuing with oesophagectomy. The stomach can be mobilized laparoscopically, or a gastric tube can be fashioned, but this is very time-consuming. If one wishes to mobilize the stomach laparoscopically, as soon as the hiatus is opened, the pneumoperitoneum will escape. Therefore, it is my practice to perform laparoscopy, turn the patient on to the left side and do the thoracoscopic mobilization of the oesophagus, and then turn the patient back to perform the abdominocervical mobilization.

Minimal access surgery has had a tremendous impact on both the patient and the surgeon. Thoracotomy has always been a painful incision to heal and has kept patients in hospital for a week to 10 days, depending on which operation has been performed. Less invasive thoracic surgery performed thoracoscopically, results in less pain because of the smaller scars, and therefore reduced hospitalization and an earlier return to normal activities.

Thoracoscopy and thoracoscopic procedures have proved themselves extremely quickly. However, thoracic surgeons have been slow to follow the lead given by gynaecologists and surgeons for this minimal access type of surgery. In the fullness of time, thoracotomy may prove to be an operation of the past.

References

Buess G et al., (1991) Endoscopic oesophagectomy without thoracotomy. *Problems in General Surgery.* 8: 486–487.

Cooper J (1986) *Thoracic surgery*, 4 ed. Butterworth-Heinemann, Oxford.

Edmondson RA, Banerjee AK and Rennie JA (1992) Endoscopic transthoracic sympathectomy in the treatment of hyperhidrosis. *Am. Surg.* 215: 289–293.

Jacobaeus HC (1910) Uber die Moglichkeit, die Zystoskopie bei Untersuchung seroser Hohlungen anzuwenden. *Munch. Med. Wochenschr.* 57: 2090–2092.

Orringer MB and Sloan H (1978) Esophagectomy without thoracotomy. *Thor. Cardiovasc. Surg.* 76: 643–654.

Ear, Nose and Throat

JOHN WALDRON

12

Introduction

The upper respiratory tract is not readily accessible to direct examination and manipulation. Traditional methods of inspection, using a headlight and a combination of mirrors and speculae, allow a variable amount of the upper respiratory tract to be examined in different patients. The ease of examination depends on variations in anatomy, the presence of obstructive pathology, and the sensitivity of the patient's gag reflex. The nose and paranasal sinuses can only be crudely assessed by routine inspection, and the posterior nasal cavity and nasopharynx are difficult to examine, even indirectly using a mirror. Examination of the larynx and hypopharynx using a mirror provides a satisfactory view in many, but not all, cases.

The development of flexible and rigid endoscopes, with high quality illumination and optics, has greatly facilitated examination of the upper respiratory tract. This improved visualization has increased our ability to perform surgical procedures under direct vision, using minimal access approaches and techniques. The main areas of otolaryngology in which minimal access techniques have found application are the nose and paranasal sinuses, and the larynx, pharynx and upper trachea.

Nose and paranasal sinuses

Prior to the development of flexible fibre-optic and rigid Hopkins rod endoscopes, examination of the nose and sinuses was limited to direct inspection with a headlight anteriorly, and indirect inspection with a mirror of the nasopharynx and posterior nasal cavity. The sinuses could not be directly assessed by these techniques, only the mucosa around their ostea draining into the nasal cavity could be inspected. Surgery of the sinuses could be carried out either transnasally, using unaided vision with a headlight and nasal speculum for access and illumination, or via an external approach using an external incision and bone removal for access to the sinus.

The development of small nasal endoscopes has greatly improved the ability to diagnose nasal and sinus pathology accurately. The small (2.8 mm diameter) flexible endoscopes, such as the Olympus ENF-P series, allow a good view of the entire upper respiratory tract in the great majority of patients using topical anaesthesia. A range of narrow diameter (2.8 mm and 4 mm) rigid endoscopes are available with different fields of view (0°, 30°, 70°, 120°). These allow excellent visualization of the nasal cavity and nasopharynx, and can also be used, in conjunction with a trochar and cannula, to enter into the maxillary sinus and directly inspect this area which had previously been impossible without performing open surgery. The improved visualization and instrumentation has allowed the development of two new areas in rhinology which utilize minimal access techniques – sinoscopy and functional endoscopic sinus surgery.

Sinoscopy

Sinoscopy of the maxillary sinus may be performed using local anaesthesia in an out-patient setting, or using general anaesthesia. The sinus is entered using a trochar and cannula, designed so that the standard rigid endoscopes can be passed through the cannula. The trochar and cannula may be passed transnasally via the inferior meatus of the lateral nasal wall, or sublabially through the canine fossa and anterior wall of the sinus (Figure 12.1). Both routes allow inspection of the entire maxillary antrum by using endoscopes with different fields of view.

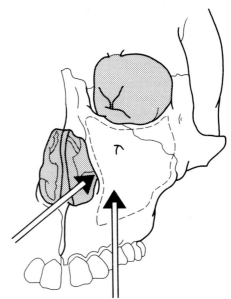

Figure 12.1: Sublabial and inferior meatal approaches to the maximillary antrum.

Using local anaesthesia, the patient may be placed supine, or in the sitting position. Local anaesthesia for the inferior meatal approach may be obtained using 10% cocaine solution (maximum dose 3 mg/kg). This is initially sprayed into the nasal cavity, and then placed on to pledglets which are placed in the inferior meatus at the position of the intended antrostomy. This lies at the highest point of the inferior meatus, under the inferior turbinate, approximately 1.5 cm back from the anterior end of the turbinate. A combination of 4% xylocaine and 1:1000 adrenaline solution may be substituted for cocaine. Anaesthesia for the sublabial approach is obtained using submucosal infiltration of xylocaine 2% with 1:80 000 adrenaline, administered via a 23 French dental syringe, into the canine fossa, which lies immediately lateral to the prominent ridge of the canine tooth.

The trochar and cannula are then passed into the sinus by the intended route, using a rotating motion to bore through the bone of the antral wall. The cannula is held with the index finger along its length, to within 2 cm of the tip. This prevents accidental damage to the far wall of the sinus if the entry is sudden. Once the sinus is entered, the trochar is withdrawn, a suction catheter is used to clear any blood and secretions, and the endoscope is inserted.

Studies comparing the information obtained from plain radiographs of the sinuses to that obtained at sinoscopy, show sinoscopy to be markedly superior in assessing inflammatory disease of the maxillary sinus (Pfleiderer et al., 1986). In addition to providing diagnostic information, sinoscopy can also be used to biopsy and remove abnormal mucosa and to treat some conditions such as foreign bodies and mucosal cysts (Fisher et al., 1989).

Surgical instruments may be passed into the maxillary sinus by these routes, and biopsies taken and procedures performed under endoscopic control (Draf, 1983). If necessary, the rigid endoscope may be inserted via the sublabial route, whilst the instruments are passed via the transnasal route through the inferior meatal antrostomy.

Functional endoscopic sinus surgery

The development of nasal endoscopy and sinoscopy has allowed more accurate assessment of the extent of disease, particularly in inflammatory conditions, to be made. In conjunction with coronal tomograms, utilizing either plain X-ray, or preferably computed tomography, a precise assessment of nasal anatomy and the extent of disease can be made (Bolger et al., 1991). This has resulted in the concept being advanced by Messerclinger that most inflammatory sinus disease originates from the nose (Messerclinger, 1985; Kennedy et al., 1985). Although the symptoms may arise predominately from the diseased maxillary or frontal sinuses, the underlying cause is thought to be in the clefts of the lateral nasal wall. The frontal, anterior and middle ethmoid and maxillary sinuses drain into the middle meatus of the lateral nasal wall, in close relation to certain of the anterior ethmoidal air cells (Figures 12.2 and 12.3). The sphenoid and posterior air cells drain into the superior meatus. These ethmoid air cells are considered to be prechambers, providing ventilation and drainage for the corresponding sinuses. This area of the lateral nasal wall, containing the ostea of the sinuses and their corresponding prechamber air cells, is known as the osteomeatal complex.

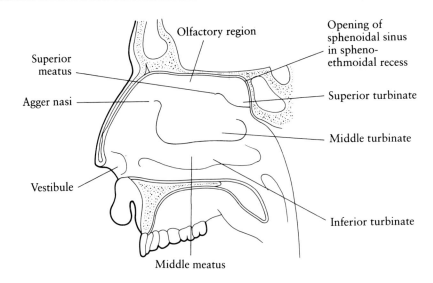

Figure 12.2: Anatomy of the lateral wall of the nose.

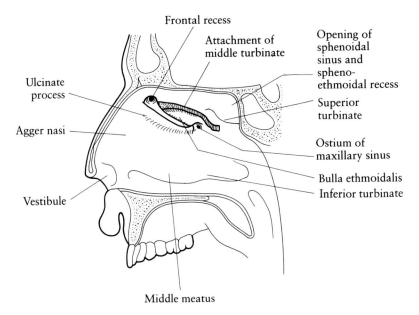

Figure 12.3: The lateral nasal wall. The middle turbinate has been removed, and the underlying structures are shown.

These prechambers are narrow clefts, which may be readily obstructed by mucosal swelling. They may also predispose to obstruction if they are narrowed by anatomical variations.

The fundamental premise of the Messerclinger technique of 'functional endoscopic sinus surgery', is that inflammatory disease in the sinuses will return to normal if the problems in the osteomeatal complex are treated.

Thus, the surgery is directed to the anterior ethmoidal cells, in the region of the osteomeatal complex. This surgical approach is a minimal access one for two reasons: the approach is entirely transnasal, using endoscopic visualization to guide the surgery, and only the minimum surgery necessary to correct abnormalities in the osteomeatal complex is performed. This is in contrast to the approach of traditional sinus surgery in which the sinus is usually entered by an external approach and all the diseased mucosa is exenterated.

There are probably no absolute contraindications to the use of functional endoscopic sinus surgery as an approach to inflammatory sinus disease, except complicated frontal sinus problems, which may be more adequately dealt with via an external approach. However, the individual surgeon's experience with this approach is an important factor in deciding whether to use this method of surgery or other more conventional techniques. Severe and occasionally fatal complications have occurred, and the operator should confine himself to cases in which he is confident of the anatomy. At all times he must be prepared to abandon the procedure temporarily if haemorrhage prevents adequate visualization or to revert to an external approach if it is felt that an orbital complication may have been produced.

Functional endoscopic sinus surgery can be performed using local or general anaesthesia. Local anaesthesia is obtained using cocaine (10%) solution or xylocaine 4% with adrenaline 1:1000, to decongest and anaesthetize the nasal mucosa. This is initially sprayed into the nasal cavity and then applied on pledglets. This is supplemented by infiltration of 1–1.5 ml of 1% xylocaine with 1:200 000 adrenaline submucosally over the uncinate process of the middle meatus of the lateral nasal wall. Sedation, using a benzodiazepine, or equivalent, is a useful adjunct to local anaesthesia, and may be given as an oral premedication or intravenously, at the time of surgery. When general anaesthesia is used, the nose is prepared in the same manner, with topical application and infiltration to produce vasoconstriction and mucosal shrinkage. Ten minutes are allowed to permit mucosal shrinkage, and the nose then inspected systematically using the 0° or 30° rigid endoscopes. If necessary, sinoscopy is performed at this time. If there are large obstructing nasal polyps, these are removed with a cutting snare, and further topical anaesthesia is applied to the mucosa exposed by their removal. If deviation of the nasal septum prevents adequate access to the nasal cavity, it is corrected with a submucosal resection or septoplasty at this time. Instrumentation for functional endoscopic sinus surgery consists of straight, angle punch and cupped forceps, periosteal elevators and nasal suckers. Most of these are standard nasal instruments used in open sinus surgery, although the larger instruments are less suitable as it may not be possible to pass them alongside the endoscope into a narrow area of the nose. When general anaesthesia is being used, a combined suction irrigation apparatus may be employed, incorporated into a sheath with the endoscope, and mounted on a pistolgrip handle. The suction in this apparatus is continuous, whilst the irrigation is controlled by a trigger on the handle.

Functional endoscopic sinus surgery is then started under direct vision using the 0° or 30° endoscope. The actual procedure performed will depend on the nasal anatomy and the type and extent of disease. Typically, the anterior ethmoid air cells within the uncinate process are opened initially. These cells are then resected to expose the ethmoidal infundibulum, and allow the ethmoidal bulla to be visualized. The bulla is then resected in the same way. This dissection is carried out using punch forceps and elevators. The maxillary sinus ostium lies at the posterior end of the infundibulum in the middle meatus just above the inferior turbinate. It can be probed with an angled instrument if it is not seen directly. If necessary, it can be enlarged to improve drainage of the maxillary sinus. Care must be taken when entering to keep just above the inferior turbinate. Entry at a higher level may result in penetration into the orbit rather than the maxillary antrum. The ostium is enlarged to 1.5–2.0 cm, largely in an anterior direction, using back-biting forceps. It is important not to enlarge the ostium too far anteriorly, as this may damage the nasolacrimal duct. If the patient has frontal sinus disease, the air cells of the frontal recess and agger nasi are resected, to improve drainage of the frontal sinus.

If it is necessary to open the sphenoid and posterior ethmoid air cells, then the sphenoid ostium should be sought at an early stage. This lies at an angle of 30° from the nasal floor, 7 cm from the anterior maxillary spine. A calibrated probe can be used to measure the distance. Once the ostium is identified, the anterior wall of the sphenoid inferior and medial to the ostium, is removed. The roof and lateral wall of the sphenoid are vital landmarks, and define respectively the planes of the upper and lateral limits of dissection in the posterior ethmoids. Failure to appreciate this may lead to penetration into the anterior fossa or orbit. Once these landmarks are found, the dissection is carried anteriorly through the ethmoid air cells.

If there is significant bleeding at the completion of the procedure, nasal packing may be inserted. If not, an antibiotic ointment is applied to the operated area. The patient is seen at frequent intervals after surgery, starting on the second postoperative day, to remove crusts and prevent adhesions forming which may delay healing.

Whilst there are no controlled studies available comparing functional endoscopic sinus surgery with traditional sinus surgery, the results of treating inflammatory nasal disease using functional endoscopic sinus surgery are good in experienced hands (Schaefer, 1989).

Increasing experience of functional endoscopic sinus surgery has lead to an increase in the range of conditions which have been treated by this approach. Severe nasal polyposis, frontal sinus mucoceles, antrochonal polyps, orbital decompression and dacrocystorhinostomy have all been dealt with using these techniques. However, severe complications have been reported, and sinus surgery is currently the most common cause of litigation in otolaryngology in the United States (Stankiewicz, 1989; Maniglia, 1991). The close relationship of the sinuses to the orbit and optic nerves, and to the dura, place these structures at risk of damage, particularly in revision cases where surgical landmarks may be obscured. The most dangerous complications are cerebrospinal fluid (CSF) leak and intracranial haemorrhage, and orbital complications involving either the optic nerve or orbital contents.

These complications can be minimized by adequate surgical training, careful patient selection and assessment, and meticulous surgical technique. The reported complication rates vary from 2–17%, and this may represent different levels of surgical experience (Stankiewicz, 1989). As with other sinus surgery, a thorough knowledge of anatomy is vital before such procedures are undertaken, and a practical 'hands-on' course using cadaver dissection is an excellent way of gaining experience in the surgical anatomy before this is applied to patients.

The larynx and pharynx

Tracheostomy

Tracheostomy may be performed to bypass upper airway obstruction, to allow long-term ventilation, to reduce the dead space, and to allow clearing of secretions from the tracheobronchial tree. A formal tracheostomy is performed through a horizontal or vertical incision and involves dissection of tissues down on to the trachea which is opened under direct vision. This usually entails separation of the strap muscle and retraction, or transfixion and division, of the thyroid isthmus, and removal of a window from the anterior tracheal wall.

Two recent minimal access techniques have been developed as alternatives to this approach. The first, cricothyrotomy, allows insertion of a small tube which permits easy aspiration of secretions in the tracheobronchial tree. However, the narrow diameter of the tube used does not allow this to be used as an alternative airway for more than a very short period of time. The second, percutaneous tracheostomy, is an alternative method of performing a tracheostomy using a guidewire and dilators rather than a formal dissection.

Cricothyrotomy

The cricothyroid membrane joins the cricoid and thyroid cartilages and lies in the mid-line just below the prominence of the thyroid notch (Figure 12.4). It lies deep to the skin and a thin layer of subcutaneous tissue. The easily palpable landmarks of the thyroid and cricoid cartilages, and the superficial position of the larynx at this point, allow relatively easy access to the airway through the cricothyroid membrane. However, if a large opening is made through the cricothyroid membrane, there is a high risk of a resultant sub-glottic stenosis. For this reason, only a small bore tube should be used when performing a cricothyrotomy. The main use of cricothyrotomy is to allow access for aspiration of secretions from the tracheobronchial tree. It is an excellent technique for this situation in which it represents a good alternative to a conventional tracheostomy.

In cases of acute upper airway obstruction, a cricothyrotomy may be used to secure an emergency airway, and oxygenate the patient. It has the advantage that it is quick and easy to perform, and it requires less surgical ability than an emergency tracheostomy. In addition, kits are widely available specifically designed for this purpose. However, the resistance to air flow down the thin (4 mm) tube makes it unsuitable for longer term use, and in

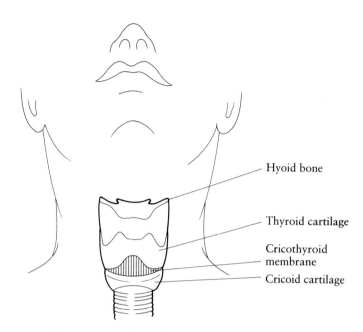

Hyoid bone

Thyroid cartilage

Cricothyroid membrane

Cricoid cartilage

Figure 12.4: Position of the cricothyroid membrane.

these situations a conventional tracheostomy must be performed as soon as possible.

Cricothyrotomy is usually performed using local anaesthesia and may be carried out as a bedside procedure. The head and neck are extended and kept in the mid-line. The cricothyroid membrane is palpated and a small amount of local anaesthetic is infiltrated subcutaneously. If there is any doubt as to the anatomy, the needle can be advanced through the membrane and air aspirated to confirm entry into the airway. The skin is then stretched over the larynx and maintained under tension by the assistant. A vertical slab incision is made through the skin and cricothyroid membrane. Care must be taken to avoid damage to the cricoid cartilage, and to limit the depth of penetration of the blade to prevent injury to the posterior wall of the trachea (proprietary sets contain a guarded blade for this purpose). The introducer is then passed through the incision into the airway and down the trachea, and the tube is advanced over this. Secretions and any blood may be aspirated using a fine suction catheter passed through the tube. The tube is then secured in place using sutures or tapes. The main complication of this procedure is haemorrhage which is occasionally profuse, and may arise from branches of the cricothyroid arteries, or associated veins, which lie in close proximity to the membrane. The only other major difficulty is incorrect placement of the tube in some cases, particularly in patients with short, obese necks (Russell, 1989). For these reasons, it would seem advisable to perform the procedure in a setting where open exploration of the wound can be performed should complication be encountered. Although the incidence of subglottic stenosis is low when using small bore tubes, one long-term complication may be a change in the quality of voice, which has been reported in up to 70% of patients who undergo cricothyrotomy (Gleeson *et al.*, 1985).

Percutaneous tracheostomy

Variations of the Seldinger guidewire technique have been used to allow a tracheostomy to be performed via a minimal access approach. In this technique, a 1.5 cm incision is made in the skin overlying the second or third tracheal rings, and a needle is passed percutaneously into the trachea between the first and second, second and third, or third and fourth tracheal rings. Air is aspirated into the syringe to confirm entry into the trachea. A guidewire is then passed through the needle into the lumen of the trachea. In one technique, a graded series of dilators is then passed along the guidewire, to dilate the the tract up to a size which allows a tracheostomy tube to be inserted (Cook and Callanan, 1989). An alternative technique uses a speculum passed over the guidewire rather than graded dilators to dilate the tract (Schakner *et al.*, 1990). The tracheostomy tube is then inserted into the trachea and the cuff inflated.

This technique is said to be quicker, easier to perform and more suitable as a bedside or ITU procedure (Hazard *et al.*, 1988; Schakner *et al.*, 1990). Although there have been positive reports of this technique, they are not without problems. Haemorrhage, the formation of false passages with failure to maintain the airway, and damage to the posterior tracheal wall and oesophagus have all been reported (Hutchinson and Mitchell, 1991; Hazard *et al.*, 1988). Variations of the technique are being used, but it has not yet received widespread acceptance. Controlled trials evaluating the results and complications are necessary before the true value of percutaneous tracheostomy can be determined. At the present time, it would appear wise to ensure that personnel and facilities for exploration of the neck, and conversion of the procedure to a formal tracheostomy are present, before embarking on a percutaneous tracheostomy.

Endoscopic surgery of the larynx and pharynx

Direct examination of the larynx and pharynx using rigid endoscopes was developed around the turn of this century by pioneers such as Chevalier Jackson. Since that time, steady improvement has been made in light sources, instrumentation and anaesthesia. The addition of the operating microscope with a 400 mm objective allows magnified binocular vision to be used. The carbon dioxide (CO_2) laser may be attached to the operating microscope, and directed with a micromanipulator. This allows accurate dissection of the tissue combined with haemostasis. This is a considerable advantage when operating in the airway, where any bleeding is hazardous. Such precise dissection is vital in the larynx, where unnecessary tissue removal or scar formation may have adverse effects on the voice or airway.

Many benign laryngeal disorders, such as vocal cord nodules, polyps, and submucosal oedema are treated with endoscopic resection if they fail to respond to conservative treatment. These procedures have been established for many years and will not be discussed further. However, there are a number of conditions in which minimal access endoscopic approaches have been developed as an alternative to external approaches through the neck. Some examples of these illustrate the advantages, and limitations, of the endoscopic treatment of laryngeal and pharyngeal disorders.

Tumours of the larynx

Premalignant changes are not infrequently seen in the laryngeal mucosa, particularly that overlying the true vocal cords. Management of these lesions is by excision biopsy, 'stripping' the abnormal areas of mucosa, and submitting them for histological examination. Both dysplasia and carcinoma *in situ* may be managed in this way, with repeated procedures if necessary. The technique of removal of mucosa, or 'stripping' of the vocal cord, requires removal of all of the abnormal mucosa as precisely as possible. This causes minimal disruption to the laryngeal anatomy, and careful handling of the specimen allows accurate histological examination, particularly of the depth of invasion. This is most easily accomplished using the operating microscope and fine microlaryngoscopy instruments. The excision may be performed using the laser by sharp dissection with microscissors or a sickle knife.

Traditional treatment of laryngeal carcinoma has usually consisted of radiotherapy, or partial or total laryngectomy. Recently, some surgeons have shown that small T1 carcinomas of the vocal cord may be treated by endoscopic laser resection with equivalent results to those obtained with radiotherapy or partial laryngectomy. Blakeslee et al., (1984) report the results of endoscopic laser resection of small T1 cord lesions which did not involve the anterior commissure or the arytenoid, and did not extend into the subglottis, or into the supraglottis beyond the floor of the vestibule. Their three year recurrence-free rate was 90%. However, if these strict criteria are not met, the recurrence rate using this type of minimal access approach is greatly increased. Although similar results are obtained conventionally using radiotherapy, or with vertical partial laryngectomy, it is argued that this type of excision allows radiotherapy to be held in reserve for any subsequent tumour in the head and neck region, and produces a better voice than does vertical hemilaryngectomy (Ossoff et al., 1985). It must be stressed that this approach is not yet universally accepted; accurate pretreatment staging and histological examination of the resected specimen, are vital to ensure that more advanced tumours are not treated in this fashion, which would be inappropriate.

In larger squamous carcinomas of the larynx, minimal access approaches are not appropriate for curative treatment. There is, however, one situation with an advanced tumour obstructing the airway where an endoscopic resection of a tumour using the laser may be of value. Patients with advanced tumours may present with stridor due to obstruction of the laryngeal airway. This is most easily dealt with by performing a tracheostomy. However, patients who have a tracheostomy prior to a laryngectomy for resection of carcinoma are thought to be at greater risk of peristomal recurrence of tumour (Klein et al., 1965). In this situation, the laser may be used to debulk the tumour at presentation and improve the airway (Davis and Sharpshay,

1981). This may allow time for the definitive histology to be obtained and for the patient to be prepared physically and psychologically for a laryngectomy. In this situation, the minimal access surgery is a temporary measure to avoid a tracheostomy in order to improve the patient's prognosis after definitive treatment.

One specific type of laryngeal tumour, verrucous carcinoma, is suitable for primary endoscopic resection. The well-differentiated verrucous carcinomas have 'pushing' margins and do not usually invade deeply into the surrounding tissues. They may therefore be treated by endoscopic resection, with careful analysis of the resection margins to ensure complete removal. The CO_2 laser and operating microscope allow accurate resection of these tumours with good haemostasis, and avoid the necessity for more aggressive surgery (Sharpshay and Rebeiz, 1990).

Bilateral vocal cord paralysis

Bilateral vocal cord paralysis may result in a compromised airway due to the vocal cords lying in the adducted position close to the midline and failing to abduct on inspiration. The patient typically has stridor, and dyspnoea on exertion. To improve the airway, it is necessary to lateralize one vocal cord. This has traditionally been performed using Woodman's procedure or a variation of this (Woodman, 1946). This involves an external approach through the neck, resection of the arytenoid, and lateralization of the vocal ligament, with a non-absorbable suture encircling it from outside by simultaneous direct laryngoscopy. The risk of oedema compromising the airway postoperatively following this procedure necessitates a covering tracheostomy.

The use of the CO_2 laser has allowed improvement of the airway by endoscopic resection of part of the vocal cord and/or resection of the arytenoid. This removes the need for open exploration of the neck and for a covering tracheostomy. It therefore greatly reduces the morbidity and length of hospitalization of the patient, and is the procedure of choice in many centres (Howard, 1987), (Figure 12.5).

Pharyngeal pouch

Unlike the other examples given above, both open and minimal access techniques have been used to treat pharyngeal pouches from the beginning of this century. In 1906, Mosher first divided the wall between the pouch and the lumen of the oesophagus (Dohlman and Mattsson, 1960). Dohlman used diathermy to divide the wall, and reported a 7% recurrence rate in a series of 100 patients. In this technique, a special oesophagoscope is positioned with its long blade in the oesophagus, and the shorter blade in the pouch. Diathermy forceps are clamped across the wall separating the pouch from the oesophagus, and the area is diathermized. The wall is then divided with a cutting diathermy. A more recent development has been the use of the CO_2 laser to divide the wall (Van Overbeek et al., 1984). The advantage of the endoscopic Dohlman's procedure is that it is quicker, and carries a

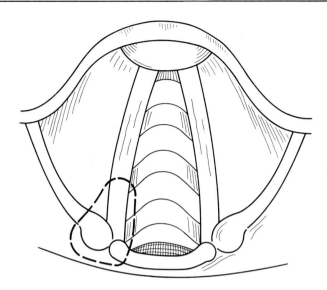

Figure 12.5: A larynx showing the extent of resection with a laser arytenoidectomy.

lower morbidity than an open exploration and excision, or inversion, of the sac. However, it requires considerable operative experience, and symptoms are more likely to return following a Dohlman's procedure, than if a formal excision of the sac is performed. In addition, most exponents of Dohlman's procedure would only divide a limited length of the wall at one time. This necessitates repeated procedures in patients with larger pouches, which negates the advantages of reduced morbidity and shorter hospitalization. Most surgeons favour open surgery for a symptomatic pouch in fit patients, but there may still be a role for an endoscopic procedure in selected symptomatic elderly patients with a moderate sized pouch (Doyle and Stevens, 1985).

References

Blakesee D, Vaughan CW and Sharpshay SM (1984) Excision biopsy in the selective management of T1 glottic cancer: a three year follow-up study. *Laryngoscope.* **94:** 488–493.

Bolger WE, Butzin CA and Parsons DS (1991) Paranasal sinus boney anatomic variations and mucosal abnormalities: CT analysis for endoscopic sinus surgery. *Laryngoscope.* **101:** 56–64.

Cook PD and Callanan VI (1989) Percutaneous dilational tracheostomy technique and experience. *Anaesthesia and Intensive Care.* **17:** 456–457.

Davis RK and Sharpshay SM (1981) Pretreatment airway management in obstructing carcinoma of the larynx. *Otolaryngology Head and Neck Surgery.* **89:** 209–211.

Draf W (1983) *Endoscopy of the paranasal sinuses.* Springer-Verlag, Berlin.

Dohlman G and Mattsson L (1960) The endoscopic operation for hypopharyngeal diverticula: a roentgencinematographic study. *Arch. Otolaryng.* 71: 744–752.

Doyle JD and Stevens HE (1986) Esophageal diverticula. In: *Otolaryngology – head and neck surgery, Vol 3.* Ed. Cummings CW. Mosby, St Louis.

Fisher EW, Whittet HB and Croft CB (1989) Symptomatic mucosal cysts of the maxillary sinus: antroscopic removal. *J. Laryngol. Otol.* 103: 1184–1186.

Gleeson MJ *et al.*, (1984) Voice changes following cricothyroidotomy. *J. Laryngol. Otol.* 98: 1015–1019.

Hazard PB, Garrett HE and Adams JW (1988) Beside percutaneous tracheostomy: experience with 55 elective procedures. *Ann. Thor. Surg.* 46: 63–67.

Howard D (1987) Neurological affectations of the larynx and pharynx. In: *Scott-Brown's Otolaryngology, Vol 5.* Butterworths, London.

Hutchinson RC and Mitchell RD (1991) Life threatening complications from percutaneous dilational tracheostomy. *Critical Care Medicine.* 19: 118–120.

Kennedy DW *et al.*, (1985) Functional endoscopic sinus surgery, theory and diagnostic evaluation. *Arch. Otolaryng.* 111: 576–582.

Klein WF, Shapiro MJ and Rosin HD (1965) Study of postlaryngectomy stoma recurrence. *Arch. Otolaryng.* 81: 183–186.

Maniglia AJ (1991) Fatal and other major complications of endoscopic sinus surgery. *Laryngoscope.* 101: 349–354.

Messerklinger W (1985) Endoskopische diagnose und chirurgie der rezidivierenden sinusitis. In: Krajina Z (Ed.) *Advances in nose and sinus surgery.* Zagreb University Press, Zagreb.

Ossoff RH, Sisson GA and Sharpshay SM (1985) Endoscopic management of selected early vocal cord carcinomas. *Ann. Otol. Rhinol. Laryngol.* 94: 560–566.

Pfleiderer AG, Croft CB and Lloyd GAS (1986) Antroscopy: its place in clinical practice: a comparison of antroscopic findings with radiological appearances of the maxillary sinus. *Clin. Otolaryng.* 11: 455–461.

Russell WC (1989) Complications and inappropriate use of minitracheostomy. *Anaes. Intensive Care.* 17: 513.

Schachner A *et al.*, (1990) Rapid percutaneous tracheostomy. *Chest.* 98: 1266 – 1270.

Schaefer SD (1989) Endoscopic total sphenoethmoidectomy. *Otolaryng. Clin. N. Amer.* 22: 727–732.

Sharpshay SM and Rebeiz EE (1990) Uses and abuses of lasers for treatment of laryngeal carcinoma. In: *Otolaryngology–head and neck surgery, Update II.* Ed. Cummings E. Mosby, St Louis.

Stammberger H (1985) Endoscopic surgery for mycotic and recurring sinusitis. *Ann. Otol. Rhinol. Laryngol.* 94: Supplement 119.

Stankiewicz JA (1989) Complications of endoscopic sinus surgery. *Otolaryngol. Clin. N. Amer.* 22: 749–758.

Van Overbeek JJM, Hoeksema PE and Edens ET (1984) Microendoscopic surgery of hypopharyngeal diverticulum using electrocoagulation or carbon dioxide laser. *Ann. Otol. Rhinol. Laryngol.* 93: 34–39.

Woodman DG (1946) A modification of the extralaryngeal approach to arytenoidectomy for bilateral abductor paralysis. *Arch. Otolaryng.* 48: 63–65.

Index